Compendium medicine

Pocket
Gastroenterology and Hepatology

Romée Snijders & Veerle Smit
Suzanne Anjie

Together for Healthcare

Want to know more about Compendium Medicine? Check out our website!

www.compendiummedicine.com

First edition, 2025

Neither the publisher nor any authors, contributors, or other representatives of Compendium Medicine assume any liability for any injury and/or damage to persons and property, as a matter of products liability, negligence or otherwise, or from any use or operation of any methods, products, instructions, or ideas in this book. This is a comprehensive limitation of liability that applies to all damages of any kind, including (without limitation) compensatory; direct, indirect, or consequential damages; loss of data, income, or profit; loss of or damage to property and claims of third parties. Links to third-party websites are provided by the publisher in good faith and for information only. The publisher disclaims any responsibility for the materials contained in any third-party website referenced in this work.

This book contains information contained from authentic and highly regarded sources. Every effort has been made to trace copyright holders and obtain their permission for the use of copyright material. Reprinted material is quoted with permission, and sources are indicated. The publisher does not provide medical advice or guidance and this work is merely a reference tool. Healthcare professionals, and not the publisher, are solely responsible for the use of this work including all medical judgments, and for any resulting diagnosis and treatments.

With respect to any pharmaceutical product identified, readers are urged to check the most current information provided on procedures featured by the manufacturer of each product to be administered, to verify the recommended dose or formula, the method, and duration of administration and contraindications. It is the responsibility of practitioners, relying on their own experience and knowledge of their patients, to make diagnoses, determine dosages and the best treatment for each patient, and take all appropriate safety precautions. Compendium Medicine does not accept responsibility or legal liability for any errors in the text, or for the misuse or misapplication of material in this work.

ISBN 9789083374086
BISAC MED031000
Thema MJH

MIX
Paper | Supporting responsible forestry
FSC® C118234
www.fsc.org

Preface

Welcome to the *Compendium Community!*

'Together for Healthcare' – these three simple words encapsulate the spirit of the collective mission and underscore the essence of *Compendium Medicine*. In an era where the complexity of healthcare is becoming increasingly interconnected, collaboration is not merely an option but an imperative. These books symbolise the effectiveness of collaboration, knowledge sharing, and a joint commitment to improve and interconnect healthcare.

We proudly present the first edition of our pocket *Gastroenterology and Hepatology*, designed to provide all the essential information you need at your fingertips. This comprehensive guide covers a wide range of clinical topics that will prove invaluable during your internship, residency, and on-call shifts. Chapters include endoscopy, frequently encountered acute scenarios, gastroenterology and hepatology conditions, and practical appendices featuring commonly used calculators and reference tools.

The innovative *Compendium Method©*, designed for medical students and doctors, employs comprehensible illustrations for every medical condition, straightforward tables, icons, and useful mnemonics. It is visually appealing, to the point, and concise. We only focus on the essentials and make sure all the content is comprehensively presented.

Our strength lies in the diverse expertise of our close-knit medical team, consisting of students, medical doctors, and medical specialists. This collaborative approach ensures that our content is comprehensive and accurate.

We are committed to inclusivity and aim to make our texts and images a reflection of the diversity of patients our readers provide care for. We aspire for every (future) doctor and patient to find themselves reflected in our books. Our team works continuously to improve and expand the selection of books. We welcome readers to share their feedback and suggestions, contributing to the continual improvement of our pocket series.

We are grateful for the interdisciplinary collaboration reflected in this pocket, shaped through contributions from radiology, surgery, internal medicine, pharmacotherapy, and more, mirroring real-life clinical practice. The outstanding result is this extraordinary pocket – a pocket for everybody in healthcare.

Enjoy reading and enjoy working, and we hope to hear from you soon!

Amsterdam, November 2025

Veerle Smit, MD & Romée Snijders, MD, PhD
Doctors and founders *Compendium Medicine*

Editorial staff

Want to know more about us?
Scan this QR code.

Editorial board

Romée J.A.L.M. Snijders, MD, PhD & Veerle L. Smit, MD

Chief editor

Gwendolyn Vuurberg, MD, PhD

Pocket editor

Current edition

Suzanne I. Anjie, MD, PhD Candidate, Amsterdam University Medical Center, Amsterdam
Romée J.A.L.M. Snijders, MD, PhD, Jeroen Bosch Hospital, 's Hertogenbosch

Previous edition

Suzanne I. Anjie, MD, PhD Candidate, Amsterdam University Medical Center, Amsterdam
Romée J.A.L.M. Snijders, MD, PhD Candidate, Radboud University Medical Center, Nijmegen

Authors

Current edition

Niels (L.D.) Broekman, MD, PhD Candidate, Amsterdam University Medical Center, Amsterdam
Jessica van der Weijden, MD, PhD, Flevoziekenhuis, Almere

Previous edition

Niels (L.D.) Broekman, BSc, Leiden University Medical Center, Leiden
Veronique Goudberg, BSc, Leiden University Medical Center, Leiden
Linde Verbugh, BSc, University of Amsterdam, Amsterdam
Jessica van der Weijden, BSc, University Medical Center Groningen, Groningen

Acknowledgements

Content quality assurance

The editorial board extends its sincere appreciation to the many contributions of doctors, specialists, and professors from around the world who played a pivotal role in crafting this pocket. We wish to express our thanks to the entire international team for their dedicated efforts and invaluable expertise. Special appreciation is also extended to the team of specialists who actively participated in shaping the previous edition.

Current edition

S. Amber Ali, MD, Basildon University Hospital, Basildon
Rianne C.J. Beckers, MD, PhD, Maastricht University Medical Center, Maastricht
Lucas H.P. Bernts, MD, PhD, Radboud University Medical Center, Nijmegen
Alessio Gerussi, MD, PhD, University of Milano-Bicocca, Milan
Tom van Gils, MD, PhD, University of Gothenburg, Gothenburg
Daisy de Groot, MD, Amsterdam University Medical Center, Amsterdam
Thomas J. Konturek, MD, UCI Health - Placentia Linda Hospital, Placentia
Rose Leijdesdorff, MD, PhD Candidate, Amsterdam University Medical Center, Amsterdam
Assoc. Prof. Manuel Mendizabal, MD, PhD Candidate, Austral University Hospital, Pilar
Antonio Molinaro, MD, PhD, University of Gothenburg, Gothenburg
Miki Scaravaglio, MD, University of Milano-Bicocca, Milan
Robbert W Schouten, MD, PhD, Amsterdam University Medical Center, Amsterdam
Bas J.J.W. Schouwenberg, MD, PhD, Radboud University Medical Center, Nijmegen
B.W. Marcel Spanier, MD, PhD, Rijnstate Hospital, Arnhem
Vicky Tallentire, MD, PhD, University of Edinburgh, Edinburgh
Steffi E.M. van de Ven, MD, PhD, Erasmus Medical Center, Rotterdam
Evelien M. Vermeulen, MD, Amsterdam University Medical Center, Amsterdam
Rogier P. Voermans, MD, PhD, Amsterdam University Medical Center, Amsterdam

Previous edition

Rianne C.J. Beckers, MD, PhD, Maastricht University Medical Center, Maastricht
Floor A.C. Berden, MD, PhD, Radboud University Medical Center, Nijmegen
Lucas H.P. Bernts, MD, PhD, Radboud University Medical Center, Nijmegen
Sarah Bos, MD, PhD, Treant, Emmen
Prof. Danny De Looze, MD, PhD, University Hospital Ghent, Ghent
Prof. Joost P.H. Drenth, MD, PhD, Radboud University Medical Center, Nijmegen
Tom van Gils, MD, PhD, Amsterdam University Medical Center, Amsterdam
Irene E.G. van Hellemond, MD, PhD, Catharina Hospital, Eindhoven
Michael Klemt-Kropp, MD, PhD, NorthWest Hospital, Alkmaar
Mark P. Lamberts, MD, PhD, VieCuri, Venlo
B.W. Marcel Spanier, MD, PhD, Rijnstate Hospital, Arnhem
Steffi E.M. van de Ven, MD, PhD, Erasmus Medical Center, Rotterdam
Anna J. Verhulst, MD, Amsterdam University Medical Center, Amsterdam
Marijn C. Visschedijk, MD, PhD, University Medical Center Groningen, Groningen
Rogier P. Voermans, MD, PhD, Amsterdam University Medical Center, Amsterdam
Rianne A. Weersink, PharmaD, PhD, Deventer Hospital, Deventer
Esmerij P.M. van der Zanden, MD, PhD, Amstelland Hospital, Amstelveen

Sounding board

Nour Al Kahaili, BSc, Leiden University Medical Center, Leiden
Ania Sasiada, MD, El Bierzo Hospital, Ponferrada
Rosa Weel, BSc, University of Amsterdam, Amsterdam

Editorial coordinators

Laura M. Barrantes Rodríguez, MD, junior editor
Vera den Boef, MSc, project manager
Pauline Blom, final editor
Melanie Goedegebure, product manager
Delano R. Sanches, MD, BSc, illustration manager

Illustrators

Yente S. Beentjes, MD, University Medical Center Utrecht, Utrecht
Hebe T.A. Boerhout, Utrecht University, Utrecht
Dagmar Bouwer, Leiden University, Leiden
Cas van Cruchten, Maastricht University, Maastricht
Susan Deelstra, University of Groningen, Groningen
Maria van Doorn, BASc
Lotte Dupuis, Radboud University, Nijmegen
Astrid A.H. Feikema, Radboud University, Nijmegen
Iza Hogenelst, University of Applied Sciences, Amsterdam
Jasmin Kaur, BSc, Rotterdam University of Applied Sciences, Rotterdam
Koen L.C. Ketelaars, MD, GP practice De Brink, Severum
Rosalie C. Krijl, MD, Ask Arbo Artsen, Zeist
Juliëtte M.E. Linskens, MD, Maastricht University, Maastricht
Kim A.M. van den Nobelen, BSc, Radboud University, Nijmegen
Carlijn Sturm, BSc, Leiden University, Leiden
Isabel Versmissen, MD, Foundation SBOH, Eindhoven
Linda Xie, MD, Reinier de Graaf Hospital, Delft

Language support

Translation Agency Perfect
Mark Hannay, translator
Ruth Rose, editor
Merit E. Maas, MD, MSc, Centre for Youth and Family Rijnmond, Rotterdam
Nathasja van Leeuwen, MD, St. Joseph Hospital, Kagondo

Graphic designers

Maria van Doorn, BASc
Ivana Kinkel

The Compendium Method©

Manual

In *Compendium Medicine* we use the same concise, visual and schematic description of the various medical specialties. Everything is geared towards overview and structure, facilitating study and practice. We call this the *Compendium Method©*.

Fixed layout

All our medical specialties are presented in the same, recognisable way and each has its own colour and icon. The pockets have a fixed chapter structure. The table of contents of each pocket tells you exactly which topics are covered. The symbols in the corner of the page show what kind of information is being discussed.

- ATLS
- Anatomy
- Physiology
- Patient history
- Physical examination
- Diagnostics
- Treatment
- Differential diagnosis
- Conditions
- Clinical reasoning
- Appendices
- References
- Abbreviations
- Index

Illustrations

The figures provide at-a-glance insight into topics like anatomy or the typical patient. They are also intended for study and practice, such as checking whether you can identify the letters in a picture without looking at the caption.

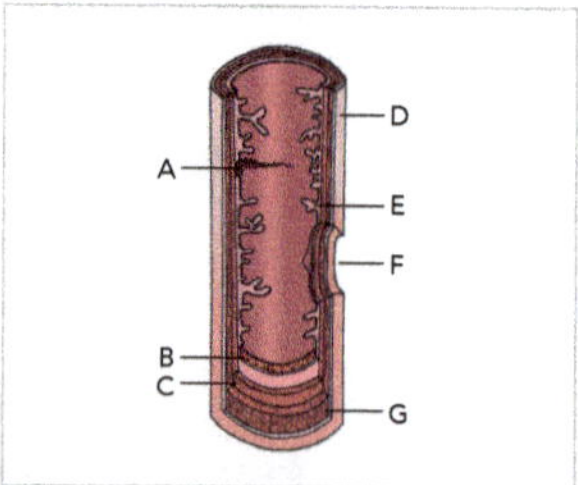

Figure 33 // Boerhaave syndrome and Mallory-Weiss syndrome

A: Mallory-Weiss syndrome (mucosal tear) **B:** Submucosa **C:** Circular muscle layer **D:** Serosa **E:** Mucosa **F:** Boerhaave syndrome (distal LES perforation) **G:** Longitudinal muscle layer

Conditions

Each condition in this pocket starts with a full-sentence definition followed by a telegram-style explanation. For each condition, the following icons (as applicable) are discussed. These visual cues that convey specific attributes or features of the condition are also useful when studying. You can cover the text and quiz yourself.

- D Definition
- E Epidemiology
- Ae Aetiology
- R Risk factors
- Hx Patient history
- PE Physical examination
- Dx Diagnostics
- Tx Treatment
  - General
  - Paramedical care
  - Pharmacological treatment
  - Invasive, non-pharmacological treatment
- P Prognosis
- ! Watch out/don´t forget

Tables

We use tables to arrange the information in a clear and structured manner, with columns representing different conditions and rows indicating features or characteristics. Centered formatting for matching features makes it easy to identify similarities and differences.

Diagrams

→ = positive/yes/+ → = negative/no/-

Diagrams help you reason clinically, starting from a particular symptom, using the green and red arrows as signposts. Always remember that the full differential diagnosis may consist of additional diagnoses.

Icons & frames

Fun fact: our founders are Dutch, and in the Netherlands, we refer to a mnemonic as a "donkey bridge". That's why the symbol for mnemonics in our books is a donkey.

Throughout this pocket you will find highlighted frames.

QR code	Mnemonic	Europe
Alarm!	Description of the typical patient	USA
Formula	Reference to another chapter	The Netherlands
Note		

Punctuation marks

The punctuation in our books also focuses on overview and ensures that the subject matters are covered concisely and effectively.

(--) Rare	(++) Most common	↓ Decrease/detoriation
(-) Uncommon	→ Consequence	♀ Female sex
(+) Very common	↑ Increase/improvement	♂ Male sex

Abbreviations

We make extensive use of abbreviations, medical terms and symbols for scientific units and quantities. Below are some examples of the abbreviations used in this pocket.

sec	second/seconds	d	day/days	min.	minimum
min	minute/minutes	wk	week/weeks	max.	maximum
h	hour/hours	mo	month/months	e.g.	for example
		y	year/years	L	litre/litres

Index

The pockets include a comprehensive and easy-to-use index. It contains all the topics covered in the books so you can quickly navigate and find the information you are looking for.

Appendices

In the pockets, you will find space for your notes, additional information, reminders, or insights. In addition, handy appendices have been added; these contain specific information that you would like to have at hand and are therefore located at the back of the pockets.

They/theirs

We realise that sex and gender identity are not binary and that there is more variation than just 'woman' or 'man'. For readability's sake (as well as for grammatical reasons) we have therefore chosen to use the pronouns 'they/theirs', regardless of sex or gender identity.

Warning

When studying this pocket, be mindful of the protocols within your own facility and adhere to the established guidelines. It is also essential to understand the circumstances under which you may or may not provide assistance in a given country, as this can potentially have legal consequences.

Want to know more about the Compendium Method©? Scan the QR code.

Table of contents
Gastroenterology and Hepatology

Table of contents
Gastroenterology and Hepatology

Table of contents
Gastroenterology and Hepatology

Reinforce your foundational knowledge with our 'Compendium Medicine' app. Available on Apple and Android app stores for daily question practice and a monthly challenge.

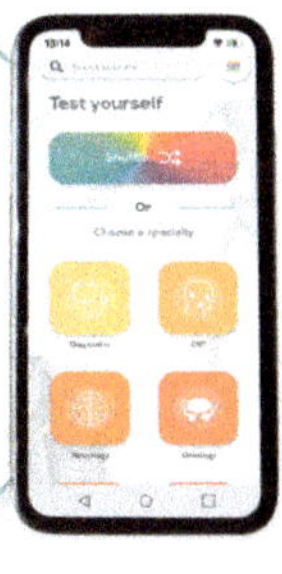

Patient history

Introduction

- Introduce yourself
- Check personal details
- Assess the patient: acute or non-acute, determine reason for consultation and/or chief complaint, nonverbal communication

→

Patient history

- General patient history
- History of presenting complaint/ current illness
- History of relevant system (full review of systems if necessary)

→

Concluding

- Summarise your findings
- Patient's remarks and/or questions
- Explain physical examination and/or indicated diagnostics

Consider psychosocial variables such as language barriers, cultural differences between patients and physicians, financial backgrounds, and addiction, which may impact disease progression.

Diagram 1 // Patient history

General patient history

Medical history, medication use (exact dosage, frequency, last dose, administration form), history of substance use (smoking, alcohol, drugs), allergies (latex, plasters, medication, contrast agents), family history (FHx), psychosocial history, travel history, social history (home situation, work, study, social support), vaccinations, ill individuals in immediate vicinity.

Taking a diligent FHx is particularly important if malignancy or inflammatory bowel disease (IBD) are suspected. In case of weight loss (intentional/unintentional), anaemia, abdominal swelling, changed bowel habits, or oesophageal dysphagia, ask specifically about any gastrointestinal (GI) malignancies in the family (who was diagnosed, at what age). With prolonged diarrhoea and bloody stools, ask about relatives with Crohn's disease and ulcerative colitis. Also, look out for hereditary causes of anaemia, e.g. hemoglobinopathies or pernicious anaemia.

- Always ask about previous endoscopies (e.g. colonoscopies, gastroscopies) and findings.
- Nutritional status and dietary habits are crucial in a patient's GI history, as it directs towards a correct diagnosis. Ask about intake (liquids and solid foods), eating habits, diet, vitamins and supplements, allergies, intolerances, weight (gain/loss, intentional/unintentional).

- Explicitly ask about over-the counter (OTC) medications, such as herbal and vitamin preparations, esp. when suspecting liver disease. Many liver enzyme disorders are caused by drug toxicity: obtain a detailed list of the patient's medications with their stop/start dates. This detailed record is also crucial for IBD and liver transplant patients. Also inquire about vaccination status.
- With abdominal symptoms or bleeding, always ask about NSAIDs (ibuprofen, naproxen, diclofenac) and use of proton pump inhibitors (PPIs).

Common medications that cause liver enzyme disorders include paracetamol (acetaminophen), statins (e.g. atorvastatin), and antibiotics (AB) (e.g. doxycycline, nitrofurantoin). Consult the Drug-Induced Liver Injury Network for a list of medications that can cause acute liver failure. Scan the QR code for more information.

Review of systems

General system

General well-being, itching, fever, chills, night sweats, appetite, weight change (deliberate/unintentional), fatigue, exercise tolerance.

Watch for red flags/B symptoms (e.g. disabling fatigue, unintentional weight loss, unexplained fever, night sweats, itching, icterus). These symptoms may be associated with a serious condition, such as malignancy.

Circulatory system

Dizziness/light-headedness (orthostatic), chest pain (on exertion or at rest), palpitations (e.g. fluttering, pounding, racing), dyspnoea (e.g. dyspnoea on exertion or at rest, orthopnoea), nycturia, intermittent claudication, cold extremities, peripheral oedema.

> Peripheral oedema is a common symptom of congestive heart failure (CHF) and can be caused by the heart's reduced ability to pump blood. Thiamine deficiency can lead to heart failure and therefore oedema (wet beriberi). Also, liver cirrhosis can lead to oedema and ascites due to portal hypertension.

Respiratory system

Dyspnoea, coughing (dry, sputum, nocturnal), audible breathing (e.g. wheezing, rhonchi), chest pain (worsens when breathing deeply), sputum (e.g. consistency, colour, blood), haemoptysis. ENT: sore throat, earache, tinnitus, voice (hoarse), recurrent respiratory infections.

> The typical patient with fluid infusion or transfusion-associated circulatory overload (e.g. a patient with acute pancreatitis receiving significant fluid resuscitation or a patient with anaemia receiving blood transfusion) has pre-existing heart failure or poor left ventricular function and presents with sudden-onset dyspnoea several hours after the start of transfusion. This can even lead to cardiac asthma.

Urogenital system

Miction (e.g. dysuria, stranguria, haematuria, pollakisuria, polyuria), bladder function, incontinence, flank pain, changes in bowel habits, sexual history. ♀: vaginal discharge, menstrual cycle, hot flashes. ♂: weak stream, feeling of incomplete emptying, dribbling, discharge, erectile dysfunction, testicular pain or swelling.

> It can be difficult to differentiate between abdominal pain secondary to GI, gynaecological, or urological pathology (e.g. sexually transmitted infection (STI), nephrolithiasis, urolithiasis, pyelonephritis, urinary tract infection (UTI)). It is therefore very important to thoroughly inquire about the urogenital system.

Endocrine system

Changes in bowel habits (e.g. diarrhoea/constipation), polydipsia, polyuria, menstrual irregularities, agitation/inertia, cold or heat intolerance, exophthalmos, enlarged thyroid, muscle problems, skin/hair changes, sweating, oedema, weight changes, mood swings, alterations in libido or sexual function.

Locomotor system

Warmth, redness, swelling, cramps, restless legs, joint pain, joint instability, morning stiffness, loss of function, action radius, muscle atrophy.

> Pancreatitis may present as back pain or pain between the shoulder blades without abdominal pain.

Haematological system

Bone pain, epistaxis, haematomas, heavy menstrual bleeding, prolonged bleeding, petechiae, lymph node swelling, night sweats, fever, fatigue.

> The liver produces vitamin K-dependent clotting factors. Cholestasis, liver failure, or dietary monotony (esp. in combination with alcohol use disorder) may therefore prompt clotting disorders.

Central nervous system

Concentration difficulties, amnesia, dizziness (spinning rotation), loss of consciousness, seizures, headache, impaired senses (e.g. hearing, smell, taste, vision), language, speech, mastication, swallowing, diplopia, abnormal sensation (e.g. numbness, tingling), loss of strength, gait disorders, balance problems, tremors or involuntary movements, psychiatric symptoms.

> Bradyphrenia, loss of consciousness, personality changes, and intellectual dysfunction are some signs of hepatic encephalopathy.

Skin and mucous membranes

Skin rash (efflorescence, redness), skin discolouration (incl. scleral icterus), nail/finger abnormalities, itching.

Mental health

Cognitive functioning, sleep problems, anxiety, depression, mood swings, delusions, hallucinations, suicidal thoughts or self-harm.

Gastrointestinal and hepatology history

Anaemia

Recent blood loss (rectal, vaginal, blood donations), diet (see nutrition), potential absorption disorder (IBD, coeliac disease, previous GI resections), chronic disease, renal insufficiency, recent infectious diseases.

Abdominal pain

Pain (nature, duration, location, timing, paroxysmal/continuous, radiating, movement-evoked), urge to move, VAS score, concomitant symptoms (e.g. nausea, vomiting, jaundice), links to pain (diet, stress, micturition, bowel movements, menstruation, sexual intercourse), alleviating actions, other relevant factors.

The essential components of a pain history can be recalled using the mnemonic SOCRATES.

Pain (SOCRATES)
Site
Onset (sudden/gradual)
Character (dull, sharp, stinging)
Radiation
Associated symptoms
Time course/duration
Exacerbating, relieving factors (urge to move, pain during transport)
Severity

Dyspepsia

Pain (nature, duration, location (epigastric, retrosternal), timing, paroxysmal/continuous), links with diet, lying down, burping, regurgitation, cramps, bloating, nausea, vomiting, weight loss.

GI bleeding

Haematemesis (colour, odour, quantity), melaena (colour, odour, consistency, quantity), rectal blood loss (colour, odour, quantity), medication use (NSAIDs (ulcer), PPIs, anticoagulants (type and time of last dose)), last meal, vomiting prior to onset of bleeding (Mallory-Weiss syndrome), B symptoms (malignancy), most recent endoscopy, PMHx (peptic ulcer disease, aortic prosthesis, liver cirrhosis, clotting disorders, alcohol consumption, diverticulosis, haemorrhoids), concomitant symptoms.

Hepatic, bile duct, and pancreatic symptoms

Abdominal pain (nature, duration, location, timing, paroxysmal/continuous (colic pain is a sign of symptomatic gallstone disease), radiating, urge to move), nausea, vomiting, discoloured stool, dark urine, jaundice, presence and possible progression of hepatic encephalopathy, changes in appetite, alcohol consumption, medication, recent endoscopic retrograde cholangiopancreatography (ERCP), sexual history.

> If hepatic encephalopathy is suspected: ask about pre-existing liver disease; sleep disorders; signs of consciousness disorders; personality changes; orientation to time, place, and person; uncoordinated muscle activity; and gait disorders.

Nausea and vomiting

Frequency, colour, blood (coffee grounds emesis, fresh blood), regurgitation and rumination, abdominal pain, links to intake, fever, fluid intake, changes in bowel habits, known or possible pregnancy, recent stay abroad, close contacts with similar symptoms, signs of dehydration.

> Dehydration is a major complication of vomiting. Elderly patients (>70y) and infants are particularly at risk. In the elderly, watch for severe thirst, dry mouth, decreased skin turgor, drowsiness, confusion, dizziness, and decreased urinary output. In infants, look for fewer wet diapers, sunken fontanelle, absence of tears when crying, and poor feeding.

Bowel habits

Frequency, quantity, shape, colour, consistency, mucus and blood loss, nocturnal bowel movements, incomplete defecation, difficult/painful passing of stools, urgency, incontinence, overflow diarrhoea, fluid and fibre intake, use of laxatives or other medications that affect bowel movements. Bowel habits are highly personal: always ask how the current situation compares to the patient's normal bowel habits.

> Opioid use is one of the most common causes of medication-related constipation in adults. Anticholinergics, antipsychotics (esp. clozapine), anti-seizure medication, bisphosphonates, calcium antagonists, and diuretics can also cause constipation.

> Medication-induced diarrhoea usually occurs as a side effect of AB, laxatives, digoxin, colchicine, metformin, beta blockers, cytostatics, and magnesium salts. Certain medications can also exacerbate the clinical course of diarrhoea, such as corticosteroids, diuretics (higher risk of dehydration), and immunosuppressants (lowered defences against infectious causes of diarrhoea).

Swallowing symptoms

Choking, dysphagia, globus sensation, heartburn, previous food impaction, regurgitation, chest pain or retrosternal pain, nausea, vomiting, signs of dehydration, coughing, vocal changes, decreased intake, weight loss.

> In case of swallowing symptoms, also ask about history of muscular diseases, stroke, Parkinson's disease, oropharyngeal carcinoma, as well as treatments (esp. radiotherapy).

> These chapters deal specifically with gastroenterological issues. See the pocket *Acute Medicine* for more information on an extended general patient history, physical examination, and diagnostics.

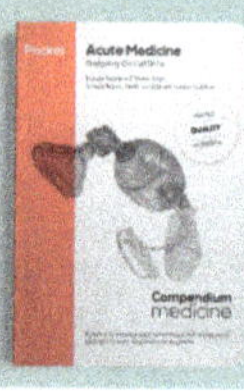

Physical examination

The next chapter provides a systematic guide to performing a general physical examination. Emphasis is placed on the importance of clear communication and patient comfort throughout the examination. The most important aspects of the abdominal examination are presented.

Introduction
- Permission (explain examination and consent)
- Wash your hands, use PPE
- Privacy
- Expose target body part

→

Physical examination
- General inspection
- Vital signs
- Target physical examination
- Tract-specific examination

→

Concluding
- Thank patient
- Dispose of PPE and wash your hands
- Summarise your findings
- Explain indicated diagnostics and/or next steps

Diagram 2 // Physical examination
PPE, personal protective equipment

General inspection

Sex, age (biological vs. calendar), state of consciousness (GCS and AVPU score, see Tables 1 and 2), mental state, posture, skin colour (e.g. pale, cyanotic, flushing/blushing, icteric), mobility, grooming, nutritional status (e.g. cachexia, BMI), and any medical equipment attached to the patient or in the bed space.

Skin colour may give an indication of underlying conditions. For example:
- Pale: anaemia
- Cyanosis: hypoxaemia
- Flushing/blushing: hormonal status, anaphylaxis
- Icteric: high bilirubin levels

Anthropometric data

Abdominal circumference, weight, height, BMI.

Vital signs

REFERENCE RANGES			
RR	9-14/min	**Diastolic BP**	60-90 mmHg
SpO_2	>95%	**CVP**	R 4-9 cm H_2O (3-8 mmHg)
HR/pulse rate	60-100/min	**T**	36-38°C / 96.8-100.4°F
Systolic BP	100-140 mmHg	**CRT**	<3 sec

Table 1 // Normal vital signs (Vx)
BP, blood pressure; CRT, capillary refill time; CVP, central venous pressure; HR, heart rate; RR, respiratory rate; SpO_2, oxygen saturation; T, temperature

A capillary refill time (CRT) ≥3 sec suggests poor peripheral perfusion (e.g. hypovolaemia, sepsis, chronic heart failure).

The first sign of a critically ill patient often is an increased respiratory rate.

Pulse

- Heart rate: 60-100 bpm
- Heart rhythm: regular or irregular rhythm (e.g. atrial fibrillation, atrioventricular blocks)
- Pulse character/pulse force: full, normal, weak, absent/non-palpable
- In emergency situations or when access to the radial artery is challenging, the carotid or femoral pulse can be palpated for assessment

MEWS

The modified early warning score (MEWS) is an objective parameter for early recognition of patients who are at risk of rapid deterioration (see Table 2). Different hospitals have different trigger scores for notifying physicians: verify that your facility uses the same point assignments listed here.

	+3	+2	+1	0	+1	+2	+3
RR (per min)		<9		9-14	15-20	21-29	≥30
Saturation (%)	<92	92-93	94-95	>95			
Supplemental O_2		Yes		No			
Temperature		<35°C/ <95°F		35.0-38.4°C/ 95-101.1°F		≥38.5°C/ 101.3°F	
Systolic BP (mmHg)	≤70	71-80	81-100	101-199		≥200	
HR (per min)		≤40	41-50	51-100	101-110	111-129	≥130
Consciousness (AVPU score)				Alert	Responds to voice	Responds to pain	Unresponsive

Table 2 // Modified early warning score
AVPU, alert verbal pain unresponsive; BP, blood pressure; HR, heart rate; RR, respiratory rate

General physical examination

Always perform the physical examination according to the patient's specific complaints and clinical history. Consider indications or any red flags for additional diagnostics. This section provides a focused exploration of the most common general and system-specific aspects of physical examination in the pocket *Gastroenterology and Hepatology* rather than attempting to cover all aspects comprehensively.

Assessment of a patient's mental state is indicated, particularly when e.g. hepatic encephalopathy is suspected. Pay attention to the presence of bradyphrenia, loss of consciousness, or personality changes.

Thorax

Lungs

Inspection

Skin abnormalities (e.g. thoracic scars, rash, peripheral and central cyanosis), breathing pattern (e.g. depth, rate, sound, posture, accessory breathing muscles, rhythm, asymmetry in the expiratory and inspiratory phases), chest wall deformities (e.g. asymmetry, pectus carinatum, pectus excavatum, hyperexpansion/ barrel chest), extremities (e.g. colour, nail clubbing), respiratory effort.

Palpation
Diaphragmatic excursions, epigastric angle, local point tenderness, vocal fremitus, subcutaneous emphysema.

Percussion
Air resonance (normal), dullness (increased tissue density, e.g. pneumonia, pleural effusion), stony dullness (e.g. pleural effusion), hyper-resonance (increased air, e.g. emphysema, pneumothorax), symmetry, lower lung border, shifting lung borders, lung-liver border, diaphragm.

Auscultation
Breathing sounds (vesicular/normal, bronchial/harsh-sounding (e.g. consolidation)), quiet/reduced breath sounds (e.g. silent chest in COPD), symmetry, vocal resonance (volume), inhalation/exhalation ratio, abnormal breath sounds (fine end-inspiratory crackles indicating opening of obstructed central bronchi, coarse crackles indicating opening of distal airways, pleural rub, rhonchi, inspiratory/ expiratory stridor, wheezing, muffles, absent breath sounds).

Heart
Inspection
Skin abnormalities (e.g. thoracic scars, rash, petechiae/Osler's node/Janeway lesion/splinter haemorrhages (e.g. endocarditis stigmata)), neck veins (pulsations, CVP ↑), peripheral pitting oedema.

Palpation
Apex beat (heaves/thrills), thrill/vibration.

Percussion
Heart borders (top, left, right).

Auscultation
Heart rate, heart sounds (S1 and S2), S2 splitting, presence of S3 (e.g. in athletes or pathological cause, e.g. post-myocardial infarction, mitral regurgitation, ven-

tricle septum defect, dilated cardiomyopathy) and/or S4 (decreased ventricular compliance, e.g. in hypertrophic cardiomyopathy, aortic stenosis), cardiac rhythm (regular/irregular, breathing-based or unrelated to breathing), murmurs (timing in systole or diastole, high/low frequency, loudness, radiation over carotid arteries, valve locations, see Figure 1 and Table 3), pericardial friction rub.

VALVE DEFECTS	PHASE OF HEART CYCLE	SHAPE	PMI	ILLUSTRATION
Aortic valve regurgitation	Diastole	Decrescendo	3 ICS left	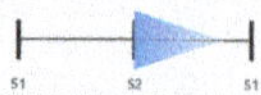
Aortic valve stenosis	Systole	Crescendo-decrescendo	• 2 ICS right • Radiation: carotid artery	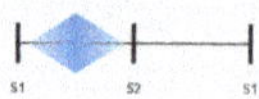
Mitral valve regurgitation	Systole	Holosystolic	• Apex • Radiation: left flank and axilla	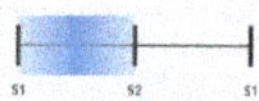
Mitral valve stenosis	Diastole	Opening snap, presystolic murmur	Apex	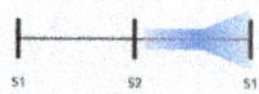
Pulmonary valve regurgitation	Diastole	Decrescendo	2 ICS left	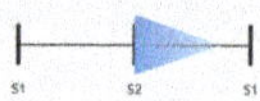
Pulmonary valve stenosis	Systole	Crescendo-decrescendo	2 ICS left	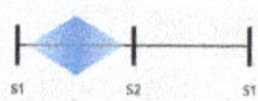
Tricuspid valve regurgitation	Systole	Holosystolic	4 ICS left	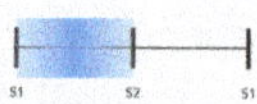

Table 3 // Characteristics of cardiac murmurs caused by valve defects
ICS, intercostal space; PMI, point of maximum intensity

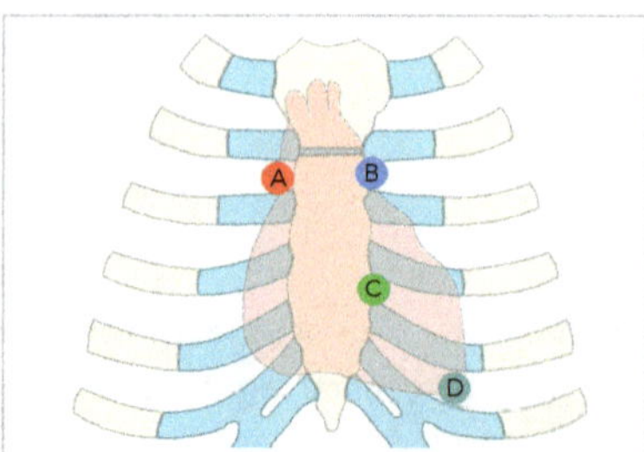

Figure 1 // Valve locations
A: Aortic valve **B:** Pulmonary valve **C:** Tricuspid valve **D:** Mitral valve

Percussion and palpation play a relatively minor role in cardiovascular examination and are not frequently utilised in clinical practice.

Abdomen

Inspection

Shape/symmetry (e.g. abdominal obesity, bulging flanks, mass (pulsatile, expansile), abdominal distension: fat, fluid, flatus, faeces, fetus, fulminant mass), navel (flat, everted), skin abnormalities (e.g. scars, striae, rash, discolouration, caput medusae, spider angioma), bruising (e.g. umbilicus (Cullen's sign) or flanks (Grey-Turner's sign) in pancreatitis-related retroperitoneal haemorrhage), abdominal hernias, visible peristalsis, visible motion with respiration.

Auscultation

Bowel sounds: normal/low-pitched (every 5-10 sec), absent (>1-2 min, indicative of ileus), tinkling/high-pitched (indicative of mechanical bowel obstruction), bruits (e.g. abdominal aorta aneurysm, renal artery stenosis).

Percussion

Quality (dullness over fluid/solid structures, tympany over air-filled structures, hypertympanic when free intraperitoneal air), organs (e.g. bladder contours, liver contours, spleen contours), pain, shifting dullness (if suspecting ascites) (see Figure 4).

Palpation

Superficial palpation: tenderness, voluntary guarding, involuntary guarding/rigidity (e.g. peritonitis), fluid thrill (if suspecting ascites) (see Figure 3).
Deep palpation: rebound tenderness (e.g. peritoneal irritation), organomegaly (liver/spleen), masses (e.g. location, size, shape, consistency, mobility), organs (aorta, bladder, colon, gallbladder, liver, spleen, kidneys).
Specific tests: McBurney's sign, Rovsing's sign and Psoas sign (all suggestive of appendicitis); Murphy's sign (suggestive of cholecystitis).

> Signs of peritoneal irritation include: sensitivity to percussion, abdominal guarding, active muscle resistance, ipsilateral or contralateral rebound tenderness, and pain during the rectal exam. Patients are often so sore that even bumping into the exam table will trigger a reaction. Peritoneal irritation is associated with e.g. appendicitis, diverticulitis, cholecystitis, and intestinal perforation. It is a reason for surgical consultation, diagnostic imaging, and other diagnostics.

During abdominal examination, it is helpful to recognise and follow the four quadrants of the abdomen i.e. the right upper quadrant (RUQ), left upper quadrant (LUQ), right lower quadrant (RLQ), and left lower quadrant (LLQ), see Figure 2.

In patients with pain, begin palpation of the abdomen in the non-painful quadrant(s). During palpation, pay close attention to the patient's face: this is an important indicator for localisation of pain and severity.

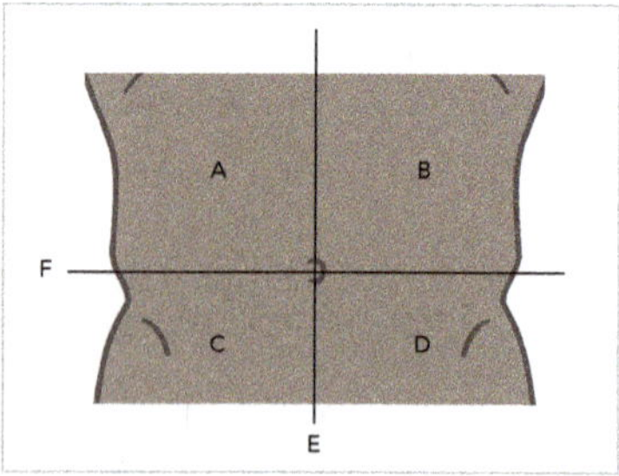

Figure 2 // Quadrants of the abdomen **A:** Right upper quadrant **B:** Left upper quadrant **C:** Right lower quadrant **D:** Left lower quadrant **E:** Medial plane **F:** Transumbilical plane

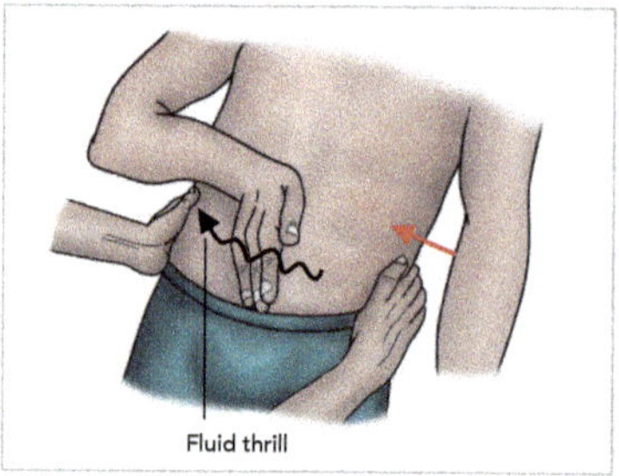

Figure 3 // Fluid thrill

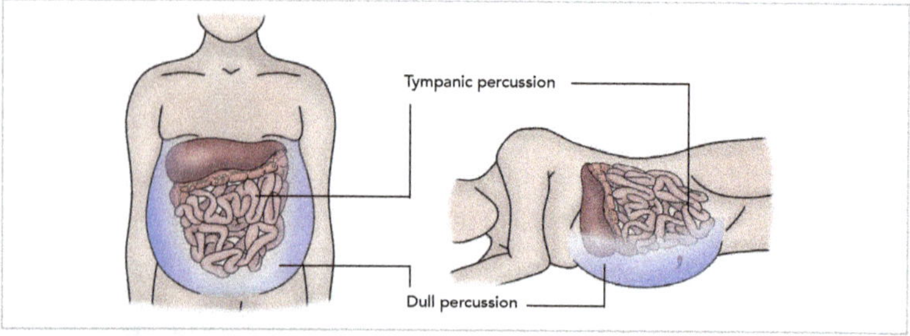

Figure 4 // Shifting dullness

Rectal examination

Inspection

Scars, prolapse (ask patient to push), skin tags, fissures (usually dorsal), fistulas (productive/non-productive, appearance of discharge), ulcers, warts, swellings, haemorrhoids.

Palpation

Sphincter tone (ask patient to squeeze), rectal mucosa (360° check for irregularities), ♀ rectouterine pouch, ♂ prostate (size, consistency, pain, nodule).

Functional pelvic floor examination: resting muscle tone, strength, relaxation, paradoxical construction.

After withdrawing: inspect the glove for stool (colour, consistency), blood, pus, mucus.

> Provide clear instructions to the patient prior to performing the exam. Use plenty of lubricant (e.g. gel, Vaseline®), and take your time to give instructions, inspect the patient, and perform the internal exam. When using a coloured glove, wipe your finger with white toilet or tissue paper.

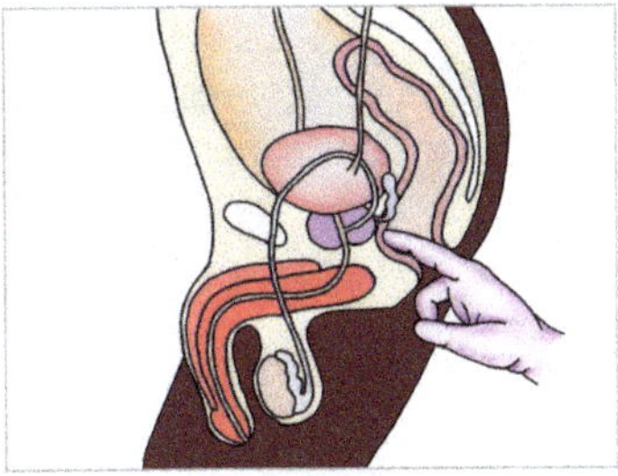

Figure 5 // Rectal examination

> **Digital rectal examination:** Ask the patient to bear down as you gently and smoothly insert the examining finger. After withdrawal, discreetly inspect the glove for blood, stool, pus, or mucus.

Extremities

Inspection

Hair growth, skin abnormalities (e.g. scars, rash, bruises), contours of arms and legs (e.g. muscle atrophy), symmetrical spacing between extremities and torso, joints (e.g. redness, position, swelling), oedema, trophic disorders (e.g. shiny skin, lack of hair, brittle nails), varicose veins, flapping tremor.

Palpation

Peripheral oedema (e.g. pitting, non-pitting), arterial pulsations (i.e. brachial, radial, femoral, popliteal, posterior tibial, dorsalis pedis arteries), reflexes (i.e. biceps, brachioradialis, triceps, quadriceps muscles, Achilles tendon), sensation, temperature, swelling, joint (e.g. ROM, stiffness, stability), muscles (e.g. tension, tenderness, eccentric and concentric strength).

Diagnostics

Lab values

Reference values may vary between laboratories. Test results should preferably be compared to previous values. Request them from the patient's GP or another hospital if necessary.

While the following section provides examples of conditions associated with altered lab values, it is essential to acknowledge that the scope of medical diagnoses is vast and varied.

When interpreting laboratory results, it is crucial to consider them in the context of all findings. For example, an isolated thrombocytopaenia has a completely different differential diagnosis than thrombocytopaenia with anaemia and leukopaenia (pancytopaenia).

General blood count

LAB VALUE	EXPLANATION	INTERPRETATION
Haemoglobin (Hb)	Protein in erythrocytes that can bind and carry oxygen	↑ Polycythaemia: • Primary polycythaemia: - Congenital - Acquired: malignant bone marrow disease • Secondary polycythaemia: - Secondary to hypoxia: e.g. COPD or smoking, sleep apnoea, high altitudes, right-to-left shunts, congestive heart failure - Secondary to kidney disease - Secondary to EPO-producing tumour - Secondary to alcohol use disorder • Secondary to dehydration ↓ Anaemia, see Table 5

Table 4A // General blood count

CMV, cytomegalovirus; COPD, chronic obstructive pulmonary disease; DIC, disseminated intravascular coagulation; EBV, Epstein-Barr virus; EDTA, Ethylenediaminetetraacetic acid; EPO, erythropoietin; HIV, human immunodeficiency virus; ITP, immune thrombocytopaenia; HELLP, haemolysis, elevated liver enzyme levels and low platelet levels

LAB VALUE	EXPLANATION	INTERPRETATION
Haematocrit (Ht)	Measure of red blood cell volume in relation to total blood volume	↑ • Dehydration • Primary or secondary polycythaemia ↓ Anaemia
Mean corpuscular volume (MCV)	Measure of the average volume of erythrocytes, see Table 5	↑ Macrocytic = Normocytic ↓ Microcytic
Platelet count (PLT)	• Platelets/thrombocytes • Are primary haemostasis by aggregation	↑ Thrombocytosis: • During/after infection/inflammation • Splenectomy/hyposplenism • Iron deficiency • Myeloproliferative disease • Paraneoplastic ↓ Thrombocytopaenia: • Synthesis ↓: bone marrow insufficiency, e.g. tumour invasion/medication-induced, deficiencies (vitamin B12, folic acid), liver disease (e.g. liver cirrhosis), hyperthyroidism/hypothyroidism • Utilisation/degradation ↑: disseminated intravascular coagulation (DIC), immune thrombocytopaenia (ITP), medication-induced immune thrombocytopaenia, post-transfusion, preeclampsia/HELLP, viral infection (e.g. CMV, EBV, hepatitis B/C, HIV), parasitic infection (malaria), idiopathic, heparin-induced thrombocytopaenia (HIT) • Loss ↑: blood loss, splenomegaly (e.g. in portal hypertension) • Other causes: gestational trombocytopenia, hereditary thrombocytopaenia (e.g. Bernard-Soulier syndrome) • Watch out for pseudothrombocytopaenia: false lower result due to agglutination in EDTA tube
Red blood cell (RBC) count	• Erythrocytes: red blood cells • Transport O_2 and CO_2 between lungs and tissue	↑ Erythrocytosis: • Primary: polycythaemia vera, see Hb • Secondary to oxygen deprivation, see Hb ↓ Erythropenia: • Reduced synthesis: - Nutritional deficiency - Disrupted production in bone marrow • Increased degradation, e.g. autoimmune haemolysis, haemoglobinopathy, DIC, valve haemolysis
Mean corpuscular haemoglobin (MCH)	Average amount of oxygen-carrying haemoglobin per erythrocyte (Hb/erythrocytes)	↑ Hyperchromic anaemia: • Vitamin B12 deficiency • Folic acid deficiency

Table 4B // General blood count

LAB VALUE	EXPLANATION	INTERPRETATION
Mean corpuscular haemoglobin concentration (MCHC)	Average haemoglobin concentration per erythrocyte (Hb/Ht)	= Normochromic anaemia ↓ Hypochromic anaemia: • Iron deficiency • Haemoglobinopathy
Red blood cell distribution width (RDW)	A measure of MCV variance	↑ In case of high MCV variance, e.g. after a blood transfusion or in combined microcytic and macrocytic anaemia (MCV may be normal)
Reticulocyte count (RTIC)	• Reticulocytes: immature erythrocytes that still have RNA • Adequacy of a reticulocyte response depends on haematocrit levels. A deep anaemia should give a marked increase in reticulocyte count.	↑ Reticulocytosis: • Increased erythrocyte synthesis, e.g. haemolytic anaemia, bleeding ↓ Reticulopenia: • Reduced erythrocyte synthesis, e.g. medication-induced myelosuppression, aplastic anaemia, aneamia of chronic disease

Table 4C // General blood count

Anaemia - interpretation

HB	MCV	DIFFERENTIAL DIAGNOSIS
↓	↓	• Iron-deficiency anaemia (chronic blood loss) • Haemoglobinopathy • Other causes: lead poisoning ⊖, sideroblastic anaemia ⊖, hookworm infection ⊖
	↓/=	Anaemia of chronic disease (e.g. infections, malignancy, autoimmune diseases)
	=	• Acute blood loss • Long-term chronic kidney disease (EPO deficiency) • Malnutrition • Mixed-aetiology anaemias • Multiple myeloma
	=/↑	• Haemolysis • Medication-induced • Thyroid dysfunction (specifically hypothyroidism) • Haematological malignancy • Bone marrow disease: - Aplastic anaemia - Bone marrow filtration - Myelodysplastic syndrome

Table 5A // Anaemia - interpretation

HB	MCV	DIFFERENTIAL DIAGNOSIS
↓	↑	• Vitamin B12 deficiency (e.g. malabsorption, HIV) • Folic acid deficiency • Pregnancy • Toxic: alcohol use disorder, medication-induced (e.g. cytostatics)

Table 5B // Anaemia - interpretation

For the differential diagnosis of anaemia, the iron panel is essential, see Iron panel.

Arterial blood gas (ABG)

LAB VALUE	EXPLANATION	INTERPRETATION
pH 7.35-7.45	Hydrogen ion concentration in the blood	↑ Alkalosis ↓ Acidosis
$PaCO_2$ 35-45 mmHg (4.7-6.0 kPa)	Partial pressure of carbon dioxide	↑ • Respiratory acidosis: hypoventilation, type II respiratory insufficiency (e.g. COPD) • Respiratory compensation in metabolic alkalosis ↓ • Respiratory alkalosis: hyperventilation • Respiratory compensation in metabolic acidosis
HCO_3^- 22-26 mmol/L (mEQ/L)	Buffer for H^+	↑ Metabolic alkalosis: • Loss of H^+: - Gastrointestinal loss (e.g. vomiting, diarrhoea (with Cl^-)) - Renal loss (e.g. activation of RAAS due to primary hyperaldosteronism, heart failure, cirrhosis) - Intracellular H^+ shift (as in hypokalaemia) • Increase in HCO_3^-: - Renal retention (e.g. loop and thiazide diuretics) - Cystic fibrosis ↓ Metabolic acidosis: • Increase in H^+: - Excessive production (e.g. ketoacidosis, lactate acidosis, rhabdomyolysis) - Renal insufficiency (impaired H^+ excretion) - Intoxications with exogenous acids (e.g. toxic alcohols, salicylates) - Hyperchloraemia • Loss of HCO_3^-: - Gastrointestinal (e.g. severe diarrhoea, laxative use, gastrointestinal fistulas) - Renal loss - Medication (e.g. spironolactone)

Table 6A // Arterial blood gas (ABG)

LAB VALUE	EXPLANATION	INTERPRETATION
Base excess (BE) -2 to +2 mmol/L	Base excess or deficit needed to get pH to 7.40	↑ • Metabolic alkalosis • Metabolic compensation in respiratory acidosis ↓ • Metabolic acidosis • Metabolic compensation in respiratory alkalosis
Anion gap (only in metabolic acidosis) 4-12 mmol/L	• Number of unmeasured anions (negatively charged particles, including albumin, SO_4^{2-} and HPO_4^{2-}) • Formula: $[Na^+]$ - ($[Cl^-]$ + $[HCO_3^-]$)	↑ Due to increase in H^+: • Endogenous: lactic acidosis, ketoacidosis, renal insufficiency • Exogenous: intoxications, e.g. ethylene glycol, methanol, salicylate = Due to loss of HCO_3^- (compensated by higher levels of chloride): • Gastrointestinal loss of HCO_3^- (urine anion gap -) (accompanied by Cl^- retention in the kidneys), e.g. diarrhoea • Renal loss (urine anion gap +), e.g. hyperchloraemia • Addison's disease
PaO_2 75-100 mmHg (10.0-13.3 kPa)	Partial pressure of oxygen	↑ Hyperventilation ↓ Type I respiratory insufficiency: • Hypoventilation • Ventilation perfusion mismatch • Diffusion disorder • Right-to-left shunt
SaO_2 ≥95%	Oxygen saturation of haemoglobin	↓ Oxygen deficiency, e.g. carbon monoxide poisoning
Lactate 0.5-1.7 mmol/L	End product of anaerobic glycolysis	↑ Diminished tissue oxygenation (lactate acidosis), e.g. sepsis, hypoxaemia

Table 6B // Arterial blood gas (ABG)

- Decreased albumin can result in a false low anion gap (AG), calculated as: AG = Na^+ - (Cl^- + HCO_3^-).
- Oxygen saturation (sO_2) measures the saturation of functional Hb = $O_2Hb/(O_2Hb$ + deoxyHb). As a result, the saturation of haemoglobinopathies such as carboxyHb, MetHb, and SulfHb is not measured. In the presence of dyshaemoglobins, oxygen saturation is an unreliable metric (overestimation) and measuring the oxygen fraction is preferred.
- An air bubble in the sample will produce anomalous pCO_2 (decreased) and pO_2 (increased) values due to gas diffusion.

In practice, a venous or capillary blood gas test usually provides the necessary information and is more comfortable for the patient. Arterial blood gas tests are only needed for measuring the Aa gradient (difference between pO_2 in alveoli vs. in arterial blood).

The common causes of anion gap acidosis can be recalled using the mnemonic MUDPILES: **m**ethanol, **u**raemia, **d**iabetic ketoacidosis, **p**ropylene glycol, **i**soniazid, **i**ron, **l**actic acidosis, **e**thylene glycol, **s**alicylates.

Blood gas - interpretation

	PH	pCO_2	HCO_3^-	ANION GAP	COMPENSATION MECHANISM
Respiratory alkalosis	↑/=	↓	↓/=		↓ Renal [HCO_3^-] reabsorption (slow)
Metabolic alkalosis	↑/=	↑/=	↑		Hypoventilation (fast)
Respiratory acidosis	↓/=	↑	↑/=		↑ Renal [HCO_3^-] reabsorption (slow)
High anion gap metabolic acidosis	↓/=	↓/=	↓	↑	Hyperventilation
Normal anion gap metabolic acidosis	↓/=	↓/=	↓	=	Hyperventilation

Table 7 // Blood gas - interpretation

Electrolytes

Ca^{2+} is partially bound to albumin. Low albumin levels may lead to a decrease in total Ca^{2+} and may be accompanied by normal ionised Ca^{2+}. Total Ca^{2+} can be corrected for the patient's albumin level using lab-specific formulas. Scan the QR code for the formula.

LAB VALUE	EXPLANATION	INTERPRETATION
Sodium (Na^+)	• Main extracellular cation • Very important in water management	↑ Hypernatraemia: • Increased water loss: - Osmotic diarrhoea or diuresis (e.g. hyperglycaemia, mannitol) - Arginine vasopressin deficiency (e.g. cranial trauma, infections, autoimmune) - Arginine vasopressin resistance (e.g. drugs, amyloidosis, hereditary) • Increased sodium retention (iatrogenic with unchecked IV drip) • Insufficient fluid intake (with or without intact thirst stimulus) ↓ Hyponatraemia: often multiple causes • Water retention: - Syndrome of inappropriate antidiuretic hormone secretion (SIADH) - Renal insufficiency stage 5 - Congestive heart failure - Liver cirrhosis - Blood loss (resulting in ADH ↑ to preserve volume) - Nephrotic syndrome • Increased sodium loss: - Gastrointestinal, e.g. diarrhoea, small bowel obstruction - Renal, e.g. diuretics, renal failure, osmotic diuresis (severe hyperglycaemia), Addison's disease - Transdermal, e.g. burns, excessive sweating • Other: - Tea & toast (malnutrition) - Polydipsia

Table 8A // Electrolytes

ACE, Angiotensin-converting enzyme; ADH, antidiuretic hormone; AST, Aspartate aminotransferase; IV, intravenous; LDH, Lactate dehydrogenase; NSAID, non-steroidal anti-inflammatory drugs; PPI, proton pump inhibitor; PTH, parathyroid hormone; SIADH, Syndrome of inappropriate antidiuretic hormone ADH release; TPN, total parenteral nutrition

LAB VALUE	EXPLANATION	INTERPRETATION
Potassium (K^+)	• Main intracellular cation • Regulates e.g. nerve impulse transmission, glycogen and protein synthesis	↑ Hyperkalaemia: • Extracellular redistribution (shift): - Metabolic or respiratory acidosis - Hyperosmolality - Insulin deficiency - Medication-induced, e.g. beta blockers, digoxin • Tissue breakdown (often in combination with LDH, AST, bilirubin): - Haemolysis - Tumor lysis syndrome - Rhabdomyolysis - Distal arterial occlusion • Impaired renal excretion: - Mineralocorticoid deficiency - Renal insufficiency - Medication-induced, e.g. ACE inhibitors, NSAIDs, potassium-sparing diuretics - Type IV renal tubular acidosis • Pseudohyperkalaemia (e.g. following blood collection) ↓ Hypokalaemia: • Intracellular redistribution: - Metabolic or respiratory alkalosis - Insulin use • Renal loss: - Renal conditions, e.g. type I and II renal tubular acidosis - Hyperaldosteronism - Medication-induced, e.g. diuretics, glucocorticoids - Hypomagnesaemia - Chronic metabolic acidosis • Extrarenal loss, e.g. gastrointestinal (diarrhoea) • Insufficient intake, e.g. chronic alcohol use disorder

Table 8B // Electrolytes

<table>
<tr><th>LAB VALUE</th><th>EXPLANATION</th><th>INTERPRETATION</th></tr>
<tr><td>Magnesium (Mg^{2+})</td><td>• 70% in bone, remainder is intracellular
• Cofactor in enzymatic processes
• Stabilises nucleic acids and ribosomes</td><td>↑ Hypermagnesaemia:
• Renal insufficiency
• Medication-induced, e.g. laxatives, lithium, antacids containing magnesium
• Other:
- Rhabdomyolysis
- Hypothyroidism
↓ Hypomagnesaemia:
• Gastrointestinal loss, e.g. diarrhoea, inadequate intake, malnutrition/malabsorption
• Medication-induced, e.g. PPIs, diuretics, cisplatina, insulin, tacrolimus, cyclosporine
• Renal loss, e.g. hyperaldosteronism, hyperthyroidism, diuretics
• Other:
- Chronic alcohol use
- Hypercalcaemia
- Hungry bone syndrome</td></tr>
<tr><td>Chloride (Cl^-)</td><td>• Main extracellular anion
• Regulation closely linked to sodium metabolism</td><td>↑ Hyperchloraemia:
• Chloride administration: secondary to administration of chloride-rich intravenous fluids
• True water loss relative to chloride:
- Renal: osmotic diuresis, postobstructive diuresis, arginine vasopressine resistance (formerly diabetes insipidus)
- Extrarenal: fever, diarrhoea, burns, dehydration
• Increase in tubular reabsorption: e.g. renal tubular acidosis, acetazolamide, neobladder
↓ Hypochloraemia:
• Increased loss:
- Gastrointestinal, e.g. vomiting
- Renal
- Ascites
- True water gain relative to chloride: congestive heart failure, syndrome of inappropriate antidiuretic hormone secretion (SIADH)
- High output stoma
• Metabolic alkalosis</td></tr>
</table>

Table 8C // Electrolytes

LAB VALUE	EXPLANATION	INTERPRETATION
Calcium (Ca^{2+})	• 99% is stored in bone as a mineral, 50% of plasma calcium is free and biologically active (ionised), 40% is bound to albumin, 10% bound to organic molecules • Regulates e.g. nerve impulse conduction, muscle contractility, enzyme functioning, and clotting	↑ Hypercalcaemia: • Primary/tertiary hyperparathyroidism • Tumour-induced, e.g. bone metastases, multiple myeloma, PTH-like peptide • Endocrine: hyperthyroidism, adrenal cortex insufficiency, pheochromocytoma • Vitamin D excessive production or intoxication (e.g. sarcoidosis, lymphoma) • Pseudohypercalcaemia ↓ Hypocalcaemia: • Primary hypoparathyroidism • PTH resistance/pseudohypoparathyroidism • Vitamin D deficiency • Chronic renal insufficiency • Hypomagnesaemia • Medication-induced, e.g. corticosteroids, diuretics, antiseizure medication • Malabsorption • Acute pancreatitis • Blood transfusions, including massive blood transfusions
Phosphate (PO_4^{3-})	• 75% in bone, remainder in muscle tissue and intracellularly • Main intracellular anion • Particularly important for cell energy metabolism	↑ Hyperphosphataemia: • Endogenous: rhabdomyolysis, haemolysis, intestinal infarction • Exogenous: supplementation, e.g. phosphate enemas • Reduced renal excretion: acute or chronic renal insufficiency, hypoparathyroidism, medication-induced (e.g. vitamin D supplementation) • Shift from intracellular: lactate acidosis, ketoacidosis • Pseudohyperphosphataemia: hyperbilirubinaemia, extreme hypertriglyceridaemia, heparin ↓ Hypophosphataemia: • Redistribution: refeeding syndrome, respiratory alkalosis, diabetic ketoacidosis, hungry bone syndrome, medication-induced (e.g. insulin) • Renal loss: hyperparathyroidism, vitamin D deficiency, medication-induced (e.g. diuretics, glucocorticoids) • Reduced absorption: TPN, malabsorption, anorexia nervosa, alcohol use disorder, chronic/non-chronic diarrhoea, vitamin D deficiency, medication-induced (e.g. overuse of antacids)
Bicarbonate (HCO_3^-)		See Arterial blood gas

Table 8D // Electrolytes

Liver tests and pancreatic tests

LAB VALUE	EXPLANATION	INTERPRETATION
Alanine transaminase (ALT)	Enzyme found primarily in hepatocytes	↑ • Liver conditions: - Hepatitis, e.g. viral, toxic, alcoholic (ALT<AST), autoimmune, ischaemic - Non-alcoholic steatohepatitis - Liver cirrhosis - Hepatocellular carcinoma/liver metastases - Medication-induced liver injury - Liver abscess - Acute liver failure - Haemochromatosis - Wilson's disease - Primary biliary cholangitis/primary sclerosing cholangitis • Bile duct obstruction, see ALP • Chronic/acute pancreatitis • Budd-Chiari syndrome • Preeclampsia/eclampsia/HELLP • Hypotension, i.e. septic shock
Aspartate aminotransferase (AST)	Enzyme found mainly in liver and striated (i.e. cardiac, skeletal) muscle tissue	↑ • In all diagnoses mentioned in ALT • May also be elevated in: - Myocardial infarction/heart failure - Muscle conditions, e.g. rhabdomyolysis, dermatomyositis
Alkaline phosphatase (ALP)	Enzyme found primarily in liver parenchyma, bile epithelium, osteoblasts, and placenta	↑ • Bile duct obstruction: - Cholelithiasis - Cholangitis - Hepatocellular carcinoma, cholangiocarcinoma, liver metastases - Pancreatic malignancy - Medication-induced - Pregnancy • Liver conditions: - Hepatitis, e.g. alcoholic - Primary biliary cholangitis - Primary sclerosing cholangitis • Bone disease (isolated elevation of ALP): - Hyperparathyroidism - Bone metastases - Paget's disease - Osteomyelitis or fractures

Table 9A // Liver tests and pancreatic tests

<table>
<tr><th>LAB VALUE</th><th>EXPLANATION</th><th>INTERPRETATION</th></tr>
<tr><td>Gamma-glutamyltransferase (GGT)</td><td>• Enzyme present in virtually all cells
• Serum GGT generally comes from the hepatobiliary system</td><td>↑ • Bile duct obstruction, see ALP
• Liver conditions:
- Primary biliary cholangitis
- Primary sclerosing cholangitis
- Hepatitis, e.g. alcoholic
• Alcohol use
• Obesity</td></tr>
<tr><td>Bilirubin</td><td>• Degradation product of haemoglobin
• Mainly formed in the spleen → conjugated in the liver → excreted with bile</td><td>↑ Hyperbilirubinaemia:
• Prehepatic (unconjugated): excessive formation of bilirubin (direct bilirubin <20%), e.g. haemolysis, haematoma resorption
• Hepatic (unconjugated and conjugated): liver disease, Gilbert's disease
• Posthepatic (conjugated): bile duct obstruction (direct bilirubin >50%, ALP ↑, GGT ↑)</td></tr>
<tr><td>Lactate dehydrogenase (LDH)</td><td>Enzyme involved in glycolysis in various tissues</td><td>↑ • Increased cellular death in:
- Liver conditions
- Myocardial infarction
- Muscle conditions
- Haemolysis
• Malignancies (specifically lymphoma, haematological malignancy)</td></tr>
<tr><td>Lipase</td><td>• Enzyme that hydrolyses triglycerides to fatty acids and glycerides
• Serum lipase is largely pancreas-specific
• Released into circulation during autolysis of pancreatic tissue
• Lipase has a higher sensitivity for pancreatitis and is released more often than amylase</td><td>↑ • Acute pancreatitis (with acute or chronic pancreatitis there might be no elevation)
• May also be elevated in:
- Renal insufficiency
- Diabetic ketoacidosis
- Bile duct disease
↓ Exocrine pancreatic insufficiency</td></tr>
<tr><td>Amylase</td><td>• Enzyme produced in the pancreas and salivary glands
• Involved in polysaccharide degradation</td><td>↑ • Acute pancreatitis
• May also be elevated in:
- Salivary gland disorders
- Renal insufficiency
- Intra-abdominal inflammation
- Bile duct disease
↓ Exocrine pancreatic insufficiency</td></tr>
</table>

Table 9B // Liver tests and pancreatic tests

A combination of elevated AST and ALT (liver enzymes) indicates hepatocellular damage. The AST/ALT ratio can provide information about the underlying condition. ALT>AST could indicate viral or autoimmune hepatitis and AST>ALT could indicate alcoholic hepatitis. A combination of bilirubin ↑, ALP ↑, and GGT ↑ indicates cholestasis.

A decrease in the synthetic function of the liver indicates severe liver disease. The common assessing liver synthetic function are albumin, PT/INR, and glucose.

Hyperbilirubinaemia - interpretation

		AETIOLOGY	CONJUGATED BILIRUBIN*	ADDITIONAL TESTS
Unconjugated/indirect	**Prehepatic**	Increased erythrocyte degradation (haemolysis)	<20%	LDH ↑, reticulocytes ↑, Hb ↓, haptoglobin ↓
	Hepatic	Disrupted transport in hepatocyte		
		Disrupted conjugation, e.g. Gilbert's disease		
Conjugated/direct	**Hepatic**	Hepatocyte damage	>40%	ALT ↑, AST ↑
		Intrahepatic cholestasis, e.g. hepatitis, liver cirrhosis	>50%	ALT ↑, AST ↑, ALP ↑, GGT ↑
	Posthepatic	Extrahepatic cholestasis, e.g. gallstones, primary sclerosing cholangitis		ALP ↑, GGT ↑

Table 10 // Hyperbilirubinaemia - interpretation *(relative to total bilirubin)

Proteins

<table>
<tr><th>LAB VALUE</th><th>EXPLANATION</th><th>INTERPRETATION</th></tr>
<tr><td>Albumin</td><td>• Half of all blood proteins
• Produced by the liver
• Main protein for osmotic pressure, also a transport protein
• Negative acute-phase protein
• Non-specific marker of liver synthetic function
• Necessary for interpretation of calcium level</td><td>↑ Hyperalbuminaemia:
• Dehydration
↓ Hypoalbuminaemia:
• Reduced synthesis:
- Liver disease (e.g. liver cirrhosis, hepatitis, malignancy)
- Inflammatory processes
- Malnutrition/malabsorption
- Hypothyroidism
• Increased degradation:
- Cushing's syndrome
- Malignancies
- Hyperthyroidism
• Increased loss:
- Renal, e.g. nephrotic syndrome
- Gastrointestinal, e.g. IBD
- Ascites (exudate)
- Burns
• Haemodilution</td></tr>
<tr><td>Total protein</td><td>Concentration of all blood proteins, e.g. proteins involved in enzymatic action, inflammatory response, immunological defense, transport, and osmotic pressure</td><td>↑ • Hyperimmunoglobulinaemia (monoclonal, e.g. multiple myeloma or polyclonal)
• Dehydration
↓ • Reduced synthesis:
- Liver conditions
- Malnutrition/malabsorption
• Increased loss:
- Renal, e.g. nephrotic syndrome
- Gastrointestinal, e.g. IBD
- Ascites (exudate)
- Burns
• Haemodilution</td></tr>
<tr><td>Haptoglobin</td><td>• Protein that binds free haemoglobin
• Positive acute-phase protein</td><td>↑ Inflammation
↓ • Utilisation in haemolysis (thus the haptoglobin is often suppressed or lowered due to haemolysis) or high cell turnover, e.g. sickle cell disease
• Also reduced in impaired synthesis, e.g. severe liver disease, severe malnutrition</td></tr>
</table>

Table 11 // Proteins

Inflammatory markers

LAB VALUE	EXPLANATION	INTERPRETATION
Erythrocyte sedimentation rate (ESR)	• Erythrocyte sedimentation rate (mm/h) • Elevated with increased concentration of acute-phase proteins and/or immunoglobulin-mediated surface charge alteration, causing erythrocytes to repel each other less and sink faster	↑ • Increased blood protein levels: - Infections - Autoimmune diseases - Rheumatic conditions - Malignancies - Monoclonal and polyclonal gammopathies - Infarction - Hypothyroidism • Anaemia • Pregnancy, obesity, older age, smoking ↓ • Abnormalities of erythrocytes, e.g. polycythaemia, sickle cell disease • Congestive heart failure • Hypogammaglobulinaemia
C-reactive protein (CRP)	• C-reactive protein • Positive acute-phase protein • Produced in the liver	↑ • Infections • Inflammation • Rheumatic conditions • Malignancies • Trauma • Thrombosis
White blood cell (WBC) count	• Leukocytes: white blood cells • Part of the immune system	↑ Leukocytosis: • Infections • Inflammatory processes • Autoimmune diseases • Myeloproliferative disease, e.g. leukaemia • Medication-induced, e.g. steroids • Smoking ↓ Leukopenia: • Infections (due to utilisation) • Medication-induced/iatrogenic, e.g. chemotherapy, immunosupressants, antibiotics • Bone marrow deficiency • Splenomegaly (e.g. in portal hypertension) • Benign leukopenia, seen in individuals of African, Middle Eastern, and West Indian descent • Other causes: B12 and folic acid deficiency

Table 12A // Inflammatory markers

LAB VALUE	EXPLANATION	INTERPRETATION
Leukocyte differential	Breakdown of total leukocytes by subtype	↑ Neutrophilia: • Bacterial infection, sepsis, myeloproliferative diseases ↓ Neutropenia: • Decreased production: severe infections, medication-induced/iatrogenic • Increased utilisation/destruction: medication-induced antibody formation ↑ Lymphocytosis: • Infection, smoking, hyposplenism, lymphoproliferative disease ↓ Lymphopaenia: • Infection, HIV, renal failure ↑ Monocytosis: • Bacterial/parasitic infection, myeloproliferative diseases, Hodgkin's disease, neutropenia, steroids ↓ Monopaenia: • In neutropenia, hairy cell leukaemia, cytotoxic agents (e.g. chemotherapy) ↑ Eosinophilia: • Parasitic infection, allergic reactions, skin diseases, myeloproliferative diseases, hypereosinophilic syndrome ↑ Basophilia: • Allergic reactions, iron deficiency, chronic myeloid leukaemia, systemic mastocytosis, allergic reaction

Table 12B // Inflammatory markers

In various inflammations, e.g. in acute pancreatitis, an elevated WBC precedes an increase in CRP (approx. 24 hours).

Renal function tests

<table>
<tr><th>LAB VALUE</th><th>EXPLANATION</th><th>INTERPRETATION</th></tr>
<tr><td>Creatinine</td><td>Degradation product of creatinine phosphate from muscle tissue, solely excreted by the kidneys (90% glomerular filtration, 10% tubular secretion)</td><td>↑ • Acute kidney injury, chronic kidney disease
• Medication-induced, e.g. trimethoprim, supplements
• Dehydration
• Muscle breakdown (e.g. rhabdomyolysis, myocardial infarction)
• Excessive meat consumption
↓ • Significant fluid overload, e.g. SIADH
• Low protein intake, e.g. malnutrition
• Reduced muscle mass, e.g. increasing age, females
• Hyperthyroidism</td></tr>
<tr><td>Creatinine-clearance</td><td>Amount of plasma filtered by the glomeruli (in mL/min). Requires plasma creatinine concentration, urine creatinine concentration, and total urine volume (in mL).</td><td rowspan="2">↓ • Prerenal kidney disease (decreased renal perfusion): e.g. hypovolaemia, hypotension, decreased circulating volume (e.g. congestive heart failure, hepatorenal syndrome), renal artery stenosis, medication-induced
• Renal kidney disease (reduced clearance due to impaired glomeruli and/or tubules): e.g. acute tubular necrosis (e.g. ischaemia, nephrotoxic drugs), acute interstitial nephritis, diabetes mellitus, medication-induced
• Postrenal kidney disease (urinary tract obstruction): e.g. urolithiasis, prostate carcinoma, benign prostatic hyperplasia, urinary retention</td></tr>
<tr><td>Estimated glomerular filtration rate (eGFR, CKD-EPI)</td><td>• Estimation of GFR based on serum creatinine, sex, and age (latter two as surrogate marker for muscle mass)
• Relevant in chronic kidney disease (stages 1-5)
• Only reliable in more or less stable kidney function</td></tr>
<tr><td>Osmolality</td><td>• Number of particles dissolved in 1 kg serum (osmolarity: in 1L)
• Formula for ´effective osmolality´: 2 × [Na^+] + [glucose]</td><td>↑ Increased level of osmoles, e.g. Na^+, glucose, urea, or exogenous osmoles, e.g. toxic alcohols
↓ Decreased level of osmoles, e.g. Na^+, glucose, urea</td></tr>
</table>

Table 13A // Renal function tests

CKD-EPI, Chronic Kidney Disease Epidemiology Collaboration

LAB VALUE	EXPLANATION	INTERPRETATION
Osmolar gap	• Measured osmolality – calculated osmolality • A high osmolar gap (>10-20 mOsm/kg) is defined as the measured osmolality minus 2 x [Na^+] + [glucose] + [urea]	↑ Increased Na^+, glucose, urea, or other osmotically active substances, e.g. toxic alcohols, ketone bodies
Urea	• Waste product of hepatic protein metabolism • Reabsorbed in the kidneys	↑ • Prerenal, renal, or postrenal kidney disease (if urea/creatinine ratio ↑: prerenal) • Dehydration • Increased protein degradation, e.g. tissue damage, upper gastrointestinal bleeding • High-protein diet ↓ • Haemodilution • Pregnancy • Malabsorption/malnutrition • Severe liver damage
Uric acid/urate	End product of purine metabolism	↑ • Increased production: - Genetic - Idiopathic - Increased tissue breakdown, e.g. infections, malignancies - Increased nucleic acid metabolism, e.g. leukaemia, lymphoma, haemolytic anaemia • Reduced renal secretion, e.g. renal insufficiency ↓ • Xanthine oxidase deficiency • Medication-induced

Table 13B // Renal function tests

Acute kidney disease - interpretation

ACUTE KIDNEY DISEASE	PRERENAL	RENAL
Osmolality (urine)	>500 mOsmol/kg	<350 mOsmol/kg
Na^+ (urine)	<20 mmol/L	>40 mmol/L
Urea/creatinine ratio (serum)	>0.1 mmol/µmol	<0.1 mmol/µmol

Table 14 // Acute kidney disease - interpretation

> The 'effective osmolality' is important because these osmotically active substances cannot pass the semi-permeable cell membrane, and thus can cause water shifts (such as cerebral oedema). Urea, for example, can pass freely through the cell membrane and is unlikely to cause water shifts.

Clotting markers

<table>
<tr><th>LAB VALUE</th><th>EXPLANATION</th><th>INTERPRETATION</th></tr>
<tr><td>International normalised ratio (INR)</td><td>• Calculation based on prothrombin time (PT)
• Measure of the extrinsic and common pathway of the coagulation cascade
• Monitoring vitamin K anticoagulant therapy
• Patient plasma PT / normalised plasma PT</td><td rowspan="2">↑ • If prolonged PT + normal aPTT:
- Use of coumarines (vitamin K antagonists) or warfarin
- Isolated factor VII deficiency
- Coagulation disorders, e.g. coagulopathy or mild vitamin K deficiency
- In acute or chronic liver failure. If chronic → progression of advanced liver cirrhosis.
- Acute disseminated intravascular coagulation (DIC)
• If prolonged PT + prolonged aPTT:
- Factor I, II, V, X, or fibrinogen deficiency, combined factor deficiencies
- Liver failure
- Acute disseminated intravascular coagulation (DIC)
- Severe vitamin K deficiency
- Anticoagulants (e.g. warfarin, direct thrombin inhibitors, others)
↓ Activation of clotting in early disseminated intravascular coagulation</td></tr>
<tr><td>Prothrombin test/ time (PT)</td><td>Test for the extrinsic and common pathway of the coagulation cascade</td></tr>
<tr><td>Activated partial thromboplastin test/time (aPTT)</td><td>• Test for the intrinsic and common pathway of the coagulation cascade
• Monitoring unfractionated heparin therapy</td><td>↑ If prolonged aPTT + normal PT:
• Factor VIII (hemophilia A), factor IX (hemophilia B), factor XI (hemophilia C) deficiency
• Factor XII deficiency
• Von Willebrand disease
• Anticoagulants (unfractionated heparin therapy)
• Lupus anticoagulant
↓ • Strong elevation one or more clotting factors (e.g. factor VIII due to stress)
• Activation of coagulation in early disseminated intravascular coagulation (DIC)
• Pregnancy (factor VIII ↑ and fibrinogen ↑)</td></tr>
</table>

Table 15 // Clotting markers

t-PA, tissue plasminogen activator

Coumarin derivative therapy can be monitored by tracking INR, heparin therapy by tracking aPTT, and LMWH therapy by tracking anti-Xa activity. Monitoring of therapy with DOACs is employed in specific cases, e.g. when using DOACs in patients with a gastric bypass. Therapy with platelet aggregation inhibitors is not monitored in practice.

Laboratories use different techniques to measure prothrombin time (PT), which makes PT values very difficult to compare. The INR is therefore used to correct for differences between labs.

Miscellaneous

LAB VALUE	EXPLANATION	INTERPRETATION
Ammonia	Degradation product of proteolysis	↑ Hyperammonaemia: • Congenital urea cycle enzyme defects • Acquired: - Liver cirrhosis (90%) - Infections - Multiple myeloma - Acute leukaemia - Medication-induced
Glucose	• Blood sugar • Main energy source for all cellular processes	↑ Hyperglycaemia: • Impaired glucose tolerance, DM, diabetes gravidarum • Acute stress: trauma, sepsis, myocardial infarction, cerebrovascular accident • Medication: corticosteroids • Endocrinopathy: Cushing's syndrome, acromegaly ↓ Hypoglycaemia: • Medication-induced, e.g. sulphonylurea derivatives, insulin • Insulinoma • Fasting/malnutrition, alcohol • Liver failure • Endocrinopathy: hypocortisolism, panhypopituitarism
Lactate	• End product of anaerobic glycolysis • Produced by muscle cells and red blood cells, esp. in hypoxic state	↑ • Hypoxic states • Dehydration • Shock • Severe anaemia • Severe liver/kidney disease • Medication-induced (e.g. metformin, propofol), toxic (e.g. methanol, carbon monoxide)

Table 16 // Miscellaneous

Iron panel

LAB VALUE	EXPLANATION	INTERPRETATION
Ferritin	• Main iron-storage protein • Most important marker for iron deficiency • Correlates with total body iron content • Positive acute-phase protein	↑ • Inflammation or infection • Haemochromatosis or iron-storage disease • Functional iron deficiency (anaemia of chronic disease) • Liver disease • Chronic kidney disease ↓ • Iron deficiency
Iron	• Measure of circulating iron (note: most iron is bound to transferrin) • Not a good parameter for iron-deficiency anaemia due to fluctuating serum levels • Component of heme in haemoglobin and myoglobin • Necessary for cellular energy metabolism, needed for the action of various enzymes (e.g. catalase, cytochrome) and neurotransmitters (e.g. serotonin, dopamine) • Absorption mainly in duodenum and jejunum	↑ • Haemochromatosis • Iron-loading anaemia (thalassaemia, haemolytic anaemia, aplastic anaemia) • Liver disease (hepatitis B or C, alcoholic liver disease) • Excess iron intake (high intake, multiple transfusion, IM/IV iron) ↓ • Iron deficiency • Anaemia of chronic disease (or inflammatory anaemia) • Polycythaemia vera
Transferrin	• Transport protein for iron and zinc • Measure of iron-binding capacity • Negative acute-phase protein	In combination with the other lab results from the iron panel
Total iron-binding capacity (TIBC)	TIBC reflects the available iron binding sites on transferrin (ratio of serum iron to serum transferrin)	↑ Iron deficiency =/↓ Anaemia of chronic disease (or inflammatory anaemia)
Transferrin saturation	• Iron-transport protein reflects both protein and iron status • Determination of iron status (deficiency or overload) • Formula: (serum iron level X 100) / total iron-binding capacity (another formula: ratio of serum iron to serum transferrin)	↑ • Iron overload • Sideroblastic anaemia ↓ • Iron deficiency (often in combination with TIBC ↑ and ferritin ↓) • Anaemia of chronic disease (TIBC =/↓) • Chronic infection or inflammation • Extensive malignancy • Kidney disease • Acute bone marrow depression (e.g. in acute inflammation) • Pregnancy

Table 17 // Iron panel

Iron status - interpretation

CONDITION	FERRITIN	MCV	TRANSFERRIN	TRANSFERRIN SATURATION
Iron-deficiency anaemia	↓	↓	↑	↓
Anaemia of chronic disease or inflammatory anaemia	=/↑	=/↓	=/↓	=/↓
Thalassaemia	↓/=/↑	↓	=	↑
Haemochromatosis	↑	=/↑	=/↓	↑ (>45%)

Table 18 // Iron status - interpretation

Nutritional panel

LAB VALUE	EXPLANATION	INTERPRETATION
Vitamin B1 (thiamine)	• Water-soluble vitamin • Involved in carbohydrate, fat and protein metabolism; cellular respiration and oxidation of fatty acids; mitochondrial energy production, protein synthesis, neurotransmitter synthesis	↓ • Poor intake: inadequate diet, chronic alcohol use disorder, bariatric surgery • Poor absorption: malabsorption syndrome, bariatric surgery, short bowel syndrome, vomiting, malnourishment • Increased utilisation: refeeding syndrome, pregnancy, breastfeeding, hyperthyroidism • Increased loss: dialysis, infection, diarrhoea, vomiting, systemic disease, medication-induced (e.g. diuretics)
Vitamin B9/B11 (folic acid)	• Water-soluble vitamin • Necessary for protein and nucleic acid synthesis	↓ • Poor intake: inadequate diet, chronic alcohol use disorder • Poor absorption: diseases involving the jejunum (e.g. celiac disease, short bowel syndrome, amyloidosis), bariatric surgery, elevated pH • Increased loss: dialysis • Medication-induced (e.g. methotrexate, phenytoin, trimethoprim) • Pregnancy • Can cause megaloblastic anaemia

Table 19A // Nutritional panel

LAB VALUE	EXPLANATION	INTERPRETATION
Vitamin B12 (cobalamin)	• Water-soluble vitamin • Cofactor in DNA, fatty and amino acid metabolisation, maturation of red blood cells and myelin synthesis	↑ Hypercobalaminaemia: • Excessive supplementation • Liver disease • Kidney disease • Diabetes mellitus • Haematological malignancy • Solid tumour ↓ • Pernicious (megaloblastic) anaemia • Poor intake: diet lacking of animal products • Poor absorption: bariatric surgery, terminal ileum disease (e.g. Crohn's disease, celiac disease, parasites, intestinal bacterial overgrowth) • Recreational use of nitrous oxide

Table 19B // Nutritional panel

When a vitamin B12 deficiency is suspected but vitamin B12 serum levels are in the low/low-normal ranges, determine its metabolites, homocysteine, and methylmalonic acid (MMA) to diagnose a functional deficiency:

- MMA: MMA needs vitamin B12 as a cofactor to be converted. If the amount of available vitamin B12 is too low, this conversion cannot take place and MMA serum levels will be higher. A combination of a low/low-normal vitamin B12 and increased MMA level indicate a functional vitamin B12 deficiency.
- Homocysteine: homocysteine breaks down into methionine and cysteine when interacting with vitamin B12. When B12 levels are in the low/low-normal range, a high level of homocysteine can be found. This indicates a functional B12 deficiency.

Tumour markers

LAB VALUE	EXPLANATION	INTERPRETATION
AFP	Alpha-fetoprotein: protein produced by a developing fetus that is not found in healthy men or non-pregnant women	↑ • Often in hepatocellular carcinoma • In scrotal or ovarian malignancies
Ca19-9	Glycolipid normally produced in healthy pancreatic tissue and gastric and gallbladder epithelium	↑ • Often in pancreatic carcinoma or cholangiocarcinoma • In gastric or colorectal carcinoma, pancreatitis, cholestasis, cystic fibrosis

Table 20A // Tumour markers

LAB VALUE	EXPLANATION	INTERPRETATION
CEA	Carcinoembryonic antigen: protein produced by a developing fetus that is only present in healthy adults in very low concentrations	↑ • Often in colorectal carcinoma • In mammary, lung, liver, pancreatic, gastric, and ovarian carcinomas • In smokers
Chromo-granin A	Protein produced by neuroendocrine cells	↑ • Often in neuroendocrine gastric, colorectal, pulmonary, or pancreatic carcinoma • In kidney or liver failure

Table 20B // Tumour markers

Tumour markers are not only used to diagnose malignancies, they are mainly used to monitor the disease process, assess the effect of treatment, estimate metastasis, and monitor recurrence.

Stool test

Microbiome

The human body is home to 10,000 different types of bacteria, as well as fungi, yeasts, and viruses. These microbiota primarily inhabit the intestines, collectively forming the microbiome. Disruptions in the microbiome can contribute to intestinal infections, alongside external pathogens.

The microbiome plays a role in **DIGEST: D**igestion, **I**mmune system, **G**ut protection, **E**nhanced motility, **S**atiety, and **T**oxin degradation.

Factors that can disrupt the microbiome balance **MINE: M**edication (antibiotics), **I**nheritance, **N**utrition, **E**nvironment (hygiene).

Bacteria

In clinical settings, patients with diarrhoea are often tested for SSYC: *Salmonella*, *Shigella*, *Yersinia*, and *Campylobacter*, the most common bacterial causes of diarrhoea. Hospitalised patients and patients recently treated with AB suffering from diarrhoea should be tested for *C. difficile*.

NAME	TRANSMISSION
***Campylobacter* species** *C. jejuni* (most common) *C. coli*	Via contaminated water/food, or direct faecal-oral contamination from animal contact
***Shigella* species** *S. sonnei* *S. flexneri* *S. dysenteriae* *S. boydii*	Faecal-oral, mainly found in surface water in the tropics. Infection by drinking contaminated water, touching contaminated objects (toilets!), or person-to-person transmission.
Yersinia enterocolitica	Found everywhere in nature, esp. in pigs
Salmonella enterica *S.* Typhi *S.* Paratyphi *S.* Enteritidis *S.* Typhimurium	Via contaminated food, water, and pets: esp. animal products (e.g. meat/eggs/dairy)
***Clostridium* species** *C. difficile* *C. perfringens*	Faecal-oral, via hands or objects. Resides in the large intestines of humans and animals.
Escherichia coli Enteroinvasive *E. coli* (EIEC) Enterotoxic *E. coli* (ETEC) Enteroaggregative *E. coli* (EAEC) Shiga-toxin-producing *E. coli* (STEC) Enterohaemorrhagic *E. coli* (EHEC)	Faecal-oral. Inhabits the large intestines of humans and animals, the most common bacterium in the intestines. Pathogenic species (EHEC, STEC) are mainly found in raw meat, vegetables, and dairy products.
***Vibrio* species** *V. cholerae* *V. parahaemolyticus* *V. vulnificus*	Via contaminated water/food or direct faecal/oral transmission. Lives in surface water. Epidemics primarily in the tropics. Non-cholera vibrio species are mainly found in salt water and seafood.

Table 21 // Most common bacterial causes of gastroenteritis

COURSE AND TREATMENT	SPECIAL FEATURES
• Relatively frequent abdominal pain and blood in stool • Flu-like prodromal syndrome in 1/3 of cases • Symptoms usually pass spontaneously after 1-7d • ABx in specific patient groups or for prolonged symptoms	• Gram-negative bacteria • May also cause extra-intestinal symptoms • IgA nephropathy is a possible post-infectious complication
• Acute onset, fever, watery diarrhoea at first, followed by a phase of slimy diarrhoea, possibly with blood in stool • Mild course: no treatment • Severe symptoms: ABx (e.g. ciprofloxacin or azithromycin)	• Tropical bacteria, can also be transmitted during oro-anal sex • Gram-negative bacteria • In most countries, shigellosis is a notifiable disease
• Usually asymptomatic course • Uncomplicated infections do not require treatment	• Symptomatic mainly in children • Gram-negative bacteria • May mimic IBD (esp. terminal ileitis)
• 6-72h after infection: abdominal cramps, nausea, vomiting, and diarrhoea. Occasionally blood or mucus in stool. • Nontyphoidal Salmonella infection: usually spontaneous recovery. ABx is not recommended due to risk of prolonging carrier status, risk of relapse, and development of resistance. • Typhoidal *Salmonella* infection: ABx (e.g. ciprofloxacin, co-trimoxazole, amoxicillin)	• Typhoidal *Salmonella* passes the intestinal mucosa and causes typhoid fever/paratyphoid fever • Relative bradycardia is common in typhoidal *Salmonella* • Nontyphoidal *Salmonella* causes gastroenteritis • Gram-negative bacteria • Notifiable disease in most countries
• Usually fever and abdominal cramps, sometimes nausea, anorexia, and occult blood in stool • Stop triggering factors (previous ABx) • In severe infections: metronidazole, vancomycin, or fidaxomicin (oral), possible faecal transplantation (oral) ⊖ • Recurrence ⊕	• Main cause of AB-associated diarrhoea, common in hospitalised patients • Gram-positive bacteria
• STEC/EHEC: may cause haemorrhagic colitis in severe cases. Some patients develop haemolytic uraemic syndrome (HUS) as a result. • No ABx in STEC/EHEC infections, symptomatic treatment only	• *E. coli* (note: not its subtypes) is the most common cause of UTIs and traveller's diarrhoea in subtropical regions • Gram-negative bacteria • STEC: notifiable disease
• Mild course in healthy travellers (++) • Heavy, odourless, watery diarrhoea ('rice water'), vomiting, usually no abdominal cramps • Greatest danger is dehydration, treatment focused on administering fluids, ABx in pregnant and severely ill patients (e.g. azithromycin)	• Gram-negative bacteria • *V. vulnificus* mainly affects men • Notifiable disease

> Notifiable diseases are diseases that require notification to public health services within one working day.

Viruses

Well-known viruses that can be found in stool and usually cause acute diarrhoea include norovirus (e.g. cruise ships, nursing homes), rotavirus (most common pathogen among children under age five before introduction of rotavirus vaccine), sapovirus, certain types of adenoviruses, and astroviruses. Complaints often arise rapidly and are usually accompanied by vomiting. In most cases, symptoms spontaneously disappear after one to four days.

Parasites

Parasites that can reside in the intestines include worms and protozoa such as *Giardia lamblia, Entamoeba histolytica, Cryptosporidium parvum,* and *Cyclospora cayetanensis*. Infections are most common in children. See Table 22.

PARASITE	TRANSMISSION AND ENDEMIC AREA	COURSE AND TREATMENT
Entamoeba histolytica	• Via contaminated water/food or direct faecal/oral transmission • Subtropical and tropical regions	• Asymptomatic (++), diarrhoea, bloody/pus/mucus stools, weight loss, abdominal pain, tenesmus • Often causes right-sided colitis • Incubation period: 1-4 wk • Complication: amoebic liver abscess (immunocompromised individuals → higher risk) Metronidazole
Giardia lamblia		• Fatty stools, foul-smelling, stomach cramps, dehydration (−) • Incubation period: 1-5 wk E.g. metronidazole, tinidazole, nitazoxanide
Cryptosporidium parvum	• Faecal/oral transmission • Worldwide	• Mild diarrhoea (severe in immunocompromised individuals) • Incubation period: 5-7d • Self-limiting (+) E.g. nitazoxanide
Cyclospora cayetanensis	Faecal/oral transmission	• Watery diarrhoea, weight loss, abdominal pain, fatigue • Incubation period: 5-7d • Self-limiting (+), immunocompromised individuals → watch for severe gastrointestinal disease E.g. trimethoprim-sulfamethoxazole (TMP-SMX)

Table 22 // Parasites

Whipple disease is a rare infection caused by Tropheryma whipplei, presenting with diarrhoea, weight loss, joint pain, and neurological symptoms. Diagnosis is made by identifying PAS-positive macrophages in duodenal biopsies. Treatment consists of IV ABx (e.g. ceftriaxone) followed by one year of oral trimethoprim-sulfamethoxazole.

Calprotectin

Calprotectin is a protein produced by neutrophilic granulocytes that is released during intestinal inflammation. It is a marker of intestinal inflammation, particularly of an inflamed colon, e.g. secondary to IBD. In addition to IBD, faecal calprotectin levels may also be elevated in gastroenteritis, malignancies, coeliac disease, or diverticulitis. Low calprotectin levels do not rule out IBD, esp. if the condition is confined to the terminal ileum in Crohn's disease. Calprotectin is used to monitor disease activity rather than as a diagnostic marker.

Elastase

Elastase is a protein-splitting enzyme made by the pancreas. The pancreas secretes the pro-enzyme pro-elastase, which is converted to elastase in the duodenum by trypsin. Faecal elastase concentrations reflect the functioning of the pancreas. Another cause of diarrhoea (e.g. infection) can result in false-low elastase levels caused by dilution of pancreatic enzymes.

Faecal Immunochemical Test (FIT)

FIT detects small amounts of blood (faecal occult blood) in stool. It is used in population screening programmes for colon cancer. This test is not intended for patients with suspected colorectal carcinoma or gastro-intestinal symptoms.

Radiology

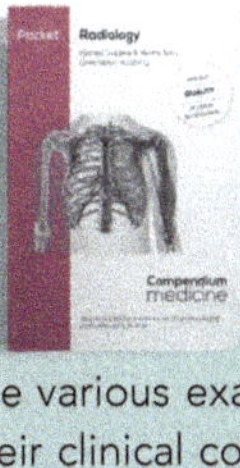

This section discusses the most commonly used radiological imaging-modalities in gastroenterology, indications, and important signs/landmarks. This is not a comprehensive list. It is important to remember that the various examples of imaging requests have been taken out of their clinical context. For more information, see the pocket *Radiology*.

A complete imaging request consists of three parts::

1 Clinical findings/details
2 Relevant medical history
3 Targeted clinical question (suspicion and differential diagnosis)

A good imaging request is essential to determine the appropriate scan phase/sequence for a CT or MRI scan and necessitates the radiologist only to open the file to correlate specific findings.

Abdominal ultrasound

TEST	INDICATIONS	EXAMPLES OF IMAGING REQUESTS
Abdominal ultrasound (US)	• Abdominal pain (e.g. appendicitis, diverticulitis, gallstones, cholangitis, kidney stones) • Abnormal blood tests (elevated inflammation markers or abnormal liver tests) • Ascites • Screening for internal bleeding/free fluid following trauma • Targeted screening for disease, e.g. hepatocellular carcinoma (HCC) in patients with liver cirrhosis, or monitoring progression of primary sclerosing cholangitis (PSC) • Screening for liver/gland metastases in oncology • Screening for intestinal abnormalities (esp. in paediatrics) or monitoring disease activity (IBD)	• Suspected gallstones: evidence of cholecystolithiasis/choledocholithiasis, dilated bile ducts, cholecystitis, or cholangitis? • Suspected ascites: ascites present? Signs of liver cirrhosis? Hepatic blood flow? Possibilities for aspiration/drainage? • Suspected/screening for liver malignancy (primary or metastatic): evidence of primary tumour/metastases in the liver? Bile duct congestion?

Table 23 // Indications for abdominal ultrasound and examples of requests

Depending on the purpose of the US, patients may be instructed to follow NPO guidelines 4 hours before the exam. This minimises disruptions caused by e.g. air in the intestines and bowel motility and ensures that the gallbladder expands for optimal assessment.

Intestinal US is a safe and non-invasive way to monitor disease activity in the colon and small intestine in patients with IBD. This exam is performed by specially trained physicians or nurses and can help minimise the need for additional endoscopies, CT scans, or MRI scans.

Conventional X-ray

Positioning of lines and tubes

Chest X-rays and abdominal X-rays can provide information on e.g. the position of lines, feeding tubes, and foreign bodies (swallowed or inserted). It is important to visualise the entire area of interest. For a nasogastric tube (NG) a part of the upper abdomen must be visible. For a duodenal tube an even larger part of the upper abdomen must be visualised. For a foreign body the entire GI tract must be imaged, including the top row of the teeth up to the pelvis. See Figure 6 for the correct position of a NG tube. Good placement of a duodenal tube is achieved when the tip first crosses the midline to the right, passing the pylorus, and continues down the duodenum to the left, again crossing the midline, reaching just below the stomach/left side of the vertebral column (Treitz's ligament).

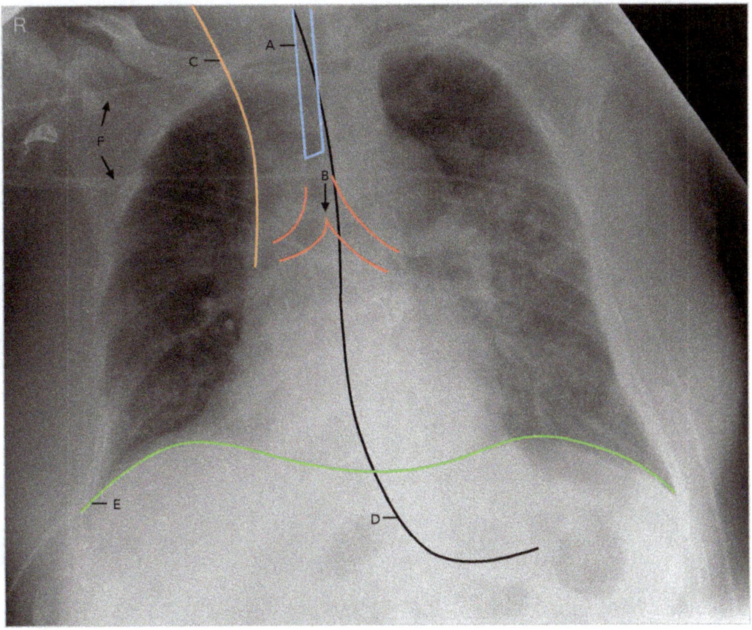

Figure 6 // Lines on chest X-ray

A: Trachea tube (optimal position: ±5 cm above the carina) **B:** Carina **C:** CVL (optimal position: tip in the superior vena cava) **D:** NG tube (optimal position: tip extends below the diaphragm) **E:** Diaphragm **F:** ECG leads

Chest and abdominal X-ray

There are many indications for chest X-rays, some of which are also relevant within gastroenterology, e.g. suspected fluid overload in the treatment of acute pancreatitis (see Figure 7) or aspiration pneumonia.

In adult patients, there is basically no indication for an abdominal X-ray, but it may provide valuable information in case of suspected volvulus (see Figure 8). On a standing, conventional chest/thoracoabdominal X-ray, subdiaphragmatic free air may be an indication of hollow viscus perforation. However, the absence of free subdiaphragmatic air on X-ray does not rule out perforation, therefore, in case of clinical suspicion, a CT is indicated.

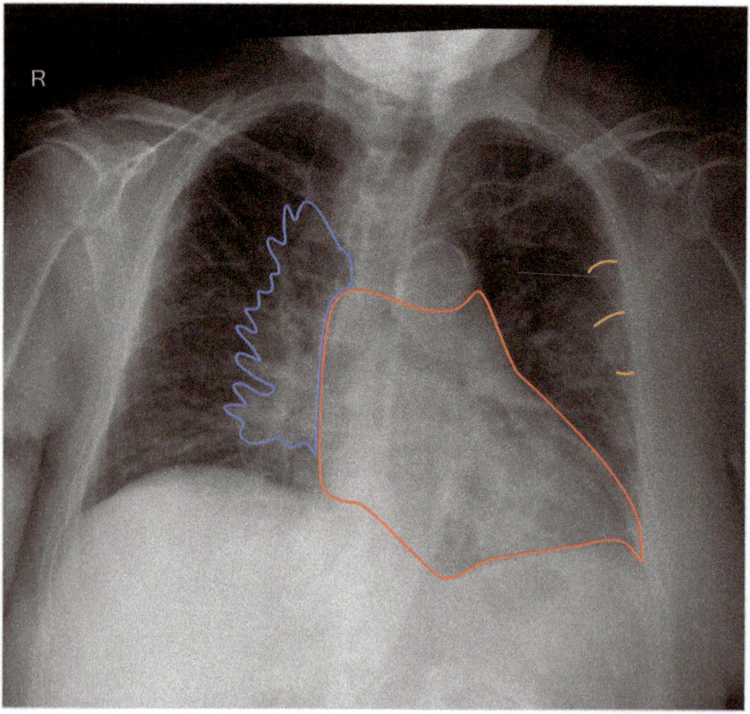

Figure 7 // Chest X-ray: congestive heart failure. Kerley lines (orange), prominent lung markings, enlarged heart (red), and perihilar consolidations (blue - batwing sign)

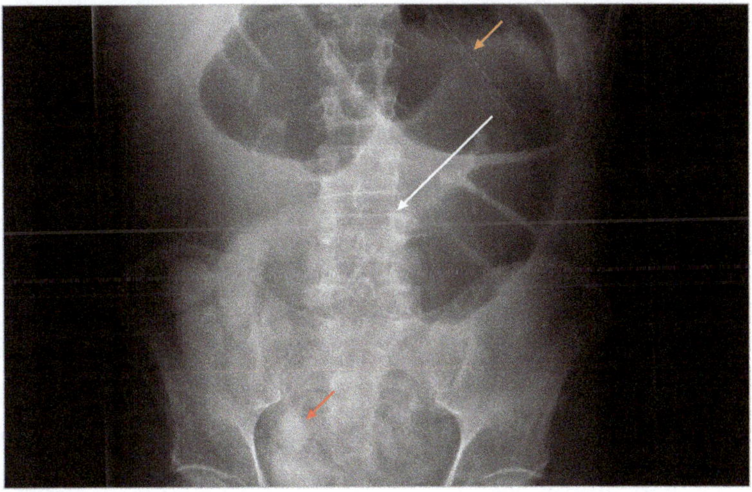

Figure 8 // Caecum volvulus with the notch of the coffee bean sign pointing to the lower right quadrant (white arrow) and an NG tube in the stomach (orange arrow). Residual contrast from a previous exam is still visible in the small intestinal lumen (red arrow) and bladder.

The notch of the coffee bean sign points to the RLQ in a caecum volvulus and to the LLQ in a sigmoid volvulus.

Abdominal CT

TYPE OF ABDOMINAL CT	INDICATIONS	EXAMPLES OF IMAGING REQUESTS
Non-contrast	Nephrolithiasis	Suspected kidney stones: nephrolithiasis? Signs of hydronephrosis?
Arterial (CTA)	• Aortic aneurysm • Arterial stenosis/occlusion • Hypervascular metastases (e.g. thyroid, sarcoma, melanoma)	Suspected aortic aneurysm: aortic aneurysm present? AAA?

Table 24A // Indications and requests for abdominal CT and CT colonography

TYPE OF ABDOMINAL CT	INDICATIONS	EXAMPLES OF IMAGING REQUESTS
Portal venous/ venous (CTV)	• General screening for abdominal abnormalities • Abscess formation • Perforation (incl. a sip of water-diluted iodinated contrast on the CT table if necessary) • Complications of pancreatitis (CT >72h, in acute phase only when in doubt about diagnosis) • Venous thrombosis	• Suspected volvulus: evidence of loop rotation/ herniation? • Suspected ileus: evidence of obstruction/distension? Cause of ileus? • Suspected GI perforation: free air? Abscess formation? Location of perforation? Suspected megacolon: dilated intestinal loops? Signs of inflammation and/or perforation? • Suspected diverticulosis: diverticula present? Complicated diverticulitis with abscess formation? • Suspected pancreatitis: necrotising pancreatitis? Evidence of complications? • Suspected liver cirrhosis: appearance and size of liver? Collateral formation? Ascites? Splenomegaly? Portal vein thrombosis?
Equilibrium delayed (wash-out phase)	• Dissection • Intestinal ischaemia • Haemorrhage, AAA	• Suspected intestinal ischaemia: perforation or free fluid? Signs of intestinal ischaemia (see Figure 9)? • Suspected haemorrhage: active intestinal/abdominal haemorrhage? Visible cause of Hb drop? Suitable for coiling?
CTA, CTV, and wash-out phase	• HCC • Hepatic metastases (liver protocol for both hyper- and hypovascular subtypes) • Pancreatic tumour	• Metastases: liver metastases? Metastases elsewhere? Evidence of primary tumour? • Pancreatic tumour: appearance of pancreas and bile ducts? Evidence of space-occupying lesion (SOL)?
CT colonography, with/without IV contrast, depending on clinical question	• Polyps • Tumours	Suspected polyps/malignancy: evidence of polyp or SOL? Evidence of metastases (on contrast CT)?

Table 24B // Indications and requests for abdominal CT and CT colonography

Relative contraindications to CT scans:

- Pregnancy
- Children
- When using iodinated contrast: allergy, severe congestive heart failure, and severe renal insufficiency (eGFR <30).

Abdominal CT always uses iodinated venous contrast through an IV unless otherwise specified. Some indications do not require IV contrast (e.g. kidney stones and some cases of renal insufficiency) or require additional contrast phases (e.g. suspected haemorrhage or intestinal ischaemia – non-contrast, CTA, and CTV preferred).

Endoscopy and biopsies are the gold standard for detecting suspected GI malignancies. Abdominal CT and CT colonography are not the first choice for detecting GI malignancies as they are suboptimal for evaluating intraluminal pathology and can therefore not be used to rule out malignancies. In addition, CT colonography requires extensive preparation on the part of the patient.

Maximum intestinal distension: 3-6-9:

- 3 cm for jejunum and ileum
- 6 cm for colon
- 9 cm for caecum

Contrast blush is active pooling of contrast agent outside the blood vessels and an indicator of an active haemorrhage (see Figure 10). A blush can usually be recognised by comparing the different scan phases (non-contrast/CTA/CTV). A blush will not necessarily appear in intermittent bleeding or at bleeding rates <0.5 ml/min. Contrast blush is most clearly visible in haemorrhage with a bleeding rate of 2-3 ml/min.

For suspected pancreatic pathology, request an abdominal CT according to a **pancreatic scan protocol**. It is important to formulate an accurate clinical question (e.g. malignancy, chronic pancreatitis) so the radiologist can decide which scan phases to include: non-contrast (e.g. calcifications), CTA, CTV, washout. Protocols may vary between hospitals.

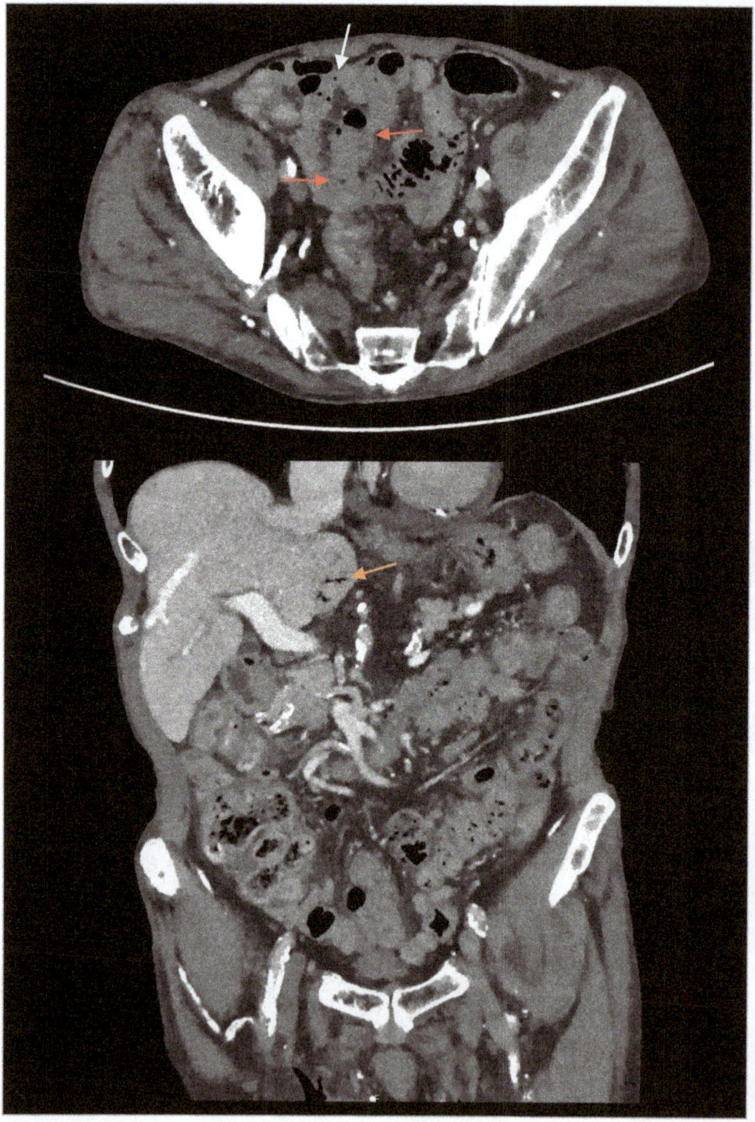

Figure 9 // Abdominal contrast CT: intestinal ischaemia with diffusely reduced enhancement of the small intestine (red arrows) with intestinal pneumatosis (white arrow) and portal gas (orange arrow)

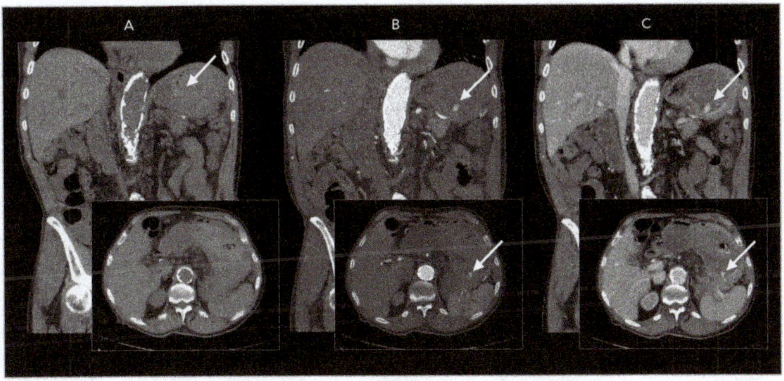

Figure 10 // Abdominal CT: gastric haemorrhage in known MALT lymphoma. The non-contrast **(A)** only reveals limited hyperdensity in the stomach (white arrow). A contrast blush is visible on the CTA **(B)** and the CTV **(C,** white arrows).

MRI

MRI scans are becoming increasingly important in diagnosing gastroenterological conditions. Different MRI sequences can be used to distinguish different types of tissue, with T1 (fat white) and T2 (fat and water white) being the most commonly used sequences. MR cholangiopancreatography (MRCP) is a commonly used technique in gastroenterology. This is a heavily T2-weighted sequence in which the bile ducts and pancreatic duct are white, with low signal of surrounding tissue (see Figure 11). MRI scans are non-invasive and use harmless electromagnetic waves instead of X-rays.

Gastroenterological indications for abdominal MRI include:

- Malignancies: pancreatic carcinoma, cholangiocarcinoma, HCC
- Pancreas: pancreas divisum, autoimmune pancreatitis, pancreatic duct injury, intraductal papillary mucinous neoplasm (IPMN)
- Intestines: fistula, intestinal wall thickening, stenosis, appendicitis (in children or pregnant patients with an inconclusive US)
- Liver: cyst, steatosis, haemochromatosis, liver lesion differentiation (e.g. malignancy, haemangioma, adenoma, focal nodular hyperplasia)
- Bile ducts (MRCP): stones in common bile duct, cholangitis (including primary sclerosing cholangitis), bile duct cyst, hamartomas

In these indications MRI is not the primary diagnostic tool of choice but follows based on findings on other imaging modalities.

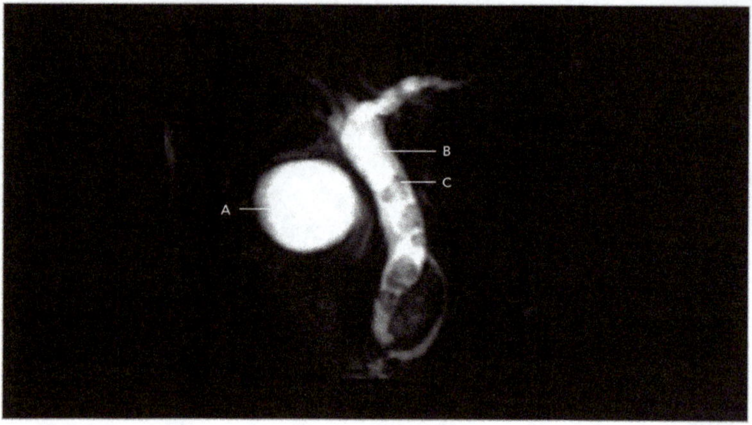

Figure 11 // MRCP: choledocholithiasis of the distal bile duct
A: Gallbladder **B:** Bile duct **C:** Gallstones

Contraindications to MRI:

- Metal in the body (e.g. metal splinters in the eye)
- Implanted devices/prosthetics (e.g. implantable cardioverter defibrillator (ICD), pacemaker, implanted insulin pump, or cochlear implant)
- Unstable patients (given the long scan duration)
- Claustrophobia
- Patients who are unable to remain still (e.g. small children).

Important: Nowadays, many prosthetics/implants are suitable for MRI. For more information, visit *www.MRIsafety.com.*

PET-CT

A PET-CT combines a PET scan and CT scan and uses a radioactive tracer to detect metabolic changes in cells. Depending on the purpose of the exam, the tracer is linked to e.g. glucose (FDG) to detect cells with an elevated metabolism. PET-CT can be used to identify hypermetabolic pathology (e.g. malignancy or infection) and pinpoint its anatomical location. Indications for a PET-CT scan include detecting metastases arising from a primary malignancy, cancer of unknown primary, setting a baseline prior to oncological treatment, and evaluating the effect of treatment.

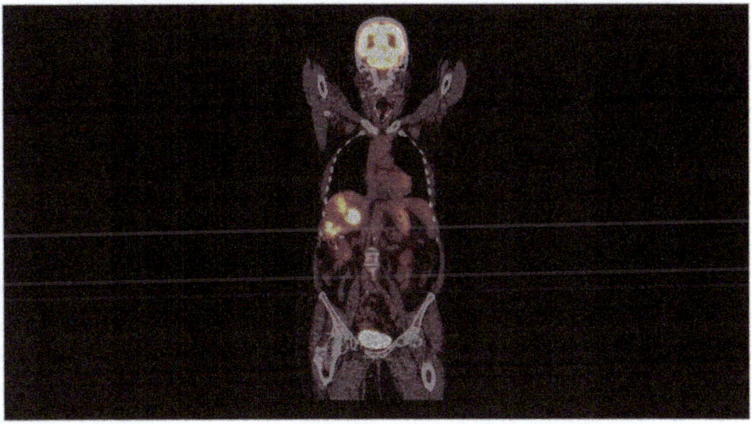

Figure 12 // PET-CT: multiple FDG-avid lesions in the liver consistent with metastases without an evident primary tumour

Elastography and hepatic fat content measurement

Elastography, or liver stiffness measurement (LSM), is an imaging technique used to determine hepatic elasticity expressed in kPa as a surrogate for fibrosis. The most commonly used modalities to measure liver elastography are vibration-controlled transient elastography (VCTE) on FibroScan®, shear wave elastography (SWE) on conventional abdominal ultrasound, and magnetic resonance elastography (MRE). Next to liver stiffness, hepatic fat content can be measured on elastography using the CAP score expressed in dB/m, and on MRI using the proton density fat fraction (PDFF). Higher CAP or PDFF scores correspond to higher hepatic fat content (see Table 25), and higher elastography scores correspond to higher F stages (see Table 26). Indications for elastography measurement include suspected liver fibrosis or cirrhosis of any aetiology, chronic HCV/HBV infection, follow-up for chronic intestinal failure, and total parenteral nutrition (TPN). Indications for hepatic fat content measurement include steatotic or suspected steatotic liver diseases such as metabolic dysfunction-associated steatotic liver disease (MASLD) and alcohol-related liver disease (ALD). Factors affecting measurement accuracy (generally overestimating the degree of fibrosis) include ascites, obesity, right-sided CHF, acute inflammation of the liver, cholestasis, and hepatic tumours. Patients should fast for three hours prior to the test.

CAP SCORE	GRADE OF STEATOSIS	FAT PERCENTAGE
238-259 dB/m	S1	11-33%
260-289 dB/m	S2	34-66%
≥290 dB/m	S3	≥67%

Table 25 // CAP score for steatosis

CONDITION	F0-F1	F2	F3	F4
Hepatitis B	2-7 kPa	8-9 kPa	10-17 kPa	≥18 kPa
Hepatitis C	2-7 kPa	8-9 kPa	10-13 kPa	≥14 kPa
HIV/HCV co-infection	2-7 kPa	8-10 kPa	11-13 kPa	≥14 kPa
Cholestasis	2-7 kPa	8-9 kPa	10-16 kPa	≥17 kPa
MASLD/MASH	2-7 kPa	8-9 kPa	10-13 kPa	≥14 kPa
Alcohol-related liver disease	2-7 kPa	8-10 kPa	11-18 kPa	≥19 kPa
Autoimmune hepatitis	2-5,7 kPa	5,8-10,4 kPa	10,5-15 kPa	≥16 kPa

Table 26 // Liver stiffness measurement (LSM) on elastography in kPa as a measure of liver cirrhosis secondary to various pathologies, F4 fits liver cirrhosis (in the absence of overestimating factors)

Endoscopy

See section *Treatment - Anticoagulants* for the management of anticoagulants around endoscopic procedures.

General

An endoscopy is a procedure used to visualise the digestive tract or a part of it. Prior to an endoscopy, the patient must undergo preparation to ensure the area to be examined is free of food remnants and/or faeces. Endoscopies can be used to perform diagnostic and therapeutic procedures, such as polyp removal, stent placement, and haemostasis. During the procedure, patients are monitored with oximetry, blood pressure, and telemetry.

Informed consent

All endoscopic procedures are invasive and carry risk. The procedure should be preceded by a shared decision-making process that includes individualisation of patient-specific risk factors, patient preferences, possible need for sedation, and alternatives. The endoscopist should discuss potential complications and obtain informed consent.

Sedation

Depending on the type of procedure, comorbidity, facility preference, resource availability, local protocols, doctor, and patient preferences, the examination is performed without sedation, with minimal or moderate sedation (midazolam), with deep sedation (propofol), or under general anaesthesia. Procedural sedation for endoscopy is to relieve patient anxiety and pain, improve the outcome of the examination, and fade the patient's memory of the event. Endoscopists commonly administer minimal or moderate sedation during non-advanced endoscopic procedures.

Upper endoscopy

An upper endoscopy, also called gastroscopy, is an endoscopic technique that involves inserting an endoscope orally to examine the upper digestive tract. Patient preparation consists of fasting. Benzocaine or lidocaine spray or gel is used in some endoscopy centres for topical pharyngeal anaesthesia and a mouth guard to protect the teeth and the endoscope.

Indications for upper endoscopy include oesophageal dysphagia, melaena, haematemesis, food impaction, or suspected pathology (e.g. peptic ulcer, malignancy, coeliac disease). Risks of upper endoscopy include bleeding (<0.5%), perforation (<0.1%), infection, and sedation-related complications such as aspiration. Risks are more common in therapeutic procedures and in patients with oesophageal diverticula.

> Indications for short-term upper endoscopy are haematemesis, melaena, and/or food impaction with excessive salivation. Specific alarm symptoms include oesophageal dysphagia, signs of GI bleeding, and cachexia. Upper endoscopy can reveal serious conditions such as malignancies, complicated ulcer disease, and variceal haemorrhage.

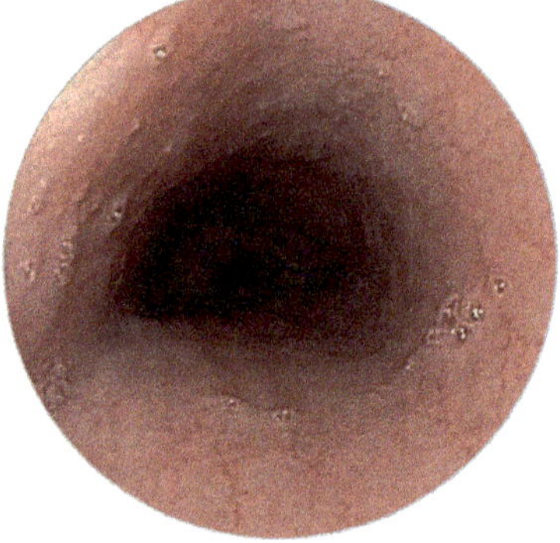

Figure 13 // Upper endoscopy: normal mucosa of the mid- oesophagus

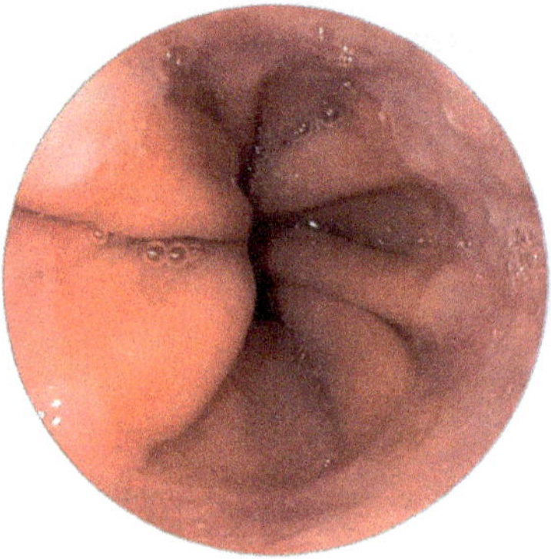

Figure 14 // Upper endoscopy: distal oesophagus with sharp Z-line (transition area from squamous epithelium of the oesophagus to columnar epithelium of the stomach)

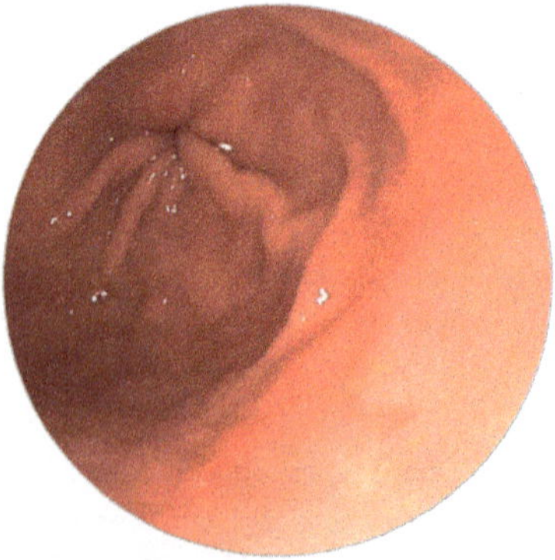

Figure 15 // Upper endoscopy: normal mucosa of the gastric antrum and pylorus.

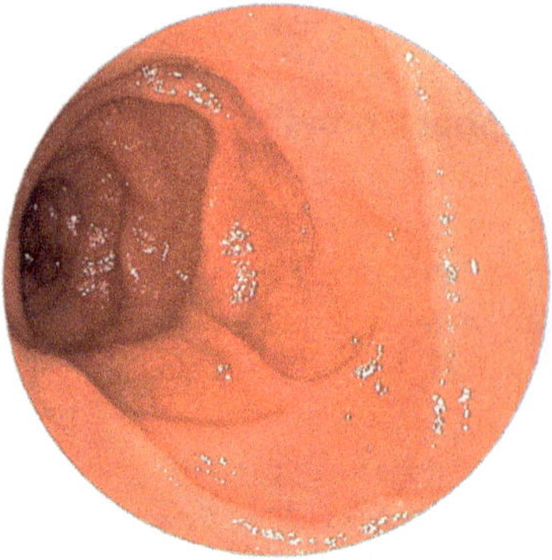

Figure 16 // Upper endoscopy: normal mucosa and haustra of the duodenum

Upper endoscopy in young patients (age <50) with gastric symptoms without alarm symptoms very rarely produces clinically relevant findings (0.3%), yet is still performed relatively often and thus unnecessarily. Consider less invasive options first, e.g. a stool test for a suspected *H. pylori* infection, more extensive patient education, or consider lifestyle education.

Example of preparing a patient for upper endoscopy:

- >6h before the exam, light breakfast only
- >2h before the exam, clear drinks only (black coffee, tea, water, apple juice)
- <2h before admission, no more fluids
- Patients can still take their scheduled medication with a little sip of water

Colonoscopy

A colonoscopy is an endoscopic technique that involves anally inserting an endoscope to examine the lower digestive tract. Colonoscopies often include ileocolonoscopies too, in which the endoscope is used to intubate the terminal ileum if possible. In some cases, for example in ulcerative colitis patients, only the distal part of the colon needs to be visualised. In that case, a sigmoidoscopy is performed. Patient preparation for a colonoscopy involves eating a low-fibre diet for several days before the procedure and taking bowel-cleansing laxatives. Indications for a colonoscopy include changes in bowel habits (esp. after age 50), chronic or episodic diarrhoea, rectal bleeding, iron deficiency anaemia, suspected IBD, suspected colorectal carcinoma, abnormal PET or CT findings, or a positive FIT as part of a colorectal cancer screening programme. Risks of colonoscopy include bleeding (0.1-0.6%), bowel perforation (0.2%), and sedation-related risks. CT colonography may be considered if the intestines cannot be properly visualised with endoscopy due to anatomical or patient-related factors.

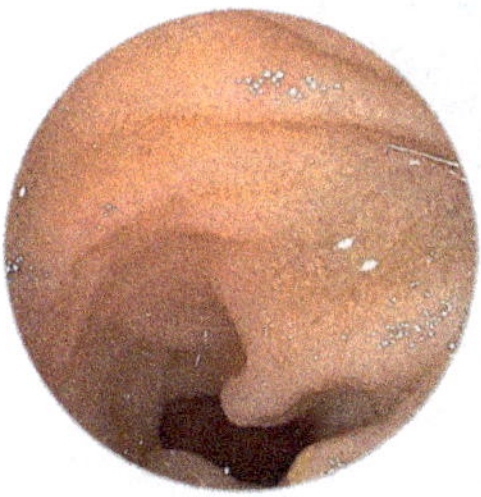

Figure 17 // Colonoscopy: normal mucosa with villi in the terminal ileum

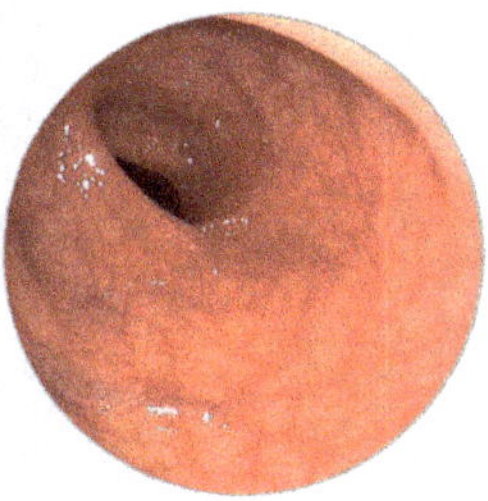

Figure 18 // Colonoscopy: normal mucosa and vascular pattern of the distal colon

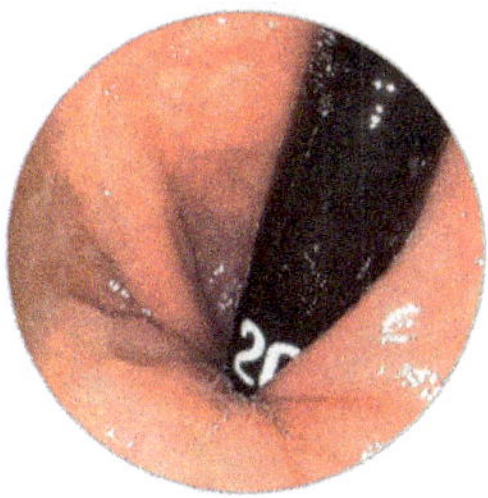

Figure 19 // Colonoscopy in retroflexion (the endoscope is turned back in a U-bend): normal mucosa of the rectum

Patients often experience mild/moderate abdominal pain, cramps, bloating, and flatulence after the exam. These symptoms are normal and are caused by CO_2 insufflation during the colonoscopy. Patients with severe, sudden abdominal pain, fever, or rectal bleeding should contact the treating physician.

Endoscopic retrograde cholangiopancreatography (ERCP)

ERCP is an endoscopic procedure used to examine the bile ducts and pancreas. The endoscope is inserted orally and advanced until it reaches the ampulla of Vater, which is located in the duodenum. The ampulla is then intubated and contrast is injected into the bile ducts (see Figures 20, 21, and 22). Various other interventions can also be performed simultaneously (e.g. stent placement, cytology brushing, balloon dilatation, gallstone removal). Patient preparation consists of fasting. They are given a rectal NSAID before the exam and a mouth guard immediately prior to the ERCP to protect their teeth and the endoscope. As a rule, propofol sedation is used for an ERCP. Indications for an ERCP include choledocholithiasis, cholangitis, removal of malignant/non-malignant biliary obstructions (e.g. pancreatic carcinoma, cholangiocarcinoma, or stenosis (primary sclerosing cholangitis (PSC)). The complications of an ERCP depend on the intervention performed during the exam. Complications include pancreatitis (post-ERCP pancreatitis approx. 5%), cholangitis (3%), bleeding (2%), perforation (<1%), and stent infection (<1%).

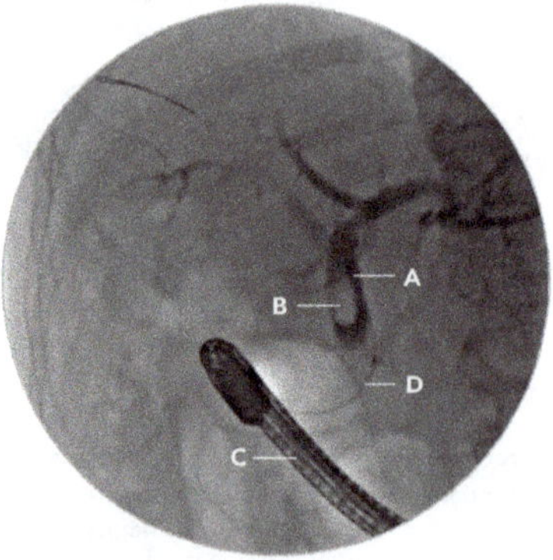

Figure 20 // ERCP: choledocholithiasis
A: Common bile duct **B:** Stone (filling defect) **C:** Endoscope **D:** Guidewire

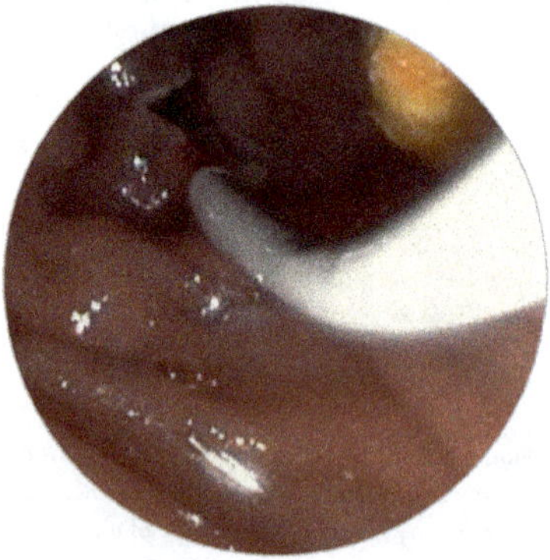

Figure 21 // Endoscopic view of the duodenum after removal of a gallstone from the common bile duct

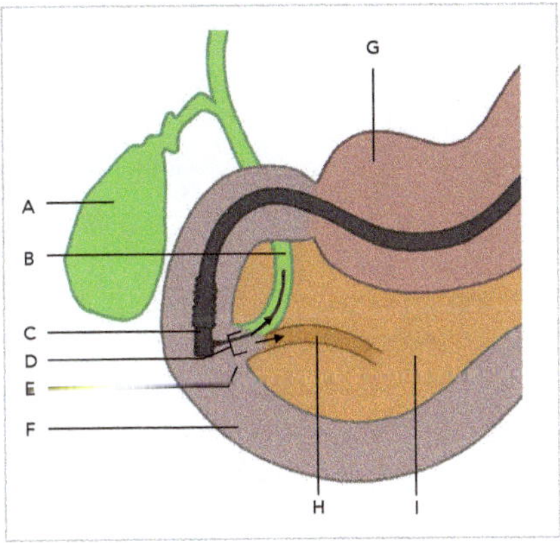

Figure 22 // ERCP

A: Gallbladder **B:** Common bile duct **C:** Endoscope tip with side viewer **D:** Contrast administration, optional intervention **E:** Ampulla of Vater **F:** Duodenum **G:** Stomach **H:** Pancreatic duct **I:** Pancreas

Endoscopic ultrasound (EUS)

EUS is an internal US exam performed with an oral or anal endoscope. An US transducer is attached to the end of the endoscope to visualise surrounding organs. Indications for EUS include detecting stones in the bile ducts, suspected malignancy (e.g. pancreas), and drainage in case of an infected fluid collection in pancreatitis. Interventions may be performed during an EUS, such as biopsy (e.g. of a suspected pancreatic malignancy), stent placement, fluid collection, or abscess drainage. Preparation depends on the type of procedure (fasting or bowel-cleansing). The most common complications are post-procedure bleeding (1-4%), infection (<1%), and perforation (<0.5%). These mainly occur during interventional procedures.

Video capsule endoscopy

Video capsule endoscopy allows visualisation of the GI tract using a camera inside a capsule. The patient swallows the capsule, which is after moved distally by peristalsis. This exam is mainly used to study the small intestine, as conventional endoscopies are often unable to reach this part of the GI tract. The primary disadvantage of this exam is that it does not allow for simultaneous interventions. Preparation varies by protocol and may include fasting or bowel-cleansing. Indications for video capsule endoscopy include iron deficiency anaemia, unexplained rectal blood loss with negative upper endoscopy or colonoscopy, or detecting disease activity proximal to the small intestine in Crohn's disease. Contraindications include stenosis, surgical resection, and altered anatomy. To reduce the risk of capsule retention, a patency capsule may be used first to confirm GI tract patency.

Treatment

General

Lifestyle management

Lifestyle interventions play a major role in improving overall health, esp. in terms of cardiovascular and malignancy-related events and outcomes. To achieve weight loss, lifestyle modification remains a first-line intervention in patients with MASLD/MASH. The most important modifiable risk factors are alcohol use, hypertension, smoking, DM, overweight, physical inactivity, and dyslipidaemia.

Smoking

Smoking cessation should be advised to all patients. Individual follow-up support, stop-smoking support programmes, nicotine replacement therapy, varenicline, and bupropion can be offered.

Physical activity

Physical activity is recommended to perform at least 150-300 min a week of moderate-intensity physical activity (e.g. walking at a brisk pace, slow cycling), or 75-150 min of vigorous-intensity physical activity (e.g. jogging, cycling, heavy gardening).

Alcohol

Alcohol consumption is completely discouraged. All adults should be routinely screened to detect and manage unhealthy alcohol use in an early stage. If screening indicates an alcohol use disorder, assess for alcohol-related complications (e.g. chronic liver disease, cancers, cardiovascular disease) at diagnosis to enable timely treatment.

BMI

Weight reduction improves dyslipidaemia, blood pressure, glucose intolerance, and liver steatosis. A BMI of 18-25 kg/m^2 should be pursued by a maintainable wholesome diet in combination with physical activity.

Mental disorders are associated with an increased risk of gastrointestinal and liver disease, partly through lifestyle factors and comorbidities. Patients with mental disorders require intensified attention and support in changing their lifestyle. These patients should be offered evidence-based mental healthcare and interdisciplinary guidance.

For specific lifestyle recommendations see the conditions in this pocket, for example head-of-bed elevation and avoiding meals within 2-3 hours of bedtime in gastro-oesophageal reflux disease.

Nutrition

Tube feeding

Enteral feeding is always the first choice for patients with a functional GI system of sufficient length and absorption capacity. The purpose of tube feeding is to optimise patients' nutritional status. Indications include patients who cannot or do not want to eat (e.g. due to neurological impairment, severe loss of appetite, or anorexia nervosa), patients who are not allowed to eat (e.g. oesophageal perforation), and patients with a poor nutritional status and/or clinical condition. Feeding tubes can be inserted in different ways; see Table 27 and Figure 23 for different types of feeding tubes.

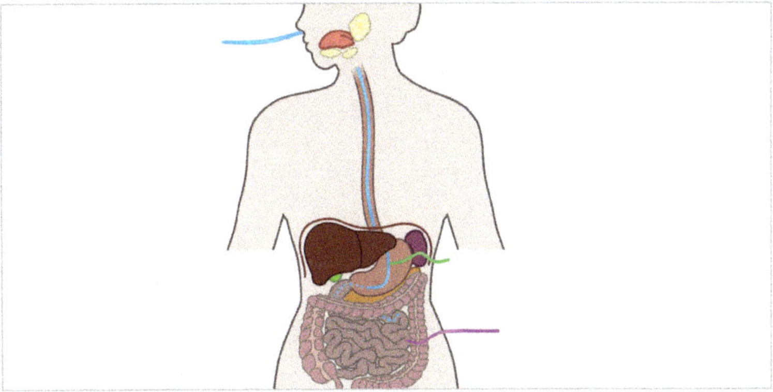

Figure 23 // Feeding tubes
Blue: nasogastric tube, blue dotted line: nasoduodenal tube, green: gastrostomy, purple: jejunostomy

TUBE TYPE	PLACEMENT
Nasogastric (NG) tube	• Tube is inserted manually through the nasal cavity, through the oesophagus, and down to the stomach • Usually placed by a ward nurse without anaesthesia
Nasoduodenal (ND) tube	• Tube is inserted endoscopically through the nose into the duodenum using a guidewire • Tube is advanced through the mouth into the duodenum, after which the endoscope is removed and the tube is guided out through the nose • Placement both under and without anaesthesia
Cortrak tube	• Tube is inserted into the duodenum through the nose using an electromagnetic system • Usually placed without anaesthesia by a specially trained GI nurse
Nasojejunal (NJ) tube	In some centres, if a NG tube cannot be tolerated, then a NJ tube is typically advanced into the proximal jejunum beyond the ligament of Treitz, rather than using a ND tube.
Percutaneous endoscopic gastrostomy (PEG) tube	There are two specific techniques for placing a PEG tube: the push technique and pull technique. An extension can be advanced to the jejunum (PEGJ), or a tube can be placed directly in the jejunum by means of a direct percutaneous endoscopic jejunostomy (DPEJ), often by a surgeon.
PEG pull	A wire is inserted through an incision in the abdominal wall, which is attached to the gastroscope and then withdrawn (pull). The PEG tube is attached to the wire, then the wire and PEG tube are pulled back out, see Figure 24.
PEG push	The stomach is punctured with a needle and the stomach is anchored to the abdominal wall. A fistula tract is made in the middle of the triangle (push), through which the gastrostomy catheter is placed in the stomach, see Figure 25.
Percutaneous radiological gastrostomy (PRG) tube	Radiology-guided equivalent of PEG tube, techniques are identical

Table 27 // Different types of feeding tubes
CI, contraindication

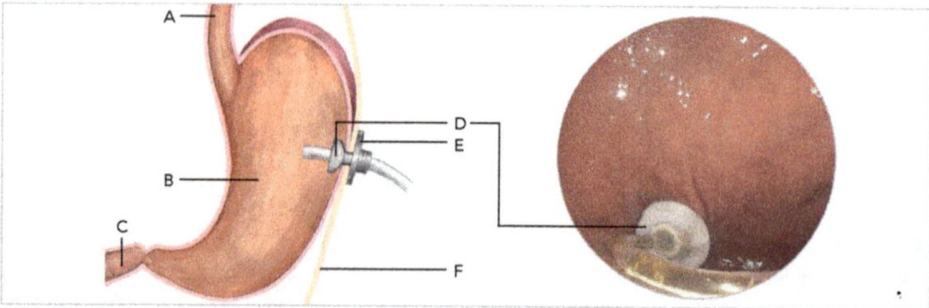

Figure 24 // Percutaneous endoscopic gastrostomy (PEG) tube: PEG pull with gastroscopic view
A: Oesophagus **B:** Stomach **C:** Small intestine **D:** Internal fixation plate **E:** External fixation plate **F:** Abdominal wall

INDICATION	NOTES
• Tube feeding • Gastric suction (e.g. in case of ileus) • Gastric lavage (e.g. in case of an overdose)	⊗ CI: Severe clotting disorders, obstruction, anatomic abnormalities, craniofacial abnormalities, recent bleeding or surgery along the pathway of the nasogastric tube
Tube feeding (alternative to NG tube, e.g. in case of impaired gastric emptying as in gastroparesis)	💡 To prevent dumping, tube feeds are given continuously by a feeding pump, rather than in discrete doses 💡 Also known as a postpyloric tube or duodenal tube
Tube feeding (alternative to NG tubes in some centres, e.g. pancreatitis)	⊗ Absolute CI: bowel obstruction distal the site of tube implantation, perforation, ischaemic bowel Relative CI: uncorrected clotting disorders
• Long-term dependence (often ≥3 mo) on tube feeding (e.g. neurogenic dysphagia) • Long-term dependence (often ≥3 mo) on parenteral medication (e.g. levodopa in Parkinson's disease)	⊗ CI: peritonitis, ascites, intestinal ischaemia, obstruction, varices, severe ulcers, tumour infiltration, ascites, coagulopathy, or artificial material and devices around the puncture site 💡 PEG tubes have several complications ranging from mild to life-threatening. These complications should be discussed and alternatives considered prior to placement. Complications include perforation (e.g. when puncturing an organ during placement), bleeding, dislocation, leakage, infection, buried bumper, and a persistent fistula. 💡 Interventional radiology guided placement of feeding tubes in patients who have CI's for PEGs, e.g. oesophageal malignancy anc varices (risk of bleeding), unsafe anatomy for PEG (no transillumination or finger indentation during upper endoscopy, interposed organs).
See indications for PEG probe, preferred if oesophageal stenosis rules out PEG pull and in patients with an oropharyngeal, laryngeal, or hypopharyngeal tumour	
Preferred for patients who cannot be sedated or patients with CI for PEGs (e.g. oesophageal malignancy, varices, unsafe anatomy for PEG)	

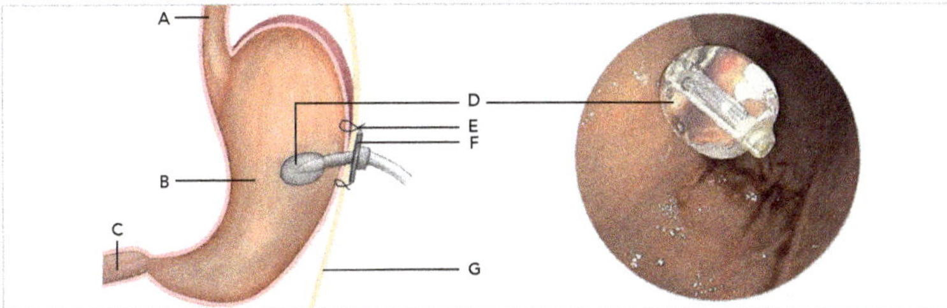

Figure 25 // Percutaneous endoscopic gastrostomy (PEG) tube: PEG push with gastroscopic view
A: Oesophagus **B:** Stomach **C:** Small intestine **D:** Balloon **E:** Suture **F:** External fixation plate **G:** Abdominal wall

Total parenteral nutrition (TPN)

TPN involves the direct delivery of nutrients into the bloodstream via e.g. a tunnelled central venous line, bypassing the intestines (parenteral) (see Figure 26). TPN provides all necessary nutrients, including carbohydrates, amino acids, fats, vitamins, minerals, and dissolved trace elements. Indications for TPN are inaccessible intestines (e.g. in ileus or active Crohn's disease) or absorption disorders such as short bowel syndrome, enteritis after radiotherapy, or a high-output stoma. Complications of TPN include infection, thrombosis, liver enzyme disorders, gallstones, kidney stones, and osteoporosis. For frequent infections, consider administering TPN through a shunt. Patients who need TPN for more than one year can take a TPN training course (if available in their area) to learn how to administer TPN independently.

Definitions of intestinal failure:

- Type I: acute, <28 days of TPN, usually self-limiting, e.g. after surgery
- Type II: medium-term, >28 days of TPN (weeks to months), e.g. when waiting for a fistula to close
- Type III: chronic, long-term TPN (months to years), e.g. short bowel syndrome or motility disorders

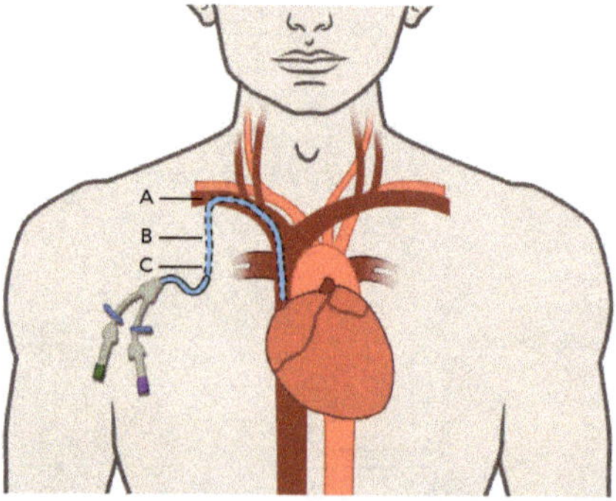

Figure 26 // Central venous line (CVL), tunnelled, through which TPN can be administered
A: V. subclavia **B:** Tunnelled central venous line **C:** Insertion site

Pharmacological treatment

Legend

- = Additional information
- = Indication for prescribing medication
- ⇔ = Interaction with drugs or high-risk groups
- = Indication for stopping with medication
- = Intoxication management
- CI = Contraindication

Anticoagulants

Anticoagulant management may differ across hospitals, so always make sure to check the local protocols when starting at a new hospital.

The management of anticoagulants depends on the bleeding risk associated with the endoscopic procedure and interventions performed.

All antiplatelet drugs require an initial loading dose, often higher, followed by a lower maintenance dose for continued treatment.

LMWHs have a longer $t_{1/2}$ and more stable serum levels, and no anti-Xa activity monitoring is needed. In case of reduced LMWH renal clearance, the dose should be adjusted based on anti-Xa levels.

DOACs are taken orally and do not require routine INR monitoring, reducing patient burden. DOAC treatment is as effective as VKA treatment, with comparable risk of stroke, cardiovascular death, and other causes of mortality. DOACs are additionally associated with a reduced risk of major bleeding, including intracranial bleeding, compared to VKAs.

DOACs are not indicated in patients with mechanical heart valves. These patients should be treated with vitamin K antagonists.

	MEDICATION	MECHANISM OF ACTION	INDICATIONS
PLATELET AGGREGATION INHIBITORS	**Acetylsalicylic acid** (aspirin)	ASA irreversibly inhibits the COX enzyme (→ production of platelet aggregation-stimulating thromboxane A2 ↓)	Treatment of ACS, AP and PAD, treatment of MI, CABG, TIA, and ischaemic stroke
	P2Y12 inhibitors (e.g. clopidogrel, prasugrel, ticagrelor)	P2Y12 inhibitors irreversibly inhibit activation via the ADP receptor on the platelet preventing aggregation	ACS, TIA or ischaemic stroke. Often used in combination with ASA as dual antiplatelet therapy (DAPT).
	Glycoprotein IIb/IIIa inhibitors (e.g. abciximab, tirofiban, eptifibatide)	Glycoprotein IIb/IIIa receptor inhibition → inhibits binding fibrinogen and von Willebrand Factor → platelet aggregation ↓	Acute coronary syndromes
VKA	**Vitamin K antagonists** (e.g. acenocoumarol, phenprocoumon, warfarin)	Inhibition of vitamin K reductase and with it the synthesis of coagulation factors II/VII/IX/X: • Acenocoumarol has a $t_{1/2}$ of 8-11h, an onset of action of 36-72h and a duration of action of 2d • Phenprocoumon has a $t_{1/2}$ of 160h, an onset of action of 48-72h and a duration of action of 1-2wk	Indicated for: • AF (CHA_2DS_2-VA >1) • Mechanical valve prosthesis • Venous thromboembolism (VTE) (DVT, pulmonary embolism); duration: 3 mo (1st VTE episode provoked by transient risk factor), 6 mo (first idiopathic VTE), >1y (recurring VTE)
HEPARIN GROUP	**Factor Xa inhibitors** (e.g. fondaparinux)	Binding to antithrombin III → factor Xa inhibition	• Used to treat venous and arterial thromboembolic disorders before starting OAC, also used as prophylaxis for surgical patients and for bridging. Therapeutic (6 mo) in VTE secondary to malignancy. • Fondaparinux: Halal alternative to LMWH
	Heparin	Heparin (SC/IV) activates antithrombin (factor III) and thus indirectly inactivates factors Xa and IIa (thrombin)	
	LMWH (e.g. nadroparin, enoxaparin)	LMWHs SC contain fragments of heparin with higher anti-Xa activity and lower anti-IIa activity. LMWHs are renally cleared.	

Table 28A // Anticoagulants

ACS, acute coronary syndrome; ADP, adenosine diphosphate; AF, atrial fibrillation; AP, angina pectoris; CABG, coronary artery bypass graft; DOAC, direct oral anticoagulants; DVT, deep vein thrombosis; LMWH, low-molecular-weight heparin; OAC, oral anticoagulation; PAD, peripheral arterial disease; PCI, percutaneous coronary intervention; Pgp, P-glycoprotein; TIA, transient ischaemic attack; VKA, vitamin K antagonists; VTE, venous thromboembolism

ADVERSE EFFECTS	NOTES
• Hypersensitivity (urticaria, exanthema, angioedema) • Bleeding risk ↑ (haematoma, epistaxis, GI bleeding) • GI (stomach problems)	⇔ Bleeding risk ↑ in the elderly and patients using corticosteroids, other NSAIDs and SSRIs ↑ ⊗ Prior to procedures with a high risk of bleeding complications, such as neurosurgery: stop ASA/clopidogrel 5-7d in advance. Due to irreversible binding, the duration of action of both drugs is 3-10d. ● Perioperative platelet transfusion as intoxication management in case of acute haemorrhage secondary to ASA or clopidogrel use
• Bleeding risk ↑ (haematoma, epistaxis, GI bleeding) • Abdominal pain, diarrhoea, dyspepsia • PPIs ↓ action of P2Y12 inhibitors	
• Bleeding risk ↑ • Thrombocytopaenia, arrhythmias, CHF	● Can be indicated after PCI in the case of no/inadequate reperfusion
Bleeding risk ↑	⇔ Bleeding risk ↑ due to: • Corticosteroids and NSAIDs (ulcerogenic) • SSRIs combined with platelet aggregation inhibitor (thrombocytopathy) • Nonadherence • Alcohol consumption • Low vitamin K intake • Febrile illness • Enhanced action of VKA due to co-trimoxazole, or after sudden discontinuation of carbamazepine or rifampicin 💡 For haemorrhage management: see following pages
• Bleeding risk ↑ • Heparin-induced thrombocytopenia (HIT) type I/II • Anaphylaxis • Transaminases ↑ • Adjust dose based on anti-Xa levels in reduced renal clearance	💡 Bridging: before any invasive procedure with bleeding risk, a short-acting medication (LMWH/ heparin) is administered to bridge the discontinuation of the OAC ▲ Following acute haemorrhaging, discontinue heparin/LMWH and administer protamine (partially inhibits anti-Xa activity, less so with LMWH!) IV as an antidote 💡 For more information on therapeutic blood monitoring, see the following pages

The efficacy of **vitamin K antagonists** (coumarin derivatives) depends on the INR. In case of haemorrhage or INR overshoots, vitamin K can be given orally (effect >8h) or intravenously (>6h). Vitamin K treatment lasts 24h and must be repeated, certainly with phenprocoumon (long $t_{1/2}$). In life-threatening situations like intracranial haemorrhages a four-factor prothrombin complex concentrate (II, VII, IX, X) should also be administered.

	MEDICATION	MECHANISM OF ACTION	INDICATIONS
DOAC	**Direct IIa inhibitors** (e.g. dagibatran)	Competitive and reversible inhibition of activated factor II	• Prevention of stroke and systemic embolism in nonvalvular atrial fibrillation • Treatment of DVT and pulmonary embolism and prevention of recurrent VTE • DOACs can not be used as anticoagulant for mechanical heart valves, and moderate to severe mitral valve stenosis
	Factor Xa inhibitors (e.g. rivaroxaban, apixaban, edoxaban)	Selective inhibition of activated factor X, preventing the conversion of prothrombin to thrombin	

Table 28B // Anticoagulants

INR

The international normalised ratio (INR) is the rate at which blood clots. The physiological INR is 1. An INR of 2 means that blood clots twice as slowly. The target value of INR is between 2.0-3.5, depending on the thrombotic risk.

Bridging

Bridging involves temporarily administering a short-acting agent (LMWH or occasionally unfractionated heparin) to bridge the time without VKA. Coumarin derivatives must be discontinued prior to any invasive procedure with a high bleeding risk. Due to their respective elimination half-lives, acenocoumarol should be discontinued three to four days and phenprocoumon five to seven days prior to surgery.

Bridging is indicated in patients with an increased risk of thrombosis. This risk can be estimated with the CHA_2DS_2-VA score, which uses validated risk factors to evaluate ischaemic stroke risk in patients with AF. Preoperative discontinuation of DOACs is not an indication for bridging because of the short $t_{1/2}$.

Bridging with LMWH is indicated for:

- Very high arterial thromboembolism risk: AF with CHA_2DS_2-VA score 8-9, mechanical or bioprosthetic heart valve, or a stroke/TIA <6 months ago.
- Very high venous thromboembolism (VTE) risk: <3 months after first or recurrent idiopathic DVT/pulmonary embolism.

ADVERSE EFFECTS	NOTES
• Bleeding risk ↑ • Anaemia • GI: dyspepsia, diarrhoea, nausea, vomiting	⇔ Bleeding risk ↑: • Corticosteroids and NSAIDs • Platelet aggregation inhibitors combined with SSRIs • Thrombolytics • Nonadherence • Alcohol consumption • Febrile illness • Pgp inhibitors such as ciclosporin, itraconazole, ketoconazole, amiodarone and verapamil ⚠ In case of active haemorrhaging on dabigatran, idaruzicimab can be administered as an antidote. In case of direct Xa inhibitors, andexanet alpha can be administered.

The **CHA_2DS_2-VA score** can be used to assess stroke risk in patients with AF.

Criterium	**Points**
Congestive HF	1 point
Hypertension	1 point
Age ≥75	2 points
Diabetes mellitus	1 point
Stroke/TIA/arterial thromboembolism	2 points
Vascular disease	1 point
Age 65-74	1 point

The **HAS-BLED score** can be used to assess bleeding risk.

Criterium	**Points**
Hypertension	1 point
Abnormal renal or liver function	1 point each
Stroke	1 point
Bleeding	1 point
Labile INRs	1 point
Elderly (>65)	1 point
Drugs or alcohol	1 point each

Laxatives

	MEDICATION	POSSIBLE INDICATIONS	ADVERSE EFFECTS
LAXATIVES	**Bisacodyl** (oral, rectal)	• Contact laxative: intestinal fluids and electrolytes ↑ → peristalsis ↑ → stool water content ↑ • Onset of action: oral >6-12h, rectal >20-45 min	• IBS with constipation • Rectal and bowel cleansing before surgery, after surgery
	Lactulose (powder, syrup, enema)	• Converted to natural acids in the colon ↑ intestinal water absorption ↑ → softer stools and volume ↑ → peristalsis ↑ • Inhibits ammonia-producing intestinal bacteria → pH ↓ → conversion of ammonia to ammonium → serum ammonia ↓ • Onset of action: 8-12h	• IBS with constipation, abdominal cramps • Hepatic encephalopathy (prevention and treatment)
	Linaclotide	Inhibits nociceptor activity, increases intestinal fluid, and accelerates transit time → peristalsis ↑, intestinal cramps ↓	Symptomatic treatment of adults with moderate/serious IBS with constipation
	Macrogol with or without electrolytes	• Intestinal water retention ↑ softer stools and volume ↑ → peristalsis ↑ • Onset of action after 1-2h or after 1-2 days (low-dose medications)	• IBS with constipation • Colon lavage prior to diagnostic exams or surgical procedures involving the colon • Treatment and prevention of faecal impaction in adults and children aged >2
	Methylnaltrexone	• Opioid receptor antagonist: selective action on μ-receptor (reversible, competitive binding) → intestinal motility ↑ → peristalsis ↑ • Onset of action <30-60 min, duration of action approx. 4h	Opioid-induced constipation in adults unresponsive to conventional laxatives
	Sodium phosphate enema	• Osmotic action of phosphate ions → water absorption in the intestinal lumen ↑ → softer stools and stool volume ↑ • Onset of action <5 min	• Emptying the rectum, sigmoid, and lower descending colon in occasional constipation • In preparation for medical and diagnostic procedures and childbirth

Table 29A // Laxatives
IBS, irritable bowel syndrome

NOTES

💡 May cause a mild, usually transient form of haematochezia (bright red blood in or with stools)
⊗ CI: Acute inflammation, ileus, intestinal obstruction

💡 Due to the presence of free sugars (fructose, galactose, and lactose), caution is advised in DM when using lactulose in high doses, e.g. for hepatic encephalopathy
⊗ CI: Galactosaemia, ileus, intestinal obstruction or perforation

💡 Increased risk of intestinal perforation
⊗ CI: Obstruction, children aged <18 due to lack of safety data

💡 Klean-Prep® is preferred for pre-colonoscopy bowel preparation in patients with severe heart failure
⇔ May reduce absorption of other medication
⊗ CI: Toxic megacolon, ileus, intestinal obstruction or perforation, severe IBD

⇔ Does not affect centrally acting analgesics because it is virtually unable to cross the blood-brain barrier
⊗ CI: Intestinal perforation or obstruction

💡 Increased risk of rectal perforation
⊗ CI: Acute infections, megacolon, GI haemorrhage, episodes of renal dysfunction, electrolyte imbalance, dehydration, heart failure

	MEDICATION	POSSIBLE INDICATIONS	ADVERSE EFFECTS
LAXATIVES	**Prucalopride**	• Selective serotonin receptor agonist with prokinetic activity in GI system → peristalsis ↑ • Onset of action <1-2d	Symptomatic treatment of chronic constipation in adults unresponsive to laxatives
	Psyllium fibre	• Bulking agent → intestinal water absorption ↑ → softer stool and stool volume ↑ → peristalsis ↑ • Onset of action 12-24h	• IBS with constipation • IBS with diarrhoea

Table 29B // Laxatives
IBS, irritable bowel syndrome

> The adverse effects of laxatives include abdominal pain, abdominal cramps, bloating, nausea, diarrhoea, flatulence. Enemas can also cause rectal discomfort and a burning sensation in the anus.

Antiemetics

	MEDICATION	MECHANISM OF ACTION	POSSIBLE INDICATIONS
ANTIEMETICS	**Domperidone**	• Dopamine antagonist that accelerates gastric emptying: • Gastric and duodenal peristalsis ↑ • Gastroesophageal sphincter pressure ↑ • Pyloric relaxation	• Symptomatic treatment for nausea and vomiting • Nausea and vomiting in migraine episodes
	Metoclopramide		• Symptomatic treatment for nausea and vomiting • Prevention of nausea and vomiting associated with chemotherapy and radiotherapy
	Ondansetron	Blocks $5HT_3$ receptors in GI tract and central and peripheral nervous system	Prevention and treatment of nausea and vomiting postoperatively and associated with chemotherapy and radiotherapy

Table 30A // Antiemetics

NOTES
Prucalopride, unlike many other laxatives, is absorbed systemically → can cause adverse systemic effects ⇔ Dose modification needed in patients with a creatinine clearance of 10-30 ml/min (1x/d 1 mg) CI: Intestinal perforation or obstruction, obstructive ileus, Crohn's disease, ulcerative colitis, toxic megacolon/megarectum
For constipation, take with plenty of water. For diarrhoea, take with little water or a more viscous liquid such as yoghurt so that the fibres can bind a lot of fluids.

When using laxatives, exercise caution with risk factors for electrolyte disturbances (e.g. heart failure, impaired renal or hepatic function, diuretic use, frail elderly patients) and dehydration. The potassium loss caused by other medications may also exacerbate, increasing the risk of toxic effects, so monitor electrolytes and renal function as needed.

ADVERSE EFFECTS	NOTES
Diarrhoea, abdominal pain, dry mouth, headache	Domperidone can lead to sore/tender breasts or galactorrhoea by stimulating prolactin release CI: Moderate and severe episodes of hepatic dysfunction (Child-Pugh C cirrhosis, 1/3 of usual dose in Child-Pugh B cirrhosis) and situations where stimulation is risky: GI haemorrhage, mechanical obstruction, perforation
Diarrhoea, drowsiness, asthenia, extrapyramidal disorders	Monitor renal function, reduce dose by 50% in patients with an eGFR of 10-50 ml/min ⇔ Avoid in patients with Parkinson's disease, counteracts the effect of levodopa. Domperidone is a suitable alternative, as it doesn't cross the blood-brain barrier. ⇔ Metoclopramide potentiates the sedative effect of central depressants and vice versa
Headache, constipation, chest pain	⇔ Antagonism of $5HT_3$ receptors decreases intestinal motility and intestinal secretion, exercise caution with signs of subacute intestinal obstruction

	MEDICATION	MECHANISM OF ACTION	POSSIBLE INDICATIONS
ANTIEMETICS	**Erythromycin**	Inhibits smooth muscle cells and the myenteric plexus by stimulating motilin receptors. Accelerates gastric emptying due to reduced fundus relaxation.	• Patients with idiopathic, diabetic, and postsurgical gastroparesis • Prior to upper endoscopy to promote gastric emptying for improved visibility (e.g. in case of upper GI haemorrhage)

Table 30B // Antiemetics

Antiemetics may prolong the QTc interval, increasing the risk of severe arrhythmias when combined with other QTc-prolonging agents. Be mindful of this and perform an ECG if necessary.

Antibiotics

	MEDICATION	MECHANISM OF ACTION	COVERAGE
ANTIBIOTICS (AB)	**Penicillins** • Penicillinase-resistant (e.g. flucloxacillin) • Broad-spectrum (e.g. amoxicillin, piperacillin)	The three groups of beta-lactam antibiotics inhibit the synthesis of bacterial cell wall peptidoglycan and derive their names from their characteristic beta-lactam ring. In combination with a beta-lactamase inhibitor such as clavulanic acid or tazobactam, they can also be used to treat beta-lactamase-forming bacteria.	• Predominantly active against G+ pathogens; flucloxacillin and augmentin are also active against beta-lactamase-producing pathogens, such as *Staphylococcus aureus* • Broad-spectrum: also active against some G- bacteria • Piperacillin-tazobactam is an example of a treatment option for cholangitis
	Cephalosporins • 1st generation: e.g. cefazolin • 2nd generation: e.g. cefuroxime • 3rd generation: e.g. ceftazidime, ceftriaxone • 4th generation: e.g. cefepime		• Cefazolin: narrow spectrum (G+) • Cefuroxime: more active against G- pathogens (beta-lactamase insensitivity) • Ceftazidime/ceftriaxone: broader spectrum, esp. effective against G- bacteria • Ceftriaxone is an example of antibiotic prophylaxis in an upper GI bleeding and as treatment for spontaneous bacterial peritonitis
	Carbapenems (e.g. meropenem)		• Very broad-spectrum AB used primarily to treat highly resistant G- bacteria, e.g. ESBL • Meropenem is an example of a treatment option for infected necrotising pancreatitis

Table 31A // Antibiotics
AB, antibiotics; ESBL, extended spectrum beta-lactamase; G+, gram-positive; G-, gram-negative; UTIs, urinary tract infections

ADVERSE EFFECTS	NOTES
Pseudomembranous colitis, transient confusion, convulsions	Usually prescribed only as a short-term prokinetic due to its antibiotic effect ⇔ Erythromycin is a moderately strong inhibitor of CYP3A4 and a substrate for CYP3A4

ADVERSE EFFECTS	NOTES
• GI: nausea, abdominal pain, diarrhoea • Toxicodermies (7-8% with amoxicillin) • Hypersensitivity (1%) • Anaphylactic shock (0.01-0.04%)	⇔ There is cross-sensitivity between different types of penicillins. Cross-sensitivity with cephalosporins is much less common. Risk of pseudomembranous colitis (*Clostridium difficile*)
• GI: nausea, abdominal pain, diarrhoea • Bone marrow depression (thrombocytopaenia, leukopenia, granulocytopenia) • Haemolytic anaemia	⇔ Cross-sensitivity with penicillins (10-15%) ⇔ No simultaneous parenteral administration with solutions containing calcium → precipitation
• GI: nausea, abdominal pain, diarrhoea • Bone marrow depression (thrombocytopaenia, leukopenia, granulocytopenia) • Haemolytic anaemia • Risk of C. difficile infection ↑	⇔ Concomitant use of bacteriostatic AB → bactericidal activity of carbapenems ↓ (also applies to other beta-lactam ABs)

	MEDICATION	MECHANISM OF ACTION	COVERAGE
ANTIBIOTICS (AB)	**Quinolones** (e.g. ciprofloxacin, levofloxacin)	Inhibition of DNA transcription and replication by inhibiting DNA gyrase	• Broad spectrum (esp. active against G- (enterocolic) bacteria, also *Haemophilus influenzae*, *Campylobacter* and *Pseudomonas*) • Ciprofloxacin is the 1st choice for treating complicated UTIs. High oral availability.
	Aminoglycosides (e.g. gentamicin)	Block the initiation of protein synthesis	• Mainly active against aerobic G- rods, as well as various G+ organisms • Synergy with beta-lactam antibiotics
	Macrolides (e.g. azithromycin, clarithromycin)	Bacteriostatic action through protein synthesis inhibition	Similar to penicillins, but with a broader spectrum (*Mycoplasma pneumoniae, Legionella pneumophila, Mycobacterium avium*); use in cases of penicillin resistance/ sensitivity.
	Tetracyclines (e.g. doxycycline, tetracycline)	Bacteriostatic action due to protein synthesis inhibition	Very broad spectrum, covering *Mycoplasma, Rickettsia, Chlamydia, Borrelia*, spirochetes and protozoa
	Sulfonamides (e.g. co-trimoxazole: sulfonamide + trimethoprim)	Synergistic inhibition of folic acid synthesis and therefore of bacterial DNA/RNA	Most G+ and G- microorganisms, as well as *Pneumocystis jirovecii* (pneumonia in HIV) and *Toxoplasma gondii* (toxoplasmosis)

Table 31B // Antibiotics

Antibiotic resistancy can be region or even hospital-specific. Always check your local antibiotic protocol for the first choice antibiotic in specific situations.

Causes of lack of response to treatment: resistance, pathogen falls outside AB spectrum, non-infectious underlying cause (e.g. autoimmune disease, malignancy or drug fever), focus of infection is not/ hardly reached (e.g. abscess, empyema, prosthesis/catheter), poor local circulation (DM, peripheral vascular disease).

ADVERSE EFFECTS	NOTES
• GI: nausea, abdominal pain, diarrhoea • Hypersensitivity • Achilles tendon rupture (with prolonged use)	⇔ Complex formation with calcium, magnesium, zinc, iron → strong absorption ↓ (antacids, milk, iron preparations)
• Ototoxicity (vertigo, ataxia, deafness; irreversible) • Nephrotoxicity (reversible)	⇔ Ototoxicity: risk ↑ with loop diuretics ⇔ Nephrotoxicity: risk ↑ in renal insufficiency 💡 Therapeutic drug monitoring necessary when administering repeated doses due to narrow therapeutic index
• GI: nausea, abdominal pain, diarrhoea • Hypersensitivity	⇔ Macrolides are potent CYP3A4 inhibitors (increased risk of adverse effects when used concomitantly with statins, e.g. myopathy and rhabdomyolysis) 💡 Risk of QT prolongation ↑
• Photosensitivity (photodermatitis, photoonycholysis) • Calcium chelation: dental discoloration, dental hypoplasia and delayed osteogenesis	💡 Chelation of metal ions: see Quinolones ⊗ Tooth discoloration/reduced osteogenesis: do not prescribe for pregnant women from week 16 or for children younger than age 8 ⇔ Enhanced action of oral anticoagulants
• GI: nausea, abdominal pain, diarrhoea • Hypersensitivity • Bone marrow suppression	⇔ Methotrexate potentiates bone marrow suppression, HIV is a risk factor ⇔ Via CYP2C9 inhibition → VKA action ↑ (risk of bleeding and INR elevation)

Bridging and switch therapy
As soon as the pathogen and sensitivity pattern are known, a narrower, more targeted treatment should be chosen to replace the initial broad-spectrum therapy (lower risk of resistance, less impact on endogenous flora and fewer adverse effects). If the patient's clinical status improves, it is also important to switch from IV AB to oral AB after 2-3d, or after 3-4d for more severe infections.

PACE-PM is a mnemonic for organisms with inducible beta-lactamase activity. These organisms are ***P****roteus* spp. (excl. *P. mirabilis*), ***A****eromonas* spp., ***C****itrobacter freundii*, ***E****nterobacter* spp., ***P****rovidencia* spp. and ***M****organella morganii*.

ANTIBIOTIC	GRAM-POSITIVE						
	Cocci						Anaerobic
	MRSA	*Staphylococcus epidermidis*	MSSA	*Enterococcus faecium*	*Enterococcus faecalis*	*Streptococcus*	*Clostridium, Peptostreptococcus*
Amoxicillin			■	■	■	■	
Amoxicillin / clavulanic acid			■	■	■	■	■
Azithromycin							
Cefazolin			■			■	
Cefepime			■			■	■
Ceftazidime							
Ceftriaxone			■			■	■
Cefuroxime			■			■	■
Clindamycin	■		■			■	■
Co-trimoxazole	■	■	■		■	■	■
Daptomycin	■	■	■	■	■	■	
Ertapenem		■	■			■	■
Erythromycin							
Flucloxacillin		■	■			■	
Fusidic acid	■	■	■		■		
Gentamicin	■		■	■	■		
Imipenem		■	■		■	■	■
Linezolid	■	■	■	■	■	■	
Meropenem		■	■			■	■
Metronidazole							■
Moxifloxacin		■	■		■	■	■
Penicillin				■	■	■	
Piperacillin			■		■	■	■

Table 32A // Antibiotic spectrum of activity

Please note that this is a general table, local protocols and resistance may vary

GRAM-NEGATIVE									
Anaerobic	**Cocci/coccobacilli**			**Bacilli**					
Bacteroides, Fusobacterium	***Nesseria meningitidis***	***Haemophilus influenzae***	***Moraxella***	***Escherichia coli***	***Klebsiella pneumoniae***	***Proteus, Mirabilis***	***Pseudomonas***	**PACE-PM* organisms**	***Legionella***
		■							
■	■	■	■	■	■	■			
									■
	■	■		■	■	■			
■	■	■	■	■	■	■	■	■	
		■	■	■	■	■	■		
	■	■	■	■	■	■			
	■	■	■	■	■	■			
■									
■	■	■	■	■	■	■			■
■	■	■	■	■	■	■		■	
									■
	■	■							
				■	■	■	■	■	
■	■	■	■	■	■	■	■	■	
■	■	■	■	■	■	■	■	■	
■									
■	■	■	■	■	■	■		■	■
	■								
■	■	■	■	■	■	■			

ANTIBIOTIC	GRAM-POSITIVE						
	Cocci						Anaerobic
	MRSA	*Staphylococcus epidermidis*	MSSA	*Enterococcus faecium*	*Enterococcus faecalis*	*Streptococcus*	*Clostridium, Peptostreptococcus*
Piperacillin / tazobactam			■		■	■	■
Rifampicin	■	■	■				
Teicoplanin	■	■	■	■	■	■	
Ticarcillin			■	■	■	■	■
Tigecycline	■	■	■	■	■	■	■
Tobramycin					■		
Trimethoprim				■			
Vancomycin	■	■	■	■	■	■	

Table 32B // Antibiotic spectrum of activity
Please note that this is a general table, local protocols and resistance may vary

Medication for acid reflux

	MEDICATION	MECHANISM OF ACTION	POSSIBLE INDICATIONS
MEDICATION FOR ACID REFLUX	**Antacids** (e.g. Algeldrate / magnesium hydroxide, calcium carbonate, magnesium hydroxide, magnesium carbonate)	Neutralises gastric acid, causing gastric pH to rise. Decreased pepsin activation, inhibiting proteolytic activity of pepsin.	• First episode of stomach symptoms • Stomach symptoms associated with NSAID use • GORD • Reflux oesophagitis
	H2 receptor antagonists (e.g. cimetidine, famotidine)	Inhibits gastric acid secretion by blocking histamine (H2) receptors of gastric parietal cells	• First episode of stomach symptoms • Stomach symptoms associated with NSAID use • Peptic ulcers • GORD • Reflux oesophagitis
	Proton pump inhibitors (PPIs) (e.g. esomeprazole, lansoprazole, omeprazole, pantoprazole, rabeprazole)	Inhibits H^+/K^+-ATPase in gastric parietal cells, thus inhibiting both basal and stimulated gastric acid secretion	• Prevention and treatment of duodenal or ventricular ulcers • GORD • Barrett oesophagus • Eosinophilic oesophagitis • Gastric symptoms associated with NSAIDs or oral steroids

Table 33 // Medication for acid reflux

GRAM-NEGATIVE									
Anaerobic	**Cocci/coccobacilli**			**Bacilli**					
Bacteroides, Fusobacterium	***Nesseria meningitidis***	***Haemophilus influenzae***	***Moraxella***	***Escherichia coli***	***Klebsiella pneumoniae***	***Proteus, Mirabilis***	***Pseudomonas***	**PACE-PM* organisms**	***Legionella***

ADVERSE EFFECTS	NOTES
• Diarrhoea (esp. with magnesium salts), alkalosis, urinary tract stones • Carbonates cause CO_2 to develop in the stomach	Antacids are faster and shorter-acting than acid secretion inhibitors (H2 receptor antagonists and PPIs) Magnesium hydroxide is also used as a laxative Absorption ↓ of medication for 2-4h
• Headaches, dizziness • GI symptoms include constipation, diarrhoea	Reduced uptake of vitamin B12 from food
• GI symptoms include abdominal pain, diarrhoea, benign gastric polyps, flatulence, constipation • Headache, dizziness, sleep disorder • Electrolyte disturbances (Mg ↓, Na ↓, Ca ↓, K ↓)	Reduced uptake of vitamin B12 from food Long-term use (>1y) is associated with a risk of hypomagnesaemia, possibly by inhibiting active transcellular transport. The same does not appear to be true for H2 antagonists.

Inflammatory bowel disease medication

The choice of IBD medication depends on the location, extent, and severity of the inflammation. Other important factors include response to previous medication, age, comorbidities, and patient preference.

	MEDICATION	MECHANISM OF ACTION	GASTROENTEROLOGICAL INDICATIONS
CORTICOSTEROIDS	**Prednisone** (oral, i.v.)	Glucocorticoid; converted to active ingredient prednisolone in the liver	• Remission induction in Crohn's disease and ulcerative colitis • Autoimmune hepatitis • Autoimmune pancreatitis • IgG4-mediated disease
	Budesonide (oral: dissolving tablet, tablet, capsule, granules)	Glucocorticoid with local anti-inflammatory effect	• Tablet, capsule, granules: - Remission induction in active Crohn's disease or ulcerative colitis - Maintenance treatment for microscopic colitis - Maintenance treatment for autoimmune hepatitis • Dissolving tablet: - Eosinophilic oesophagitis
	Budesonide (rectal foam, suppository, or enema)		Foam, suppository, enema: • Distal inflammation in Crohn's disease or ulcerative colitis

Table 34 // Corticosteroids

ADVERSE EFFECTS	NOTES
• The many adverse effects include fluid and electrolyte disturbances, moon face, musculoskeletal complaints, osteoporosis, GI symptoms, stomach ulcers, skin pathology; haematological, endocrine, metabolic, cardiological or neurological abnormalities; psychological symptoms • Increased susceptibility to infection and masking of clinical signs, impaired immune response	💡 After prolonged therapy, discontinuation may result in corticosteroid withdrawal syndrome/adrenal cortex insufficiency. When discontinuing, taper off gradually to prevent steroid-induced adrenal cortex insufficiency. 💡 Give prophylaxis against osteoporosis (calcium + vitamin D) when used >3 mo (dose-dependent) 💡 Patients may need a higher dose (stress dose) prior to a procedure or surgery or if severely ill ⇔ High dose (prednisone ≥15 mg) may potentiate VKAs: careful INR monitoring needed ⇔ Insulin/oral hypoglycaemic medication requirement may increase in diabetics
• Oesophageal candidiasis from dissolving tablet (in 20% of patients) • See the adverse effects of prednisone for other systemic adverse effects	💡 Increased susceptibility to infection, do not give if there is an active bacterial, viral, or fungal infection 💡 Budesonide has a high first-pass metabolism and a primarily local effect → approx. 50% fewer adverse effects than systemic corticosteroids (prednisone) ⊗ Avoid in Crohn's disease affecting the upper GI tract ⊗ Avoid in liver cirrhosis or with signs of portal hypertension due to the risk of portal vein thrombosis
Rectal administration lowers risk of adverse effects. May cause pain and a burning sensation in the rectum.	

	MEDICATION	MECHANISM OF ACTION	GASTROENTEROLOGICAL INDICATIONS
IMMUNOSUPPRESSANTS	**Azathioprine** (e.g. Imuran®) **Mercaptopurine** (e.g. Puri-Nethol®) **Tioguanine** (Thiosix®)	• Purine antagonist: cytostatic and immunosuppressant • Inhibits de novo purine synthesis and the purine nucleotide cycle • Thiopurines are inactive prodrugs that are converted into the active metabolites in the body: 6-tioguanine nucleotides (6-TGN)	• Maintenance treatment for Crohn's disease and ulcerative colitis: - Monotherapy - Combination therapy (with TNF-alpha blockers) - With corticosteroids • Maintenance treatment for autoimmune hepatitis (azathioprine = first-line therapy) • Tioguanine: indicated in patients unresponsive or intolerant to standard thiopurine treatment (with azathioprine or mercaptopurine)
	Methotrexate	• Folic acid antagonist: cytostatic and immunosuppressant • Inhibits conversion of folic acid, an essential process for nucleic acid synthesis in cell division, thus inhibiting formation of new cells.	Remission induction and maintenance treatment in Crohn's disease (esp. if joint symptoms present): • Monotherapy • Combination therapy (with TNF-alpha blockers) • With corticosteroids

Table 35 // Immunosuppressants

> In patients experiencing many or severe adverse effects from thiopurines, consider an unnoticed thiopurine methyltransferase (TPMT) deficiency. Modify dose in TPMT-deficient patients. Genetic variation in NUDT15 is also associated with adverse effects (myelosuppression).

ADVERSE EFFECTS	NOTES
	💡 Long onset of action (weeks to months) and is therefore often started with other medication in cases of severe inflammation 💡 Tioguanine, mercaptopurine: increased risk of urate nephropathy (hyperuricaemia, hyperuricosuria) ⊗ Stop in active infectious process ⇔ Exercise caution in patients on vitamin K antagonists, monitor INR after starting ⊗ Therapeutic drug monitoring of thiopurin metabolites is possible for azathioprine and mercaptopurines: 6-TGN is the active form, 6-MMP the toxic metabolite. Allopurinol can be started in preferential 6-MMP metabolisers. To prevent toxic 6-TGN levels, reduce thiopurine dose by 75% or switch to tioguanine. ⊗ Bone marrow toxicity (esp. leukopenia). Regularly monitor blood counts. ⊗ Liver toxicity: regular liver function tests (ALT, AST, bilirubin, ALP, GGT). May be associated with high levels of 6-MMP. ⊗ Increased risk of developing lymphoproliferative disorders and malignancies (esp. non-melanoma skin cancer, sarcomas, in situ cervical cancer). Lymphoproliferative diseases occur more frequently with EBV infection in patients on thiopurines. Check serology before starting therapy and exercise caution in EBV-negative patients.
• Stomatitis (inflammation of the oral mucosa) • GI symptoms include nausea, vomiting, diarrhoea • Cholestasis, pancreatitis (not with tioguanine) • Infections • Alopecia	
• GI symptoms include stomatitis, dyspepsia, appetite ↓, abdominal pain, nausea, vomiting, diarrhoea • Skin rash (exanthema, erythema, itching) • Headaches, fatigue, leukopaenia and thrombocytopaenia • Pulmonary toxicity (pneumonia, interstitial alveolitis, pneumonitis)	💡 Bone marrow toxicity: closely monitor blood counts 💡 Nephrotoxic: closely monitor renal function. Contraindicated in severely impaired renal function (eGFR <10 ml/min), an eGFR of 10-50 ml/min may require dose modification, renal function monitoring, and effect/adverse effect monitoring (blood count, ALT). 💡 Liver toxicity: closely monitor liver function. Discontinue treatment in case of abnormal liver function tests or liver biopsy. Do not use simultaneously with potentially hepatotoxic medications. Avoid alcohol. ⇔ NSAIDs, loop diuretics, and PPIs may delay hepatic clearance and increase the risk of methotrexate toxicity ⇔ Have patients take a weekly folic acid supplement 24h after methotrexate administration ⊗ Increased risk of developing malignant lymphoma, may go into remission after discontinuation ⊗ Teratogenic: pregnancy is contraindicated. Discontinue at least 3 months before conception in both men and women due to teratogenic effect.

Vaccines containing live, attenuated microorganisms are contraindicated in patients using immunosuppressants, e.g. the vaccine for yellow fever. Inactivated vaccines may potentially be less effective when used with immunosuppressants.

Biologicals

<table>
<tr><th></th><th>MEDICATION</th><th>MECHANISM OF ACTION</th><th>GASTROENTEROLOGICAL INDICATIONS</th></tr>
<tr><td rowspan="4">BIOLOGICALS</td><td>Adalimumab
(e.g. Humira®, Hyrimoz®)</td><td rowspan="2">Monoclonal antibodies block TNF-α → prevent immune system activation → inhibit inflammation</td><td rowspan="2">• Remission induction and maintenance treatment in Crohn's disease and ulcerative colitis
• Fistula formation in Crohn's disease</td></tr>
<tr><td>Infliximab
(e.g. Remicade®, Remsima®, Inflectra®)</td></tr>
<tr><td>Ustekinumab
(e.g. Stelara®)</td><td>IL-12 and IL-23 antagonist: interrupts Th1 and Th17 cytokine pathways</td><td>Remission induction and maintenance treatment in Crohn's disease and ulcerative colitis</td></tr>
<tr><td>Vedolizumab
(e.g. Entyvio®)</td><td>Integrin inhibitor: blocks leukocyte transport from bloodstream to intestinal wall</td><td>Remission induction and maintenance treatment in Crohn's disease and ulcerative colitis</td></tr>
</table>

Table 36 // Biologicals

	MEDICATION	MECHANISM OF ACTION	GASTROENTEROLOGICAL INDICATIONS
OTHER	**Ciclosporin** (e.g. Neoral®)	Calcineurin inhibitor: specifically and reversibly inhibits proliferation of T lymphocytes, potent immunosuppressive effect	Remission induction in severe flare-ups of ulcerative colitis as a bridge to other therapy

Table 37A // Other medications for IBD

ADVERSE EFFECTS	NOTES
• Infections • GI symptoms, GI haemorrhage, reflux oesophagitis • Hypertension, oedema, headaches, muscle aches or cramps, skin symptoms • Response to injection or infusion	Increased risk of infections and reactivation; esp. tuberculosis with TNF-alpha blockers, so screening is required prior to starting treatment Pretreatment screening for TB Possible formation of antibodies autoimmune to the medication may increase clearance and reduce efficacy. Consider monitoring medication levels and any antibodies. Increased risk of malignancies, esp. lymphoma or melanoma Seems to be safe in pregnancy, but consider discontinuing in the third trimester Exercise caution in patients with moderate or severe heart failure and demyelinating disorders
• GI symptoms include nausea, vomiting, diarrhoea • Musculoskeletal symptoms include muscle pain, back pain, joint pain • Headache, dizziness, fatigue, itching	Increased risk of infection and reactivation
• GI symptoms include gastroenteritis, nausea, flatulence, constipation, anal fissure/abscess, bloating, haemorrhoids • Musculoskeletal symptoms • Headache, rash, night sweats	Increased risk of infection and reactivation Not associated with increased risk of malignancies when used as monotherapy

ADVERSE EFFECTS	NOTES
• GI symptoms include nausea, vomiting, abdominal pain, diarrhoea, peptic ulcer • Impaired liver function, hyperuricaemia, hypomagnesaemia, hyperlipidaemia, leukopenia • Tremor, headache, anorexia, hypertension	Ciclosporin has many interactions with other medications, must be closely monitored Nephrotoxic: exercise caution when used alongside other nephrotoxic medications. Regularly monitor renal and hepatic function. Increased risk of malignancies (skin cancer, lymphoproliferative abnormalities). Use of sunscreen is recommended.

	MEDICATION	MECHANISM OF ACTION	GASTROENTEROLOGICAL INDICATIONS
OTHER	**Tofacitinib** (e.g. Xeljanz®)	Selectively inhibits JAK1 and JAK3, which attenuates signal transduction of interleukins and interferons and modulates the immune and inflammatory response	Moderately severe ulcerative colitis

Table 37B // Other medications for IBD

IBD treatment is rapidly evolving. Recently approved drugs include ozanimod (S1P receptor modulator), risankizumab (IL-23 inhibitor), upadacitinib and filgotinib (JAK inhibitors). New agents and targets are continuously emerging.

Invasive, non-pharmacological treatment

Ostomies

General

An ostomy, or stoma, is an artificial opening between the intestines and the abdominal wall. Indications for an ostomy include IBD, perforated diverticulitis, oncological afflictions, trauma, fistula, and congenital defects and therapy-resistant obstipation (e.g. anorectal abnormalities or Hirschsprung's disease). Patients may be given a temporary ostomy to promote intestinal recovery. Possible complications of ostomy surgery include ostomy leakage, skin irritation, stenosis, parastomal hernia, and dehiscence.

A mucous fistula consists of the most distal part of the colon, brought out through the abdominal wall as a non-functional stoma to drain mucus, serous fluid, and leftover stool. Indications include distal intestinal obstructions, e.g. secondary to tumours.

Ileostomy

An ileostomy is made from the end of the small intestine (ileum) and has a terminal (with or without a mucous fistula) and a double-barrel variety (see Figure 27). Ileostomies with a mucous fistula work the same as colostomies that leave the

ADVERSE EFFECTS	NOTES
• GI symptoms include abdominal pain, vomiting, diarrhoea, nausea, gastritis, dyspepsia • Skin rash, arthralgia, peripheral oedema, fever, fatigue, headache, hypertension, pneumonia, coughing • Diverticulitis, viral gastroenteritis, hepatic steatosis	💡 Exercise caution with risk factors for venous thromboembolism, may affect lipid spectrum (cholesterol ↑) 💡 Pretreatment screening for TB and viral hepatitis ⇔ Do not combine with TNF-alpha blockers, IL antagonists, or immunosuppressants (increased risk of immunosuppression and infection) ⊗ Increased risk of serious cardiovascular events (incl. myocardial infarction) ⊗ Increased risk of malignancies (lung cancer, lymphomas)

anus and rectum intact. Indications for an ileostomy include temporary or permanent intestinal relief after e.g. intestinal resection, chronic inflammation of the bowel, therapy-resistant perianal fistula formation, or non-functioning intestines. A disadvantage of ileostomies is excessive fluid loss (watch out for severe dehydration), as fluid resorption largely takes place in the large intestine. High-output ostomies produce at least >1.5-2 L/day.

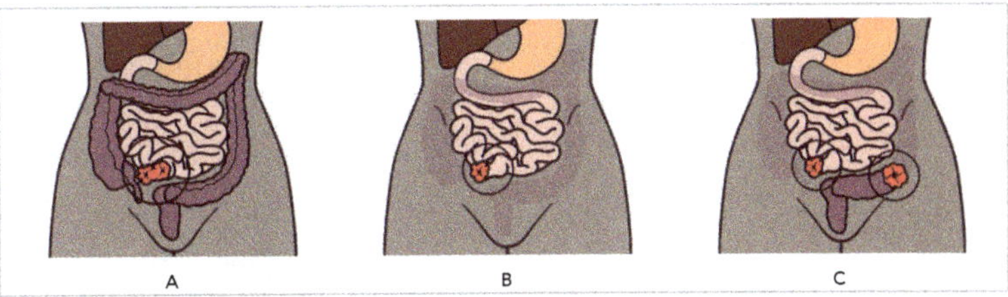

Figure 27 // Ileostomy: double-barrel **(A)**, terminal **(B)** and with mucous fistula **(C)**

Ileoanal pouch

An ileoanal pouch, or J-pouch, is a surgically created cavity between the ileum and the anus (see Figure 28). Ileoanal anastomosis is indicated after a total colectomy and involves turning part of the ileum into a reservoir connected to the anus. In the absence of the large intestine, stool thickens in the pouch before being excreted through the anus. Patients will pass stool more frequently than usual: five to six times during the day and one to two times at night. Postoperative complications include ileus, infection, strictures, anastomotic leakage, and fistula formation. Late complications include incontinence, pouchitis, cuffitis, Crohn's disease of the pouch, sinus or fistula formation, and pouch dysfunction. Metabolic complications such as anaemia, osteoporosis, and vitamin D and B12 deficiencies are also possible.

Colostomy

A colostomy is an opening in the large intestine and can be single-barrel or double-barrel (see Figure 28). A colostomy is indicated when distal continuity cannot be restored, e.g. due to chronic infections, after traumatic injury, or after tumour resection.

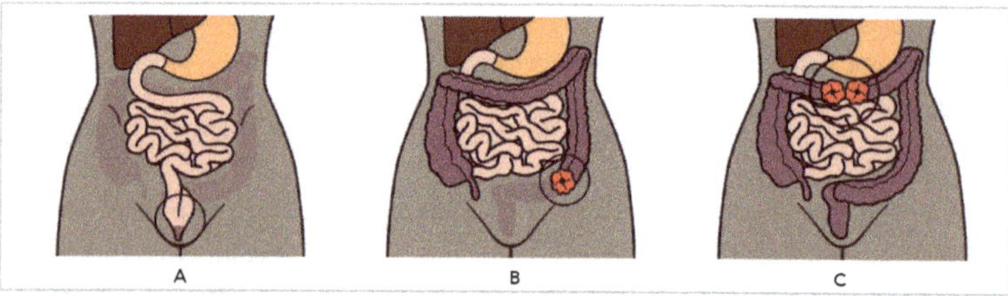

Figure 28 // Ileoanal pouch and end colostomy **(B)**: stoma in the large intestine or double-barrel **(C)**: stoma created by bringing one loop of the large intestine through an opening in the abdominal wall, opening it, and attaching it to the skin, so that the two ends are side-by-side

Endoscopic interventions

See section *Diagnostics* for an overview of endoscopic interventions.

Management of a patient with...

The diagrams presented in this section are intended as guidelines only: local protocols may vary per hospital and always take precedence. Discuss the content of this section with your supervisor and your fellow residents during your orientation period and write down points of interest for your context.

Reader's guide

- Each diagram starts with a **symptom**, followed by a **differential diagnosis**
- Next are the **primary survey instructions**
- Every diagram ends with **assessment or treatment recommendations**
- Specific treatment instructions can be found in the section *Conditions*

Management of acute abdominal pain

↓

Always consider

Abdominal

- Gastrointestinal:
  - RUQ: choledocholithiasis, cholecystolithiasis, cholecystitis, cholangitis, acute pancreatitis, biliary colic
  - RLQ: appendicitis, terminal ileitis
  - LLQ: diverticulitis, constipation, intestinal ischaemia, sigmoid volvulus
  - Epigastric region: gastritis, peptic ulcer disease, gastric perforation, pancreatitis, cholelithiasis, GORD
  - Diffuse: peritonitis, gastroenteritis, pancreatitis, IBS, portal vein thrombosis
  - Miscellaneous: perforation, mechanical/non-mechanical ileus, colon carcinoma, intestinal ischaemia, post-surgical complications
- Urogenital: renal colic, testicular torsion, acute/chronic urinary retention, UTI, pyelonephritis
- Gynaecological: acute PID, ovarian torsion, ectopic pregnancy, ovarian cyst rupture
- Vascular: AAA, aortic dissection, mesenteric ischaemia, ischaemic colitis
- Postoperatively: complications (e.g. bleeding, perforation, infection)

Extra-abdominal

- Cardiopulmonary: acute coronary syndrome, pneumonia (referred pain), pulmonary embolism
- Abdominal wall: herpes zoster, muscle haematoma, incarcerated hernia
- Metabolic: diabetic or alcoholic ketoacidosis

Note: this diagram discusses acute onset of abdominal pain and does not refer to peritoneal irritation

Diagram 3 // Management of acute abdominal pain

Primary survey instructions

- Monitor vital signs
- IV + labs if indicated: blood count, CRP, electrolytes, renal function, lactate, glucose, troponin, CK, liver enzymes, lipase, ABG, blood crossmatching, blood cultures
- ECG
- Urine sediment
- Women in fertile life stage: pregnancy test

If a patient deteriorates, contact the emergency response team (ERT) immediately and notify supervisor/gastroenterologist. Consult IC directly for specific suspicions.

↓

Assessment recommendations

- Assess patient using ABCDE approach
- Consider POCUS (assess free fluid, aneurysm, cardiac function, collapsed IVC), abdominal ultrasound, or abdominal contrast CT for underlying cause
- Consult surgeon/gynaecologist/gastroenterologist
- For specific treatment instructions, see *Conditions* for corresponding gastroenterology related causes

↓

Consult supervisor before starting treatment

Diagram 4A // Management of acute liver failure

Management of acute liver failure

↓

Definitions

- Acute liver injury: transaminases ↑ (2-3x ULN) + INR >1.5 without pre-existing liver disease
- Acute liver failure (ALF): acute liver injury with hepatic encephalopathy (HE)
- Acute liver failure: liver injury (abnormal liver tests) lasting <26 wk, coagulopathy (INR ≥1.5), and HE without pre-existing liver disease
- Acute-on-chronic liver failure: an acute deterioration of pre-existing chronic liver disease (often cirrhosis), usually related to a precipitating event (e.g. alcohol, infection), and associated with single-organ or multiple-organ failure.

Always consider

- Viral: hepatitis virus A-E, parvovirus, HZV, HSV, CMV, EBV, HIV, adenovirus, viral haemorrhagic fever
- Medication-induced: e.g. paracetamol (++), ABx (e.g. nitrofurantoin, doxycycline, azithromycin, ciprofloxacin, amoxicillin/clavulanic acid), labetalol, lisinopril, antiepileptics, thiopurines, MDMA, mushrooms (Amanita phalloides), herbs
- Vascular: right-sided heart failure, Budd-Chiari syndrome, ischaemic hepatitis
- Metabolic: acute fatty liver of pregnancy, Wilson's disease
- Autoimmune hepatitis
- Paediatric causes: Reye's syndrome, galactosaemia, hereditary fructose intolerance, tyrosinaemia
- Other: HELLP syndrome, sepsis, extensive liver surgery, overheating

↓

Primary survey instructions

- Assess hepatic encephalopathy (West Haven Criteria): ≥3 → intubation
- Determine whether patient has acute liver failure or acute-on-chronic liver failure

- Reach out to transplant centre at an early stage, determine prognosis + indication for transplantation using King's College Criteria or Clichy criteria
- Hx: see general Hx, unearth cause (PMHx, possible pregnancy, medication/intoxications, travel history, sexual history), ask about psychosocial situation, vaccinations, lifestyle habits, FHx
- Physical examination: jaundice, rash (vesicles), stigmata chronic liver disease, eyes; Kaysser-Fleischer Ring (Wilson's disease)
- Labs (severity of liver damage): blood panel (Hb, Ht, leukocytes + differentiation, thrombocytes), AST, ALT, ALP, GGT, bilirubin, creatinine, urea, Na, K, Mg, phosphate, LDH, amylase, CK, cholesterol, glucose, protein spectrum, albumin, lactate, clotting (APPT, PTT, INR, fibrinogen, factor V), ammonia blood gas, blood group, glycaemia
- Assess indication for emergency liver transplantation (depends on e.g. cause, MELD 3.0), assess: chronic liver disease, alcohol use disorder, malignancy, heart failure (King's College Criteria, see Appendix 2)
- Microbiology: blood cultures, urine cultures, sputum cultures, nasal cultures, ascites cultures
- Acute liver failure is only a relative indication for biopsy
- Stop all non-emergency medication
- Diagnostics to identify cause (depending on most likely diagnosis):
  - Labs: virus serology (hepatitis virus A-E, HIV, VZV, parvovirus, CMV, EBV, HSV) or DNA/RNA, immunology (ANA, SMA, LKM-1, AMA, IgG, IgM), blood paracetamol level, ceruloplasmin, copper, TSH, Coombs test, Ca, toxicology screening, pregnancy test
  - Imaging:
    - Chest X-ray: potential complications of liver failure (e.g. fluid overload)
    - Abdominal ultrasound or four-phase abdominal contrast CT: size of liver/spleen, appearance of liver parenchyma, infiltration, flow/patency of hepatic veins, portal vein, and hepatic artery, bile ducts, collaterals, ascites
- Hospitalisation MCU/ICU

If a patient deteriorates, contact rapid ERT immediately and notify supervisor/gastroenterologist. Consult IC directly for specific suspicions.

Diagram 4B // Management of acute liver failure

↓

Patient monitoring on MCU/ICU

- Check consciousness every 2h, neurological exam, respiration, circulation, and diuresis. Consider head CT if rapid decline in consciousness, focal neurological deficits, or seizure.
- Frequent labs: check glucose hourly, as hypoglycaemia may indicate worsening hepatic function
- Support vital organs as needed

Assessment/treatment advice

- MAP (2x diastolic + 1x systolic BP/3): aim for min. 60 mmHg
- Monitor volume status, fluid management, use vasopressors (norepinephrine)
- Place CVC and arterial line upon admission to ICU/MCU
- Prevent factors that may increase intracranial pressure: fever, seizures, hypertension, vasodilators, Valsalva manoeuvre, excitement, jugular vein compression, rotating and nodding head, endotracheal suction, fluid overload
- Correct metabolic acidosis (target pH 7.35-7.45), glucose, and electrolytes, including Ca, Na, Mg, K, P
- Optimise nutrition, e.g. with a feeding tube or parenteral nutrition (to reduce hypoglycaemia); in hypoglycaemia: glucose 10-20% or 50% IV (to prevent hypoglycaemia)
- Monitor renal function: serum creatinine, urine output, frequently measure sodium excretion → detect renal insufficiency early on (avoid potential triggers of renal insufficiency, e.g. contrast medium), start CVVH/dialysis for renal insufficiency
- Hepatic encephalopathy:
    - Assess consciousness every 2h
    - Intubation and artificial ventilation in grade 3 encephalopathy (West Haven Criteria)
- No prophylactic coagulation correction unless invasive procedure with increased risk of bleeding
- Avoid sedatives if possible
- Early initiation of N-acetylcysteine can lead to improved outcomes (also in non-paracetamol-induced ALF)

- Further treatment depends on cause/suspicion:
  - In multi-organ failure, suspected infection, or grade ≥3 hepatic encephalopathy: broad-spectrum AB + antifungal therapy in suspected infection
  - Paracetamol induced hepatotoxicity (hyperacute, marked transaminase ↑ with relatively low bilirubin): start N-acetylcysteine
  - Autoimmune hepatitis: consider a trial of corticosteroids for grade ≤2 hepatic encephalopathy
  - Amanita phalloides: activated carbon + laxative, antidote: silibinin IV
  - Budd-Chiari syndrome: consider anticoagulants and TIPS placement
  - HSV or HBV: antivirals (e.g. acyclovir IV in HSV)
  - If caused by pregnancy, consider terminating the pregnancy
  - Consider vitamin K 10 mg IV once to assess correctable deficiency and distinguish INR changes from liver dysfunction
  - Refer for liver transplant if no recovery or high risk of death (ALF or liver injury patients should be transferred to a transplant centre)
  - For specific treatment instructions of underlying cause, see *Conditions*
- Bring in appropriate specialists (e.g. ophthalmologist for suspected Wilson's disease, cardiologist for suspected heart failure, neurologist to rule out neurological causes)

↓

Consult supervisor before starting treatment

Consult the Drug-Induced Liver Injury Network for a list of medications that can cause acute liver failure. Scan the QR code for more information.

Aetiology of acute liver failure (ALF) varies geographically:
- North America, Japan, and Europe: DILI, viral hepatitis, and cryptogenic liver failure with no identifiable cause (indeterminate ALF)
- Regions with limited healthcare resources or higher prevalence of infectious diseases: acute viral hepatitis
- South America and Japan: autoimmune hepatitis

Diagram 5 // Management of alcohol-related conditions

Management of alcohol-withdrawal related conditions

Treatment advice

- Aims: reduce CNS excitability and prevent complications, quiet environment, prevent delirium, monitor vital parameters
- Fluid supplementation, refeeding lab and correct electrolyte disturbances
- Thiamine (vitamin B1), vitamin B-complex and vitamin C IV, see Diagram 5
- Consider consulting Psychiatry (for alcohol withdrawal delirium), consider consulting a dietician (for dietary plan)

Admission of a patient with an alcohol-related condition

→ Tx

- Vitamin B1 (thiamine) 1x/d 100 mg PO
- Vitamin B-complex 1x/d 1 tablet
- Vitamin C 1x/day 500 mg
- Lorazepam 2x/day 0.5 mg as needed

→ Suspected alcohol abstinence → Benzodiazepines (e.g. lorazepam): no set treatment schedule (taper guided by symptoms)

→ Increased risk of Wernicke encephalopathy → Vitamin B1 (thiamine) to 1x/day 250 mg IV/IM for 3-5d

→ Suspected Wernicke encephalopathy →

- Vitamin B1 (thiamine) to 3x/d 500 mg IV
- Vitamin B-complex to 3x/d

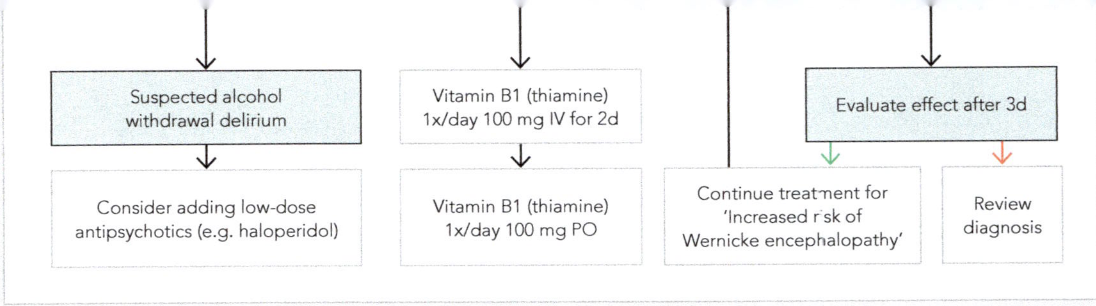

See *Alcohol-related conditions* for more information on alcohol withdrawal syndrome, alcohol withdrawal delirium, and Wernicke encephalopathy.

When administering IV glucose and thiamine, always administer thiamine first: starting with glucose increases the risk of Wernicke encephalopathy.

Haloperidol puts patients with alcohol withdrawal at increased risk of epileptic seizures.

Management of GI haemorrhage (1/2)

↓

Management of upper GI haemorrhage and/or suspected variceal haemorrhage

↓

Always consider

- Variceal haemorrhage ⊕ (PMHx varices and/or known/suspected liver cirrhosis?)
- Ulcer-related bleeding (ventricular ulcer, duodenal ulcer) ⊕
- Mallory-Weiss lesion ⊕
- Reflux oesophagitis ⊕
- Gastric and duodenal erosions-erosive defects ⊕
- Carcinoma
- Less common: arteriovenous malformation, gastrointestinal stromal tumour (GIST), angiodysplasias, aortoenteric fistula, watermelon stomach (GAVE), haemobilia, Dieulafoy lesions, Cameron lesions

Primary survey instructions

- ABCDE approach, constantly monitor vital signs (observe for pallor, clamminess, hypotension, tachycardia, consciousness, diuresis)
- Two large, functioning IVs: fluid challenge with NaCl 0.9% or Ringer's lactate. Permissive hypotension in variceal haemorrhage. For shock secondary to bleeding, consider the 'Massive Blood Loss' protocol, use of anticoagulants, and possibly treating shock.
- If haemodynamically relevant: CAD insertion + urimeter (urine output), start fluid balance
- For patients on a nursing ward: consult ERT

Diagram 6A // Management of GI haemorrhage (1/2)

Assessment recommendations

- Patient history: see general Hx, medication use (e.g. NSAIDs, anticoagulants), PMHx (e.g. liver cirrhosis, aortic prosthesis)
- Diagnostics:
  - Labs: rapid blood count (e.g. Hb from venous blood gas analysis), blood group, rhesus factor, blood crossmatching, potassium, urea, creatinine, AST, ALT, ALP, GGT, bilirubin
  - If indicated: lactate, CRP, troponin, CK, INR, ECG, chest X-ray
- Endoscopy:
  - Massive bleeding or haemodynamic instability: gastroscopy after patient stabilisation
  - Haemodynamic stability and non-threatening haemorrhage: gastroscopy <24h if clinically relevant
  - Negative gastroscopy and persistent bleeding: consider colonoscopy after appropriate bowel preparation
- Imaging:
  - 3-phase abdominal CT (incl. without contrast, CTA, and CTV) may be considered in manifest upper GI haemorrhage with non-conclusive endoscopy and in haemodynamically unstable patients with a history of central vascular reconstruction (endovascular prosthesis), suspected aortoenteric fistula, or endoscopically diagnosed haemobilia. In proven intestinal haemorrhage and dynamically unstable → selective embolisation by interventional radiologist.

If a patient deteriorates, contact ERT immediately and notify supervisor/gastroenterologist. Consult IC directly for specific suspicions.

For suspected variceal haemorrhage (1/2):

Preparation:

- Call the gastroenterologist immediately
- Find out patient's MRSA/HRMO status, use of anticoagulants, vital parameters, resuscitation instructions
- For haemodynamically unstable patients: consult with intensivist or ERT for assessment and possible readmission to ICU
- In endoscopic interventions on unstable patients or with active haematemesis: consider intubation

Suspected ulcer-related bleeding (1/2):

- IV PPI (omeprazole/pantoprazole/esomeprazole) bolus (80 mg) followed by perfusor (8 mg/h)
- If possible and indicated: treat the cause of bleeding endoscopically and locally
- During endoscopy, take biopsies for *H. pylori* (sometimes deliberately avoided in acute settings due to risk of false negative)

↓

Diagram 6B // Management of GI haemorrhage (1/2)

For suspected variceal haemorrhage (2/2):
Treatment focused on haemodynamic stabilisation:

- Transfusion policy: erythrocytes, platelet concentrate, plasma transfusion. Avoid overtransfusion, target Hb in variceal haemorrhage is 5.0-6.0 mmol/L or 6-8 g/dL.
- Correct haemostasis if indicated
- Vasoactive medication (administer ASAP after presentation, prior to procedure): octreotide 50 µg bolus followed by perfusor (25-50 µg/h) for 5d. Because of the short $t_{1/2}$, it is crucial that the administration is not interrupted. Alternative: terlipressin 2 mg 4x/d. After band ligation, terlipressin 2 mg 4x/d for 48h followed by 1 mg 4x/d the following 3d.

Primary therapy for acute variceal haemorrhage:

- Erythromycin: 250 mg IV 30-120 min before the procedure for optimal bowel clearing (in the absence of prolonged QT)
- Endoscopic treatment of oesophageal varices: rubber band ligation
- If unable to achieve haemostasis: consider temporary balloon placement or emergency TIPS
- Gastric varices: cyanoacrylate injection (USA: not FDA-approved)

Suspected ulcer-related bleeding (2/2):

- Duodenal ulcer and *H. pylori* positive: start eradication therapy
- Ventricular ulcer:
  - *H. pylori* positive : start eradication therapy
  - *H. pylori* negative: PPI 4-6 wk
  - Repeat gastroscopy indicated after several weeks due to the risk of underlying malignancy

High-risk ulcer-related bleeding (see Forrest classification below): notify interventional radiologist and/or surgeon
Recurrent bleeding: endoscopy

Glasgow-Blatchford Bleeding Score (Appendix 2): risk score used to predict the need for clinical and endoscopic treatment (higher scores → higher likelihood of interventions and mortality)

Prevention and treatment of complications:

- Renal failure: optimal volume status, avoid nephrotoxic drugs, uraemic complications are an indication for dialysis
- Ascites: watch out for SBP
- Hepatic encephalopathy: oral lactulose or rectal in case of high aspiration risk
- Secondary prophylaxis of variceal haemorrhage: rubber band ligation every 2-4 wk until varices disappear + nonselective beta blocker (target HR reduction = 25%)
- AB prophylaxis (e.g. ceftriaxone)

FORREST CLASSIFICATION	RECURRENCE RATE OF BLEEDING*
I: active bleeding	
Ia arterial or spurting haemorrhage	80-90%
Ib oozing haemorrhage	10-30%
II: stigmata of recent bleeding	
IIa visible vessel	50-60%
IIb adherent clot	25-35%
IIc dark base/haematin-covered lesion	0-8%
III: no signs of bleeding	
III Clean ulcer	0-12%

Table 38 // Forrest classification
*Without endoscopic intervention

↓

Consult supervisor before starting treatment

In patients who may need resuscitation, two large bore IV's are superior to central line placement as placement is faster, safer, and allows higher flow rates for resuscitation (14 Fr IV allows 240-300 mL/min compared to 30-60 mL/port of central line).

Diagram 6C // Management of GI haemorrhage (2/2)

Management of GI haemorrhage (2/2)

↓

Management of lower GI haemorrhages

↓

Always consider

- Diverticular haemorrhage (++)
- Angiodysplasia (+)
- Colitis (ischaemic, infectious, post-radiation)
- IBD (non-acute, persistent for several days in ulcerative colitis, Crohn's disease)
- Malignancy
- Anorectal diseases (haemorrhoids, fissure, rectal ulcer)
- Haemorrhage after endoscopic intervention
- Colon polyp (-)
- Upper GI haemorrhage (severe bleeding may be accompanied by rectal blood loss) (-)

Primary survey instructions

- ABCDE approach, constantly monitor vital signs (observe for pallor, clamminess, hypotension, tachycardia, consciousness, diuresis)
- Two large, functioning IVs: fluid challenge with NaCl 0.9% or Ringer's lactate. Permissive hypotension in variceal haemorrhage. For shock secondary to bleeding, consider the 'Massive Blood Loss' protocol, use of anticoagulants, and possibly treating shock.
- If haemodynamically relevant: CAD insertion + urimeter (urine output), start fluid balance
- For patients on a nursing ward: consult ERT

Imaging:

- 3-phase abdominal CT (incl. without contrast, CTA, and CTV) may be considered in manifest upper GI haemorrhage with non-conclusive endoscopy and in haemodynamically unstable patients with a history of central vascular reconstruction, suspected aortoenteric fistula, or endoscopically diagnosed haemobilia. In proven intestinal haemorrhage and dynamically unstable → selective embolisation by interventional radiologist.

Colonoscopy in haemodynamically stable patient with persistent blood loss after appropriate bowel preparation, preferably up to terminal ileum within 24h: identify focus of haemorrhage, possible clipping. Colonoscopies cannot be performed unprepared, e.g. in unstable patients.

- For stopping anticoagulants: see *Pharmacological treatment*

If a patient deteriorates, contact ERT immediately and notify supervisor/gastroenterologist. Consult IC directly for specific suspicions.

Assessment recommendations

- Lower GI haemorrhages are mostly venous and self-limiting and carry a lower risk of haemodynamic instability
- Patient history: see general Hx, medication use (e.g. NSAIDs, anticoagulants), PMHx (e.g. liver cirrhosis, aortic prosthesis)

- Diagnostics:
  - Labs: rapid blood count (e.g. Hb from venous blood gas analysis), blood group, rhesus factor, blood crossmatching, potassium, urea, creatinine, AST, ALT, ALP, GGT, bilirubin
  - If indicated: lactate, CRP, troponin, CK, INR, ECG, chest X-ray

Diagram 6D // Management of GI haemorrhage (2/2)

↓

- Treatment depends on underlying cause:
  - Consider temporarily pausing anticoagulants in consultation with the specialty that prescibed them
  - Visible diverticular haemorrhage: adrenaline injection, consider haemoclip. Proceed with bipolar coagulation if unable to achieve haemostasis. Watch out for diverticular perforation. Endoscopic treatment is often impossible as it requires good visibility.
  - Bleeding polyp: polypectomy
  - Angiodysplasia: coagulation
  - Bleeding tumour: coagulation or injection therapy are options, albeit often ineffective. Haemospray can provide a temporary solution. Definitive treatment is surgical resection.
  - Dieulafoy's lesion: adrenaline injection with coagulation or haemoclip
  - Post-polypectomy haemorrhage: adrenaline injection with haemoclip or coagulation. Haemorrhages after piecemeal polypectomy are often self-limiting.
  - Radiation proctitis: argon plasma coagulation or sucralfate enemas, hyperbaric oxygen therapy, formalin application
  - Haemorrhoids: Barron ligation, surgical options
  - If endoscopy remains impossible and haemorrhages keep recurring: consider angiography and coiling

! With massive anal blood loss, haemodynamic instability, and/or elevated urea creatinine ratios, consider fulminant upper GI haemorrhage

↓

Consult supervisor before starting treatment

Differential diagnosis of a patient with jaundice

↓

Always consider

Prehepatic

- Autoimmune haemolytic anaemia
- Glucose-6-phosphate dehydrogenase (G6PD) deficiency
- Hereditary spherocytosis
- Medication-induced
- Mechanical (valve defect/artificial valve)
- Malaria
- Paroxysmal nocturnal haemoglobinuria (PNH)
- Pyruvate kinase (PK) deficiency
- Sickle cell anaemia
- Thalassaemia

Hepatic

- Crigler-Najjar syndrome
- Dubin-Johnson syndrome ⊖
- Hepatitis (viral, alcoholic, infectious, autoimmune, DILI)
- Hereditary haemochromatosis
- Liver cirrhosis
- Malignancy (e.g. HCC, intrahepatic cholangiocarcinoma, or liver metastases)
- MASLD
- PBC
- Pregnancy cholestasis
- Wilson's disease

Diagram 7 // Differential diagnosis of a patient with jaundice

Posthepatic:

- Choledocholithiasis
- Bile duct obstruction/compression
  - Cholangiocarcinoma/pancreatic head carcinoma
  - Pancreatitis, cholangitis
  - Parasitic infection (Ascaris lumbricoides)
  - Stricture
- PSC

Distinction

	PREHEPATIC	HEPATIC	POSTHEPATIC
Unconjugated bilirubin in blood	↑	↑	=/↑
Conjugated bilirubin in blood	Absent	=/↑	↑
Conjugated bilirubin in urine	Absent	=/↑	↑
Urobilin in urine	↑	↑	Absent
Colour of stool	Dark	Light	Putty

Gilbert's syndrome: decreased glucuronosyltransferase activity. Gilbert's syndrome occurs in >5% of the total population, is more common in individuals of African descent, is not clinically relevant, and does not require treatment.

Diagram 8 // Management of shock symptoms

Management of shock symptoms

↓

Always consider
- Hypovolaemic shock: haemorrhage (GI haemorrhage, damage to lienal or gastroduodenal arteries in pancreatitis), severe dehydration
- Obstructive shock: abdominal compartment syndrome, tamponade, massive pulmonary embolism
- Distributive shock: SIRS or sepsis (necrotising pancreatitis, perforation secondary to ileus, ischaemic colitis, or toxic megacolon), liver failure, anaphylaxis, Addisonian crisis (long-term steroid use)
- Cardiogenic shock: myocardial infarction, arrhythmia

↓

Primary survey instructions
- ABCDE approach, constantly monitor vital signs (observe for pallor, clamminess, hypotension, tachycardia, consciousness, diuresis)
- Two large, functioning IVs: fluid challenge with NaCl 0.9% or Ringer's lactate. Permissive hypotension in variceal haemorrhage. For shock secondary to bleeding, consider the 'Massive Blood Loss' protocol, use of anticoagulants, and possibly treating shock.
- CAD insertion + urimeter (urine output), start fluid balance
- For patients on a nursing ward: consult ERT
- Labs: blood count, blood type, rhesus factor, blood crossmatching, electrolytes, renal function, lactate, CRP, lipase, arterial blood gas
- If indicated: D-dimer, troponin, CK, ECG, and chest X-ray

If a patient deteriorates, contact ERT immediately and notify supervisor/gastroenterologist. Consult IC directly for specific suspicions.

↓

Assessment recommendations

- In case of hypovolemic or distributive shock (NOT in cardiogenic shock): acute fluid resuscitation with 30mL/kg (i.e. approx. 2L in a person of 70kg). If fluid unresponsive shock, consult ICU about starting inotrophy). For haemorrhagic shock, consider the 'Massive blood loss' protocol.
- Suspected intestinal perforation: indication for emergency surgery → seek immediate assistance (surgeon)
- Suspected variceal haemorrhage: see *Management of a patient with… // Upper GI haemorrhage and/or suspected variceal haemorrhage*
- Suspected Addisonian crisis or long-term prednisone use at home (e.g. autoimmune disorder, COPD): 100 mg IV hydrocortisone
- Suspected anaphylaxis: 0.5 mg **IM** adrenaline

↓

Consult supervisor before starting treatment

Diagram 9 // Management of altered consciousness

Management of altered consciousness*

* Diminished consciousness is always altered consciousness,
but altered consciousness is not necessarily diminished consciousness!

↓

Always consider

- Delirium
- Metabolic: hepatic encephalopathy, hypoglycaemia (liver insufficiency), electrolyte disorders, hypothermia/hyperthermia, thyroid disorders
- Sepsis
- Intoxications: medications (benzodiazepines, opiates, antidepressants, paracetamol), drugs (Downers: GHB, alcohol, opiates; psychoactive drugs: LSD, magic mushrooms; Uppers: MDMA, cocaine)
- Respiratory: respiratory insufficiency (hypoxia, hypercapnia, hypoventilation secondary to intoxication)
- Neurological: subarachnoid haemorrhage, subdural haematoma, CVA, meningitis, encephalitis
- Psychiatric: psychosis, schizophrenia, personality disorders

↓

Primary survey instructions

- Assess patient using ABCDE approach. Direct bedside glucose, treat possible hypoglycaemia. Perform EMV test.
- Monitor vital signs, paying special attention the patient's airway
- Labs if indicated: blood count, CRP, lactate, electrolytes, liver enzymes, ammonia (only if indicated), toxicological screening (incl. paracetamol)

If a patient deteriorates, contact ERT immediately and notify supervisor/gastroenterologist. Consult ICU and rapid response team for specific suspicions.

↓

Assessment recommendations

- Secure airway as needed
- In severe hypoglycaemia: give IV glucose 10g as slow bolus. (10g = 100 ml glucose 10% = 20 ml glucose 50%: expected increase of 2 mmol/L per 10g). Check glucose <10 min and repeat as needed.
- Suspected hepatic encephalopathy: start lactulose immediately (enemas + orally if possible). Stage 3: pre-emptive intubation upon progression to coma (West Haven Criteria). Get help immediately: contact ERT.
- Perform Delirium Observation Screening (DOS)
- For patients on a nursing ward: bring in ERT
- For specific treatment instructions, see *Conditions*

↓

Consult supervisor before starting treatment

Conditions

Oesophagus

Achalasia

D Achalasia is a motility disorder of the oesophagus characterised by incomplete relaxation of the lower oesophageal sphincter (LES) with oesophageal dilation and decreased oesophageal peristalsis (see Figure 29).

E Incidence 2:100,000 per year, prevalence 10:100,000

Ae
- Idiopathic, neuronal inflammation and degeneration in the oesophageal wall, possibly autoimmune
- Secondary achalasia: e.g. secondary to malignancies (gastric cancer ⊕), Chagas disease, amyloidosis, sarcoidosis, neurofibromatosis

R Age at diagnosis usually 25-60

Hx Oesophageal dysphagia (solids and liquids) ⊕⊕, regurgitation ⊕, retrosternal pain ⊕, spontaneous or induced vomiting, aspiration ⊖, weight loss ⊖

PE Not contributing

Dx
- Oesophageal manometry: incomplete LES relaxation and impaired peristalsis of the distal oesophagus
- Barium oesophagram: distal oesophageal dilation, narrow gastro-oesophageal junction (bird-beak sign or rat's tail sign), absent peristalsis or tertiary contractions of the oesophagus, delayed passage of barium with stasis in the distal oesophagus, see Figure 30
- Upper endoscopy when in doubt about a possible malignancy

Tx Botox injections, oral nitrates (oesophageal spasms)
- Balloon dilatation (i.e. pneumodilatation)
- Endoscopic myotomy (per oral i.e. POEM), surgical myotomy (Heller myotomy)

P Risk of oesophageal carcinoma ↑. Up to 5% of patients have severe, disabling symptoms requiring surgical resection of the oesophagus.

! 3 subtypes
- Type 1: muscles barely contract, 100% failed peristalsis (e.g. classic achalasia)
- Type 2: pressure build-up in oesophagus → compartmentalised pressurisation
- Type 3: abnormal contractions (e.g. spastic achalasia) → pain

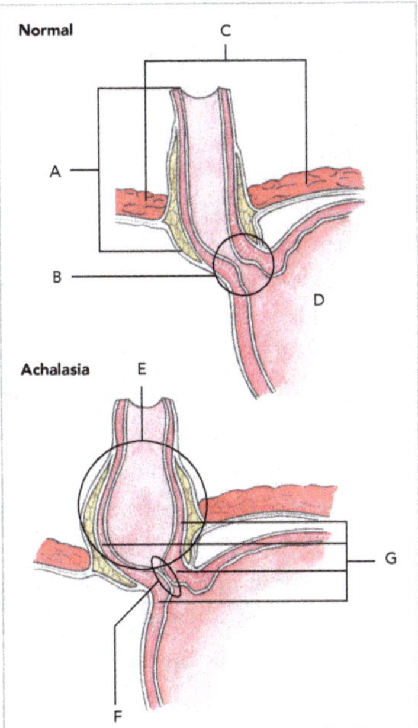

Figure 29 // Normal oesophagus and achalasia: anatomical differences
A: Oesophagus **B:** LES **C:** Diaphragm **D:** Stomach **E:** Dilated oesophagus **F:** High resting pressure in LES **G:** Oesophageal thickening due to circular muscle hypertrophy

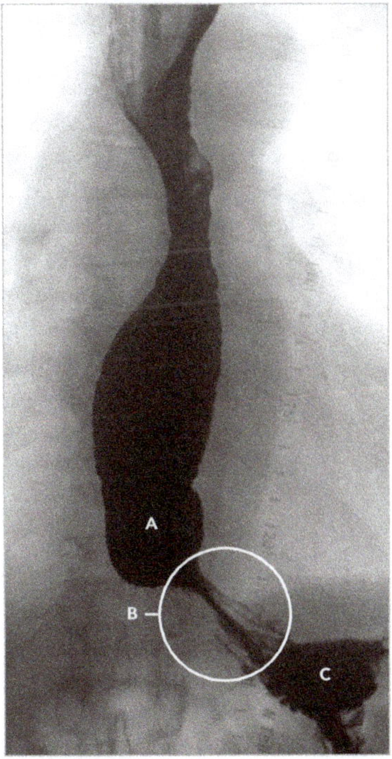

Figure 30 // Barium oesophagram for achalasia
A: Dilated oesophagus **B:** LES with 'bird-beak sign' or 'rat's tail sign' **C:** Stomach

Barrett's oesophagus

D Barrett's oesophagus is characterised by intestinal metaplasia in the distal oesophagus due to chronic gastric acid reflux.

E Incidence 1,300:100,000 per year, 6-14% of patients with gastro-oesophageal reflux disease (GORD)

Ae Chronic exposure to gastric acid → squamous epithelium changes into columnar epithelium with goblet cells (= intestinal metaplasia)

R GORD, hiatal hernia, central obesity, ♂, positive FHx, age >50, smoking

Hx Asymptomatic ⊕, may present with symptoms of GORD (e.g. heartburn or regurgitation), symptoms related to complications of Barrett's oesophagus (e.g. dysphagia, odynophagia)

PE Not contributing

Dx Upper endoscopy with distal oesophageal biopsy: endoscopic Barrett segment (columnar mucosa) >1 cm in length, intestinal metaplasia, see Figure 31 for the C&M classification and Figure 32 for the endoscopic view

Tx Smoking cessation and weight loss counseling if needed

Always: PPI

- Low-grade dysplasia (LGD): assessment by expert pathologist. In case of confirmed LGD, refer to centre of expertise. Repeat upper endoscopy in a centre of expertise after 6 mo. Persistent or progressive LGD: radiofrequency ablation (RFA).
- High-grade dysplasia (HGD) or intramucosal cancer (T1a): endoscopic eradication therapy (EET) involving at least endoscopic mucosal resection (EMR) or endoscopic submucosal dissection (ESD), consider additional RFA ⊕ or cryotherapy of the remaining Barrett epithelium
- Submucosal cancer (T1b): surgical oesophagectomy, consider EET for low-risk features
- Surveillance depending on Barrett segment length (1-3 cm: every 5y, 3-10 cm: every 3y, >10 cm: at specialised centre) and age (≤75y)

P
- Risk of oesophageal adenocarcinoma in non-dysplastic Barrett's oesophagus: 0.3-0.5% annually
- Risk of progression from histologically confirmed LGD to HGD or adenocarcinoma: 5-13% annually

! Screening for Barrett's oesophagus is recommended in individuals with symptoms of chronic GORD and >3 additional risk factors (see R, first-degree relative with Barrett's oesophagus or oesophageal adenocarcinoma)

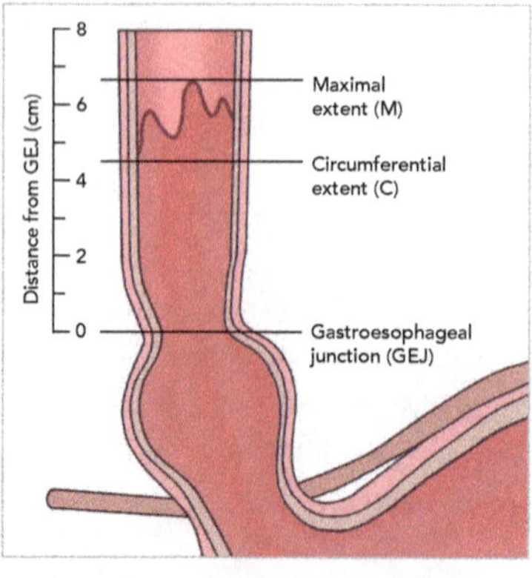

Figure 31 // C&M classification

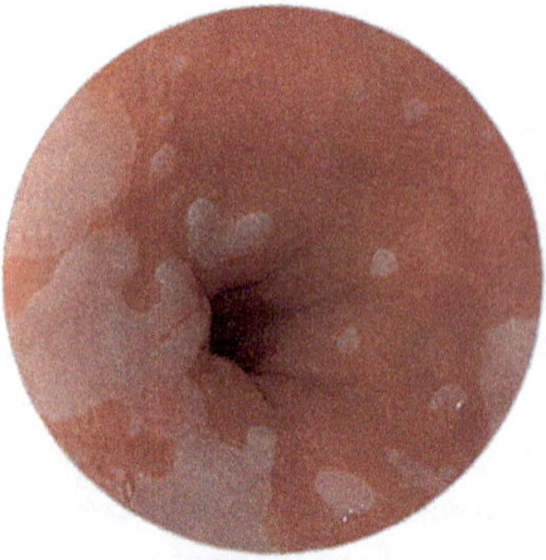

Figure 32 // Upper endoscopy: distal oesophagus with Barrett's epithelium. Islands of squamous epithelium in the middle of an area of columnar epithelium.

Boerhaave syndrome

D Boerhaave syndrome is a spontaneous perforation of the oesophagus that usually involves a longitudinal tear (also known as effort rupture) on the left posterolateral side of the distal oesophagus extending several centimetres, see Figure 33.

E
- Incidence 3:1,000,000 per year
- 15% of all oesophageal perforations occur spontaneously

Ae
- Sudden increase of intraluminal oesophageal pressure combined with negative intrathoracic pressure, e.g. with severe vomiting
- Rare aetiologies: childbirth, epileptic seizure, persistent coughing, or laughing

R Usually no relevant PMHx, patients may have eosinophilic oesophagitis, medication-induced oesophagitis, or Barrett's oesophagus

Hx
- Symptoms depend on site, degree of perforation, and time: acute and severe retrosternal, neck, or epigastric pain, possibly radiating to back or left shoulder, after a period of severe vomiting (++)
- Hours after perforation: general malaise, fever, painful swallowing, dyspnoea

PE Subcutaneous emphysema (30%). Hours after perforation: signs of hypovolemic shock (cyanosis, T ↑, BP ↓, pulse ↑, tachypnoea).

Dx
- Labs: WBC ↑, CRP ↑
- Chest/upper abdominal contrast CT: oesophageal wall thickening, mediastinal fat stranding, mediastinal free air, use of oral diluted iodinated contrast → leakage into the para-oesophageal mediastinum

Tx NPO, feeding tube or total parenteral nutrition (TPN)
PPI, broad-spectrum ABx
Depending on site, size, and time to diagnosis: endoscopy (metal stent, sponge-assisted vacuum therapy) often combined with surgery (thoracotomy with fundoplication and pleural/mediastinal drainage)

P Mortality 30% (doubles every 24h for the first 3d)

! Contamination with gastric contents → watch out for mediastinitis, pericarditis, pneumonia, empyema, sepsis

> Suspected perforation is an absolute contraindication for a barium oesophagram, as barium may cause acute mediastinitis, peritonitis, and bacteriaemia. Use water-diluted iodinated contrast instead.

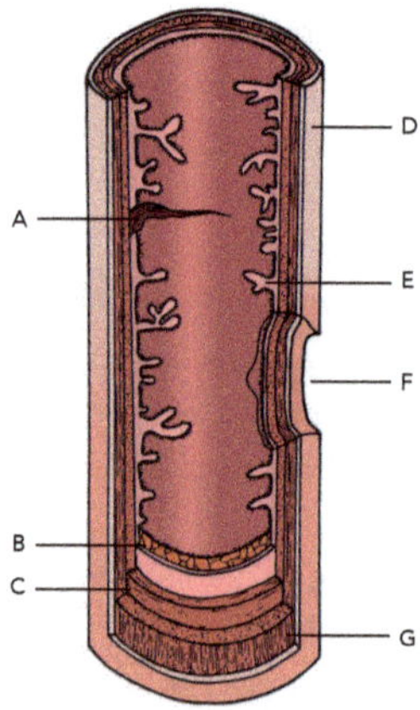

Figure 33 // Boerhaave syndrome and Mallory-Weiss syndrome
A: Mallory-Weiss syndrome (mucosal tear) **B:** Submucosa **C:** Circular muscle layer **D:** Serosa **E:** Mucosa **F:** Boerhaave syndrome (distal LES perforation) **G:** Longitudinal muscle layer

Oesophageal candidiasis

D Oesophageal candidiasis is an opportunistic infection of the oesophageal mucosa caused by Candida species (esp. Candida albicans).

E Often associated with oropharyngeal candidiasis (or vaginal/dermal candidiasis), most common infectious cause of oesophagitis

Ae Candida albicans

R Chronic use of inhalation corticosteroids or AB, immunocompromised individuals (e.g. DM, HIV, haematological malignancies, stem cell transplantation recipients, during cytotoxic chemotherapy)

Hx Asymptomatic ⊕, oesophageal dysphagia, pain swallowing, retrosternal pain

PE Painful, red oral mucosa and/or a white film on the tongue

Dx Upper endoscopy: white mucosal non-detachable oesophageal plaques (see Figure 34). Biopsy is not needed for diagnosis, in non-responsive individuals, biopsies and cultures should be obtained: pseudohyphae upon staining with hematoxylin.

Tx Antifungal therapy (first-line treatment: oral fluconazole for 2 wk)

P Often responds well to treatment

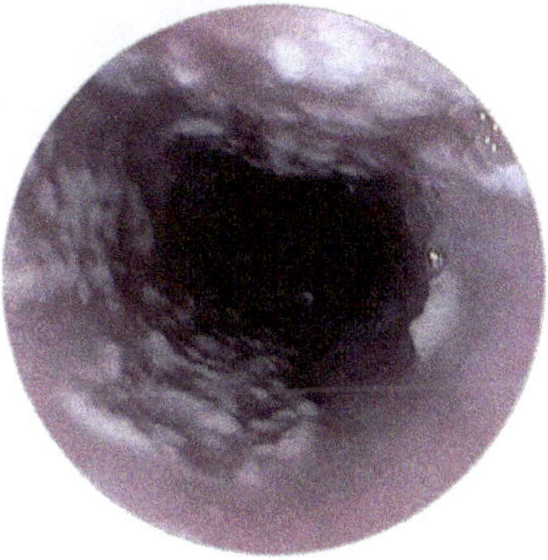

Figure 34 // Upper endoscopy: white, adherent plaques that cannot be washed off, consistent with Candida oesophagitis

Eosinophilic oesophagitis

D Eosinophilic esophagitis is a chronic allergic inflammation of the oesophagus characterised by infiltration of eosinophilic granulocytes.

E Incidence increasing, ♂:♀ 3:1

Ae Disrupted barrier function of oesophageal epithelium and food and inhalant allergens → T-helper-2-associated immune response → pro-inflammatory cytokines (IL-4, IL-5, and IL-13) ↑ → activation and recruitment of eosinophilic granulocytes and mast cells → remodelling, loss of barrier function, fibrosis, hypertrophy of oesophageal smooth muscle tissue

R Food and inhalant allergies (>70%), atopy, young adults, genetic predisposition

Hx Oesophageal dysphagia ⊕, food impaction ⊕, retrosternal or upper abdominal pain, regurgitation

PE Often not contributing

Dx
- Upper endoscopy with biopsies: oedema, concentric rings, longitudinal grooves, decreased vascularisation, white exudate (accumulation of eosinophilic granulocytes), predominantly proximal strictures (see Figure 35)
- Biopsies (proximal, distal, and mid-oesophageal): >15 eosinophils per high-power microscopy field
- Labs: serum IgE ↑

Tx
- Dietary recommendations: elemental or elimination diet
- High-dose PPI, corticosteroids (e.g. local budesonide, fluticasone), dupilumab (EoE refractory to treatment)
- Dilation for strictures

P
- PPI treatment: 50% success rate
- Dietary recommendations: 66-95% success rate, but long-term adherence is difficult

!
- Prolonged inflammation: risk of fibrotic strictures and motility disorders
- Risk of perforation in case of mechanical dilation: <1%

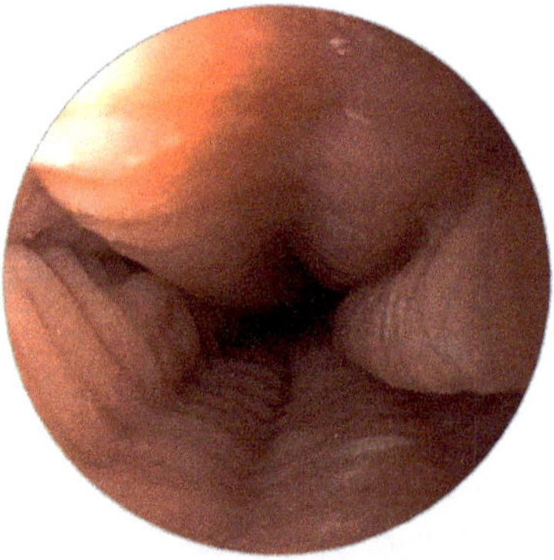

Figure 35 // Upper endoscopy: image of eosinophilic oesophagitis with oedema, concentric rings, longitudinally grooves, and white exudate

Gastro-oesophageal reflux disease (GORD)

D GORD is the intermittent reflux of gastric acid into the oesophagus and may be accompanied by erosions and ulcers of oesophageal mucosa.

E Prevalence 10-20% in the West, <5% in Asia

Ae LES relaxation or hypotonia, anatomical abnormality (e.g. diaphragmatic hernia), increased gastric acid secretion, impaired oesophageal motility, delayed gastric emptying, increased abdominal pressure (see Figure 37)

R Advanced age (++) or age <1y, hiatal hernia, obesity, pregnancy, smoking, positive FHx

Hx Typical retrosternal pain/burning sensation after eating certain foods and/or when lying flat, regurgitation, dysphagia, nausea, coughing, hoarseness, throat scraping, asthma. Pain worsens after consuming fatty or spicy foods, alcohol, caffeine, citrus products, chocolate, or large meals.

PE Not contributing

Dx
- Diagnostics are indicated for advanced age, alarm symptoms, and/or risk factors for Barrett's oesophagus:

- Upper endoscopy to rule out GORD complications (see Figure 36): basal thickening and papillary elongation (mild), erosion, ulceration, inflammation (mild), major epithelial damage (Los Angeles classification A/D for reflux oesophagitis)
- 24h pH monitoring + impedance in case of therapy resistance, preoperative settings, or difficulty diagnosing patient: differentiation between functional dyspepsia and GORD and proof of supragastric belching

Tx Lifestyle recommendations: diet, smoking cessation, head-of-bed elevation, avoid meals within 2-3h of bedtime, weight loss for overweight patients

- In patients <45y without alarm symptoms, treat pragmatically with antacids for ≤8 wk
- PPI 8 wk standard dose, in case of partial response → optimise PPI therapy

Nissen or Toupet fundoplication

P
- Anti-reflux surgery is most likely to benefit patients with Los Angeles grade C/D, prominent hiatal, and invalidating/persistent symptoms despite lifestyle adjustments and pharmacotherapy
- Risk of recurrence, oesophagitis, Barrett's oesophagus, and oesophageal carcinoma ↑

! Consider discontinuing PPI treatment in patients with non-erosive oesophagitis and without Barrett's oesophagus

The typical patient with GORD is overweight and presents with burning retrosternal pain after eating lasagna with a glass of red wine that disappears after taking antacids.

Continuous reflux of gastric acid into the oesophagus can irritate the oesophageal epithelium and cause oesophageal inflammation i.e. **reflux oesophagitis**.

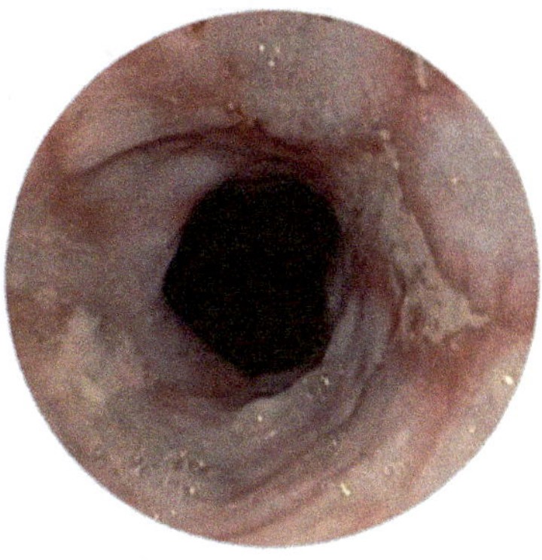

Figure 36 // Upper endoscopy: GORD with reflux oesophagitis grade C, ulcer in the distal oesophagus (>75% of the circumference) with some stenosing

Non-erosive reflux disease is a type of gastric acid-induced pathology. As the name suggests, non-erosive reflux disease is not accompanied by mucosal ulceration. This manifestation of reflux disease is more resistant to antacid therapy than the erosive counterpart.

Alarm symptoms in GORD:

- New onset of dyspepsia in patient aged ≥60
- Evidence of GI bleeding (haematemesis, melaena, haematochezia, occult blood in stool)
- Unexplained iron deficiency aneamia
- Anorexia
- Unexplained weight loss
- Dysphagia
- Odynophagia
- Persistent vomiting
- First-degree relative with GI cancer

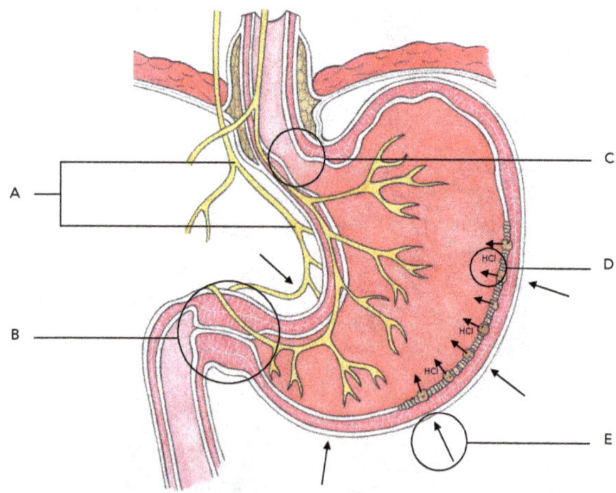

Figure 37 // GORD: causes

A: Impaired motility **B:** Delayed gastric emptying (e.g. secondary to gastroparesis or compression of adjacent structures) **C:** LES dysfunction **D:** Increased gastric acid secretion **E:** Increased abdominal pressure

Corrosive ingestion

D Corrosive ingestion is the oral intake of corrosive substances (usually liquids) that can cause serious oropharyngeal, oesophageal, and gastric injuries. The severity depends on the type of substance (acid/alkali), form (liquid/solid), and amount.

E Prevalence estimated 5,000-15,000 cases annually, most common <5y

Ae Deliberate or accidental

R Psychiatric disorder, alcohol use disorder

Hx Oropharyngeal, retrosternal, or epigastric pain, painful swallowing, oesophageal dysphagia, drooling, vomiting, haematemesis. Threatened airway: hoarseness, stridor, respiratory problems.

PE Perforation: subcutaneous emphysema, peritonitis. Severe injuries: fever, tachycardia, shock.

Dx
- Chest and abdominal CT with venous contrast: mediastinitis and extent of erosion/inflammation revealing peri-oesophageal fat stranding, possibly abscess formation and pneumomediastinum in case of perforation
- Upper endoscopy: assess severity using Zargar score (see Table 39) and place NG tube (see Figure 38)

Tx Depends on Zargar score (see Table 39)
- Consult ENT doctor
- Consult ICU in case of airway obstruction due to swelling

P
- Complications mostly occur in patients with high-grade injury (grade 2b/3): risk of bleeding, strictures (70-100% of grade 2b/3a), fistula, oesophageal squamous cell carcinoma ↑
- Strictures may still develop years after exposure
- Mortality is generally 10-20%, but depends on the grade. Early mortality rate 65% in grade 3b.

I Aspiration increases the risk of a threatened airway due to laryngeal oedema

'Acid licks the oesophagus and bites the stomach'. The oesophagus is spared due to necrotic scarring, which has a protective effect on the tissue. Increased pyloric spasms increase gastric residence time, leading to more damage. Acids tend to cause immediate pain and are therefore ingested in lesser quantities, while alkali are not immediately painful and are taken in larger quantities. Alkali causes liquefactive necrosis, leading to more extensive damage and a greater risk of perforation. Alkali are largely neutralised by low gastric pH levels.

GRADE	ENDOSCOPIC FINDING	TREATMENT
0	Normal mucosa	Wait-and-see
1	Oedema and hyperaemia	
2a	Friability, bleeding, erosions, blisters, white membranes, exudates	Modified/liquid diet
2b	Grade 2a + discrete/circumferential deep ulcerations	Endoscopic feeding tube for 1-2 wk, surveillance
3a	Multiple ulcerations and scattered areas of necrosis	Consider surgery after CT for perforation or severe transmural ischaemia/necrosis, endoscopic NG tube with tube feeding, alternatively jejunostomy or TPN, surveillance, consider broad-spectrum ABx in suspected perforation
3b	Multiple ulcerations with extensive necrosis	

Table 39 // Zargar classification

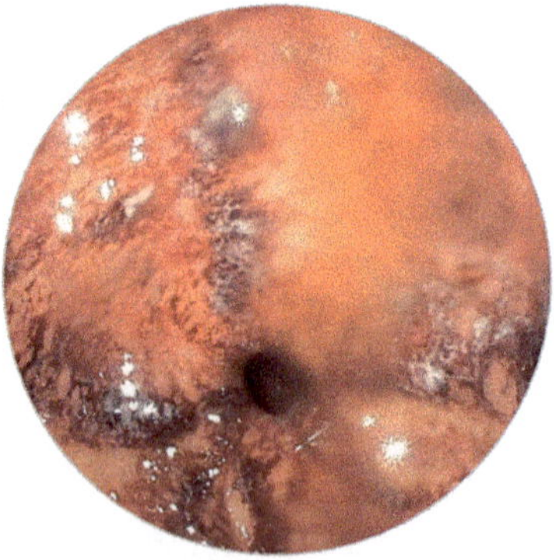

Figure 38 // Upper endoscopy: caustic gastritis (Zargar 3a) after intentional ingestion of acid

Mallory-Weiss syndrome

D Mallory-Weiss syndrome, also called Mallory-Weiss lesion, is characterised by mucosal lacerations that lead to bleeding at the gastro-oesophageal junction or proximal stomach (see Figures 33 and 39).

E Prevalence 3-15% of patients with an upper GI haemorrhage

Ae Intra-abdominal pressure ↑, often after a period of vomiting or coughing, other triggers include straining, lifting, seizures, NG tube placement

R Alcohol use, hiatal hernia, ♂, age >60, hyperemesis gravidarum

Hx Haematemesis, retrosternal/epigastric pain, melaena, after a period of heavy vomiting (+)

PE Dx See *Management of upper GI haemorrhage and/or suspected variceal haemorrhage* in case of symptoms consistent with bleeding, see *Management of shock symptoms* in case of symptoms consistent with infection/sepsis

Tx Conservative: bleeding is usually self-limiting <24h

PPI, possibly antiemetics

Active bleeding: often wait-and-see, but possible endoscopic intervention (e.g. endoscopic clipping) and/or adrenaline injection (combination therapy with both clipping and injection shows higher success rates in preventing a rebleed)

P Often self-limiting

! Beware of haemodynamic instability due to hypovolaemic shock in patients with extensive blood loss

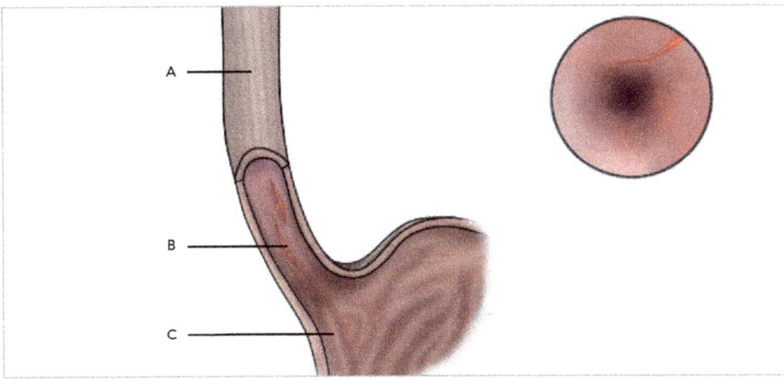

Figure 39 // Mallory-Weiss syndrome: location and upper endoscopy findings
A: Oesophagus **B:** Mallory-Weiss lesion **C:** Stomach

Oesophageal varices

D Oesophageal varices are dilated veins in the distal oesophageal submucosa. Larger varices increase the risk of variceal haemorrhage.

E Incidence unknown, occurs in 30-70% of patients with liver cirrhosis (varices are correlated with the severity of portal hypertension)

Ae
- Portal hypertension (++) secondary to liver cirrhosis (++) or portal vein/splenic vein thrombosis

- Portal vein pressure ↑ → collateral flow ↑ → oesophageal vein dilation

R Risk of variceal haemorrhage: size of varices, severity of liver disease

Hx Asymptomatic until bleeding occurs

PE
- Haemorrhage/massive blood loss: haematemesis, collapse, hypovolaemic shock
- Possible stigmata of liver cirrhosis

Dx
- See section *Management of upper GI haemorrhage and/or suspected variceal haemorrhage*
- Upper endoscopy: large/small varices (see Figure 40), sometimes active bleeding, white nipple sign (see Figure 40), red wale sign, blood clots

Tx
- Oesophageal variceal haemorrhage: see section *Management of upper GI haemorrhage and/or suspected variceal haemorrhage* (e.g. IV fluid resuscitation, vasoactive medication (octreotide), IV antibiotic prophylaxis)
- Secondary prophylaxis:
  - Non-selective beta blocker (NSBB) to prevent variceal haemorrhage in patients with compensated liver disease and portal hypertension
  - Endoscopic (prophylactic) band ligation
  - Pre-emptive transjugular intrahepatic portosystemic shunt (TIPS) in patients at high risk of recurrence

P
- 6-week mortality after acute variceal haemorrhage: 15-25%
- Risk of recurrent haemorrhages ↑

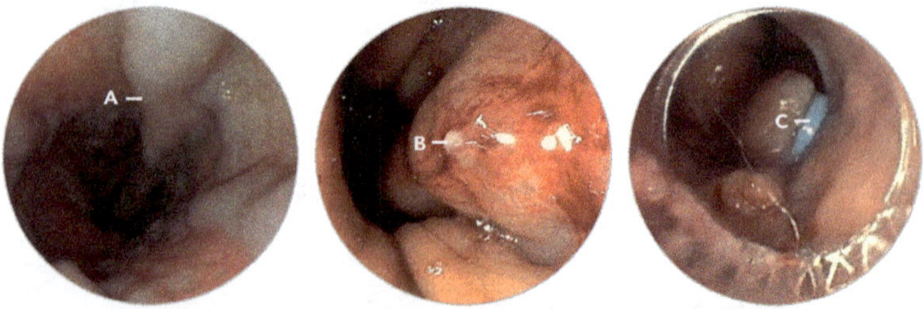

Figure 40 // Upper endoscopy: **A:** Oesophageal varices **B:** White nipple sign **C:** After rubber band ligation

> The white nipple sign is a fibrin plug on an oesophageal varix that signifies recent haemorrhage. The red wale sign, also known as a cherry red spot, is a blood blister/red spot on a varix and a sign of increased risk of bleeding.

Food impaction

D Food impaction is obstruction of the oesophagus caused by food.

E Most common cause of oesophageal obstruction, 95% of cases are accidental

Ae
- Mechanical: large/unchewed piece of food, luminal stenosis due to Schatzki's ring, strictures, or webs, eosinophilic oesophagitis, malignancy
- Motility disorders such as achalasia

R Eating meat ('steakhouse syndrome'), dental defects, eating fast, not chewing properly

Hx Retrosternal pain or fullness, drooling, unable to continue eating or drinking, regurgitation, gagging

PE Drooling patient unable to swallow saliva

Dx
- Neck/chest contrast CT: for suspected fish bone/chicken bone in proximal oesophagus and to rule out perforation and abscess formation
- Upper endoscopy: presence of food bolus in oesophagus (see Figures 41 and 42), evidence of underlying causes of obstruction

Tx Food impaction is often resolved spontaneously (80-90%) after the bolus either enters the stomach or is regurgitated. Have patients drink carbonated water or cola in case of incomplete obstruction (little evidence).

Persistent symptoms or suspected complete obstruction: upper endoscopy <24h aimed at bolus removal or manipulation into the stomach

P Follow-up to detect underlying cause, consider performing repeat upper endoscopy to take biopsies for eosinophilic oesophagitis

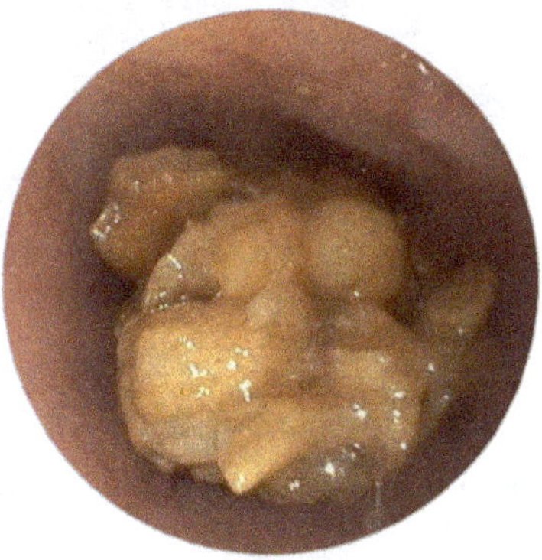

Figure 41 // Upper endoscopy: food impaction (meat) causing total oesophageal obstruction

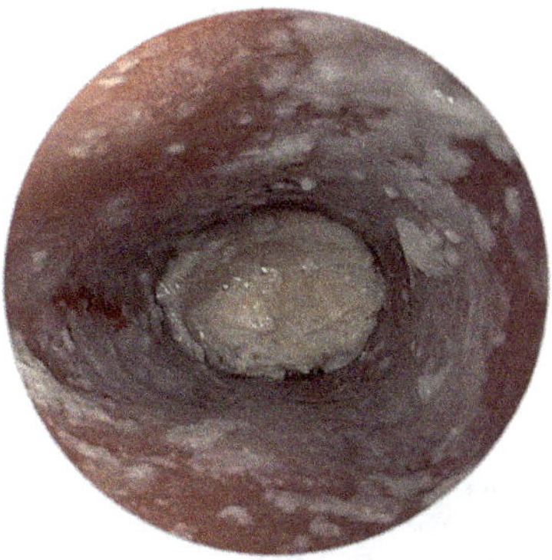

Figure 42 // Upper endoscopy: food impaction (chicken) causing total oesophageal obstruction with presence of white exudate

Zenker's diverticulum

D Zenker's diverticulum is characterised by herniation of oesophageal mucosa and submucosa through Killian's triangle due to weakness of the cricopharyngeal muscle. Zenker's diverticulum often develops near C5-C6 and bulges dorsally (see Figure 43).

E Incidence 2:100,000 per year

Ae Idiopathic, associated with spasms and impaired muscle coordination, incomplete relaxation of the inferior cricopharyngeal muscle, natural vulnerable spot in muscular wall, intra-oesophageal pressure ↑

R ♂, advanced age (muscle weakness ↑)

Hx Oesophageal dysphagia, regurgitation, globus, halitosis, coughing

PE Not contributing

Dx Barium oesophagram combined with dynamic continuous fluoroscopy or upper endoscopy: detect diverticulum

Tx If <1 cm and asymptomatic: conservative

Endoscopic (septum division, see Figure 44) or surgical (transcervical): cricopharyngeal myotomy with/without diverticulotomy

P
- Depends on age and comorbidities
- Recurrence rate 25%

! Watch out for perforation during upper endoscopy resulting in mediastinitis and empyema, risk of aspiration pneumonia ↑

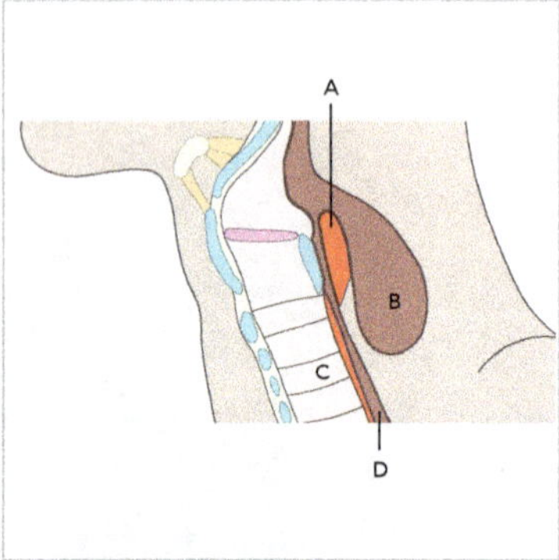

Figure 43 // Zenker's diverticulum
A: Cricopharyngeal muscle **B:** Zenker's diverticulum **C:** Trachea **D:** Oesophagus

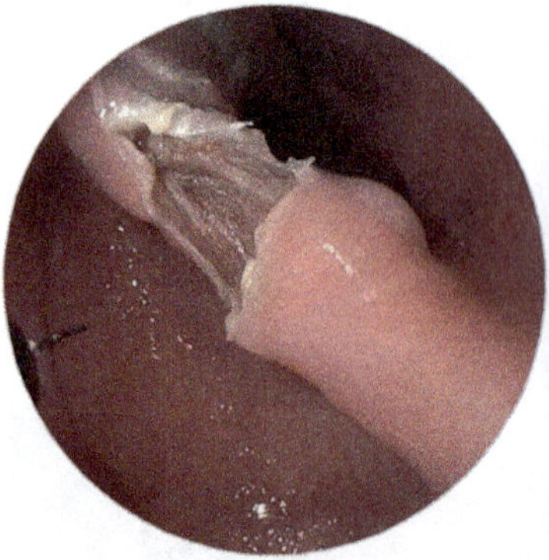

Figure 44 // Upper endoscopy: endoscopic septum division for Zenker's diverticulum

Functional dyspepsia

D Functional dyspepsia is a disorder of gut-brain interaction, characterised by dyspeptic symptoms (early satiety, bloating, pain, epigastric burning) in the absence of an apparent biochemical or organic/structural cause. The diagnosis is made using the ROME IV criteria. Postprandial distress syndrome and epigastric pain syndrome are considered subtypes of functional dyspepsia.

E Prevalence 5,000-11,000:100,000

Ae Unknown. Possible factors: motility disorder, altered microbiome, inflammation and immune activation, visceral hypersensitivity, and psychosocial dysfunction.

R ♀, psychological stress, GI infection and post-infection, smoking, NSAID use

Hx Use ROME IV criteria (see below)

PE Epigastric tenderness

Dx
- Upper endoscopy (perform only in patients aged >50-60 or in case of alarm symptoms): no obvious abnormalities
- Stool antigen assay or gastroscopic biopsy: rule out *H. pylori*
- Consider a gastric emptying exam: rule out gastroparesis

Tx
- Explain cause of symptoms, avoid stress, consider psychological counselling, hypnotherapy
- Dietary recommendations: avoid fatty meals, large servings, and trigger foods (e.g. coffee, peppermint, strong spices, carbonated drinks), avoid alcohol
- For mild symptoms: antacids, temporary H2-antagonists or PPIs. Pain/nausea or lack of improvement after PPI therapy: low-dose tricyclic antidepressants or prokinetics (e.g. metoclopramide) on trial basis.
- *H. pylori* infection: eradication

P No effect on mortality and symptoms are often self-limiting/fluctuate over time, but quality of life can be severely affected

! There is little evidence for the effect of medicated treatment and lifestyle recommendations on functional dyspepsia

ROME IV criteria for functional dyspepsia

1. One or more of the following symptoms that interfere with daily activities:
   - Postprandial fullness
   - Early satiation
   - Epigastric pain
   - Epigastric burning
2. No evidence of organ abnormalities or metabolic or structural disease that is likely to explain the symptoms
3. The symptoms must have been present at least three days a week for the past 3 months, with symptom onset at least six months ago

Alarm symptoms that indicate the need for upper endoscopy:

- Dysphagia or painful swallowing
- Food impaction with excessive salivation
- Evidence of GI bleeding (haematemesis, melaena, haematochezia, occult blood in stool)
- Unexplained iron deficiency anaemia
- Persistent vomiting
- Unexplained weight loss
- Palpable swelling or lymphadenopathy
- First-degree relative with GI cancer

Gastritis

	ACUTE GASTRITIS	CHRONIC ATROPHIC GASTRITIS
D	Inflammation of the gastric mucosa.	Atrophy of the gastric mucosa, loss of parietal and other cells, and metaplasia. A distinction is made between e.g. atrophic gastritis caused by *H. pylori* and autoimmune gastritis.
E	Prevalence 6:100,000	• Prevalence of *H. pylori* (Northern America and Europe): 20-50% • Prevalence of autoimmune gastritis: 5% of all cases of chronic gastritis
Ae	Bacterial or viral infection, drug toxicity (NSAID), autoimmune	• *H. pylori* → toxin production and immune response → chronic gastritis → mucosal immunity ↓ → mucosal damage • Autoantibody production in gastric mucosa → intrinsic factor production ↓ → vitamin B12 uptake ↓ → lack of erythrocyte building blocks → macrocytic (pernicious) anaemia (see Figure 45)

Table 40A // Different forms of gastritis

	ACUTE GASTRITIS	CHRONIC ATROPHIC GASTRITIS
R	Lowered resistance, alcohol, bile reflux, long-term NSAID use, Crohn's disease, sarcoidosis	• *H. pylori:* high salt intake, smoking, low socioeconomic status, crowded living conditions, no access to running water, educational level, ethnicity • Autoimmune: ♀, blood type A, thyroid disorders, DM type 1
Hx	• Heartburn, nausea, bloating, epigastric pain, sometimes melaena • Autoimmune: symptoms consistent with vitamin B12 deficiency (e.g. symptoms consistent with anaemia, ultimately neurological symptoms)	
PE	Not contributing	
Dx	Upper endoscopy with biopsy: erythematous oedematous mucosa, PA: gastritis	• Upper endoscopy with biopsy: pale mucosa, prominent vessels, PA: mix of mononuclear cells (lymphocytes, plasma cells, macrophages) and intestinal metaplasia, presence of *H. pylori* • Autoimmune: limited to corpus and fundus • Labs: macrocytic anaemia, if autoimmune: vitamin B12 ↓, presence of serum antibodies against intrinsic factor/parietal cells
Tx	Dietary recommendations: avoid fatty meals, large servings, and trigger foods (e.g. coffee, peppermint, strong spices (hot peppers), carbonated drinks), avoid alcohol	
	Sometimes self-limiting PPI (symptom management), stop NSAID	• *H. pylori:* eradication (ABx and PPI) followed by eradication confirmation • Autoimmune: vitamin B12 injections
P	• Intestinal metaplasia or positive family history: gastric cancer risk ↑ (surveillance may be indicated) • Chronic gastritis caused by *H. pylori*: 12-16x gastric cancer risk ↑ • Chronic autoimmune gastritis: risk ↑ of gastric neuroendocrine tumour (NET) and adenocarcinomas	

Table 40B // Different forms of gastritis

It is important to make a distinction between gastritis (primarily an inflammatory process) and gastropathy (disease of the gastric mucosa without any apparent inflammation). Histopathological evidence of inflammation is required to make a diagnosis of gastritis, endoscopic or radiological findings do not suffice.

Autoimmune gastritis is more common in patients with autoimmune disorders of the thyroid gland (up to 1/3) and in patients with DM type 1 (6-10%).

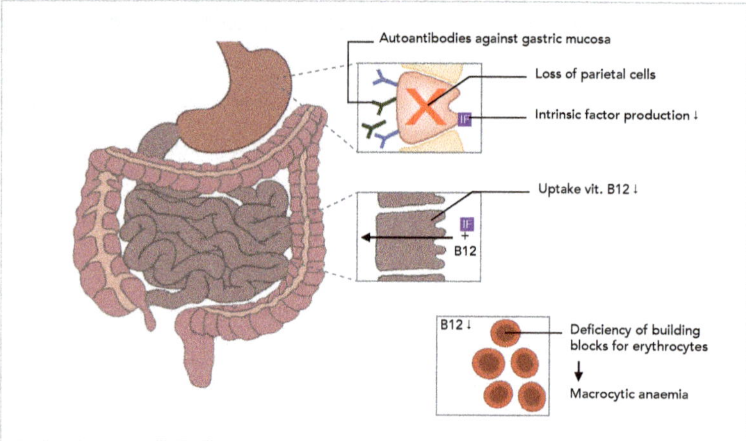

Figure 45 // Chronic atrophic gastritis

Helicobacter pylori

D *Helicobacter pylori (H. pylori)* is a gram-negative spiral-shaped flagellated bacterium that can survive in the acidic environment of the stomach. Most infected patients will have both acute and chronic features of gastritis. It is one of the main causes of peptic ulcers.

E Most common bacterial infection in humans, prevalence 50-80% and incidence 15-30% in Africa, South America, and Western Asia (see Figure 46)

Ae Infections occur mainly during childhood, route of transmission unknown (probably faecal-oral or oral-oral). The bacterium resides in gastric epithelial cells in the antral mucosa, where it increases the release of gastrin and in general increases gastric acid secretion for its own survival.

R High salt intake, smoking, low socioeconomic status, densely populated living environment, crowded living conditions, no access to running water, educational level

Hx Asymptomatic (++), heartburn, nausea, vomiting, bloating, epigastric pain, anorexia

PE No added value

Dx
- Labs: often no abnormalities, microcytic anaemia, IgG serum antibodies against *H. pylori* antigen
- Stool antigen assay: *H. pylori* positive (gold standard)
- Urea breath test: directly detects *H. pylori* urease activity

- Upper endoscopy with biopsy if indicated: pale mucosa/atrophic gastritis, active ulcer, intestinal metaplasia, *H. pylori*-positive

Tx *H. pylori* eradication: triple therapy (PPI and 2 types of ABx e.g. clarithromycin and amoxicilin/metronidazole for 14d) or quadruple therapy (triple therapy and bismuth), depending on local protocol

P Gastric cancer risk increases sixfold if left untreated

! To minimise false-negative results, always do eradication confirmation testing 4 wk after completing treatment, withholding PPIs for 14d before testing

Indications for *H. pylori* testing:
- Peptic ulcer or history of peptic ulcers without *H. pylori* eradication
- Functional dyspepsia
- Gastric MALT lymphoma
- Gastric cancer in young patients
- One-off test in patients with Lynch syndrome
- Unexplained microcytic anaemia
- Bulbitis or duodenitis revealed by upper endoscopy

If symptoms persist after eradication, consider testing for *H. pylori* again (stool antigen assay preferred). Gastric biopsy samples may have to be tested for *H. pylori* to determine antibiotic resistance, e.g. if therapy fails.

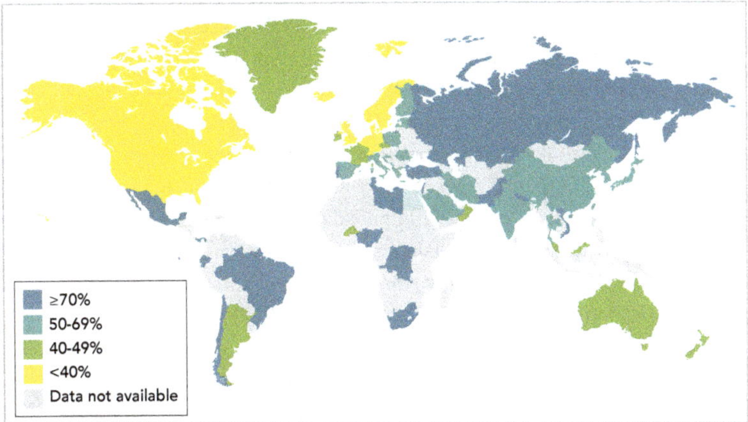

Figure 46 // Worldwide prevalence of *H. pylori* infection in adults

Stool antigen assays and breath tests that check for *H. pylori* are affected by medication use. The medications listed below should be discontinued prior to testing, to avoid a false negative result:

- ABx for 4 wk
- PPIs for 2 wk
- H2 receptor antagonists for 24h

Gastroparesis

D Gastroparesis is delayed gastric emptying which is not caused by a mechanical obstruction and results in gastric food retention.

E Prevalence ♂ 10:100,000, ♀ 40:100,000

Ae
- Idiopathic
- Vagal nerve damage (DM, iatrogenic (surgery (+)), medications) → gastric motility ↓ → gastric emptying ↓ → food retention
- Neurological disorders (i.e. Parkinson's, multiple sclerosis)

R ♀ (++), DM, abdominal surgery (e.g. gastric fundoplication), neurological disorders, smoking, alcohol, GI infection, medication (including opioids)

Hx Nausea (++), vomiting (++), abdominal pain (++), early satiety (+), bloating, weight ↓

PE Distended abdomen, epigastric tenderness, weight ↓

Dx
- Labs (for underlying cause): glucose/HbA1c, TSH
- Upper endoscopy (to rule out mechanical obstruction): gastric food stasis despite NPO protocol
- Gastric emptying test using scintigraphy (gold standard), C13-octanoic acid breath test): gastric emptying ↓, preferably tested for 4h

Tx
- Dietary recommendations: small, frequent, low-fat meals with soluble fibre only, no carbonated drinks
- Stop (and switch) drugs associated with delayed gastric emptying

Prokinetics (e.g. metoclopramide, domperidone, erythromycin), antiemetics (e.g. 5-HT3 agonists), glucose regulation in patients with DM

- Post-pyloric tube feeding: nasoduodenal tube, PEG-J (with jejunum extension), or surgical jejunostomy
- Upper endoscopy: pyloric Botox injection (not proven effective) or gastric peroral endoscopic myotomy (G-POEM)
- Surgery: near-total gastrectomy, pyloroplasty also an option

P Symptoms may persist, treatment consists of symptom management

! Symptoms have high overlap with symptoms of functional dyspepsia

Portal hypertensive gastropathy (PHG)

D PHG is characterised by the dilation of blood vessels in the gastric mucosa due to increased pressure in the portal vein (see Figure 47).

E Prevalence 20-98% in patients with liver cirrhosis

Ae Portal hypertension → delayed hepatic blood flow → splanchnic vasodilation, increasing circulating volume, and shunting → gastric mucosal blood flow ↑, dilation of blood vessels in the gastric mucosa → vulnerable gastric mucosa and delayed wound healing

R Severity of liver disease, cause of portal hypertension, oesophageal or gastric varices, previous sclerotherapy or band ligation for oesophageal varices

Hx
- Asymptomatic ⊕, often an incidental finding
- Chronic bleeding (3-60%): symptoms consistent with iron deficiency anaemia or acute (2-12%), haematemesis/melaena

PE Not contributing, possible stigmata of liver cirrhosis or signs of anaemia

Dx Upper endoscopy: 'snakeskin' (mosaic-like) gastric mucosa (see Figure 47), predominantly in fundus and corpus

Tx Primary aim of treatment is to reduce portal hypertension and prevent bleeding

Beta-blockers (NSBB), consider iron supplementation/blood transfusion (symptomatic treatment)

- No role for endoscopic treatment
- Transjugular intrahepatic portosystemic shunt (TIPS) for severe and refractory bleeding

P Long-term prognosis is determined by the severity of the underlying liver disease

I
- It is important to distinguish between PHG and gastrointestinal vascular ectasia (GAVE), given the differences in treatment goals and related therapies. For portal hypertensive gastropathy, treatment is aimed at reducing portal pressure. For GAVE, treatment consists of thermoablative therapy.
- Rule out *H. pylori* before initiating prophylactic therapy with NSBBs. NSBBs can contribute to peptic ulcer development.

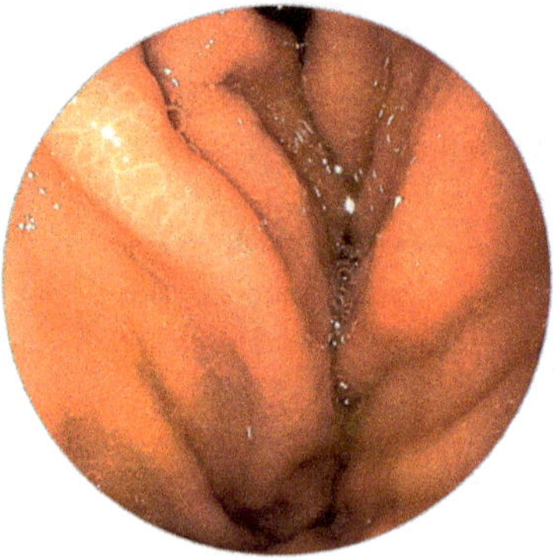

Figure 47 // Gastroscopy: portal hypertensive gastropathy and mosaic pattern in gastric mucosa

Peptic ulcer

	VENTRICULAR ULCER	DUODENAL ULCER
D	A peptic ulcer is a sore or lesion in the gastric (ventricular) and/or duodenal mucosa or submucosa, see Figure 48.	
	Located in the stomach, mostly antral	Located in the duodenum (usually in the duodenal bulb)
E	• 5% of patients with gastric symptoms >2 wk have a peptic ulcer • Duodenal ulcer: ventricular ulcer >2:1	
Ae	NSAIDs (++), *H. pylori* infection (++), other medications (e.g. corticosteroids, SSRIs, anticoagulants), stress ulcers in ICU patients, gastrinoma (−), Crohn's disease (−)	
	Malignancy	Ischaemia (+)
R	*H. pylori* (++), smoking, alcohol, advanced age, positive family history, stress, history of ulcers	
	♀:♂ = 1:1	♀:♂ = 2:1
Hx	Usually asymptomatic (70%), esp. in elderly patients. In other patients: epigastric pain (80%), acid reflux, nausea, vomiting, early satiety, symptoms consistent with anaemia.	
	• Weight ↓ • Eating → pain ↑	• Hunger pains, night pains • Eating → pain ↓
PE	• Occasional epigastric tenderness • Bleeding ulcer: haematemesis, melaena, signs of anaemia • Perforated ulcer: peritoneal irritation	

Table 41A // Peptic ulcer

	VENTRICULAR ULCER	DUODENAL ULCER
Dx	• Labs: Hb (=/↓), WBC ↑ in acute perforation • Stool antigen test: *H. pylori* • Consider upper endoscopy (see Figure 49) in advanced age and alarm symptoms • Biopsies if indicated: malignant features (e.g. ulcerated mass, irregular ulcer margins), suspicion of specific aetiology (e.g. Crohn's disease, sarcoidosis) • Abdominal contrast CT for suspected perforation: wall thickening, luminal outpouching, free gas in case of perforation, fat stranding, discontinuity of gastric/duodenal wall ⊖, abscess formation	
Tx	• Lifestyle advice: smoking cessation, quit alcohol, avoid trigger foods • Treat underlying cause PPI, *H. pylori* eradication, discontinue and avoid NSAIDs	
P	Possible complications: stenosis/gastric outlet obstruction (esp. of the duodenal bulb), haemorrhage (± 50% of patients), perforation, and fistulisation	
!	Watch out for malignancies, repeat upper endoscopy 6 wk after treatment	Low risk of carcinoma, no surveillance required

Table 41B // Peptic ulcer

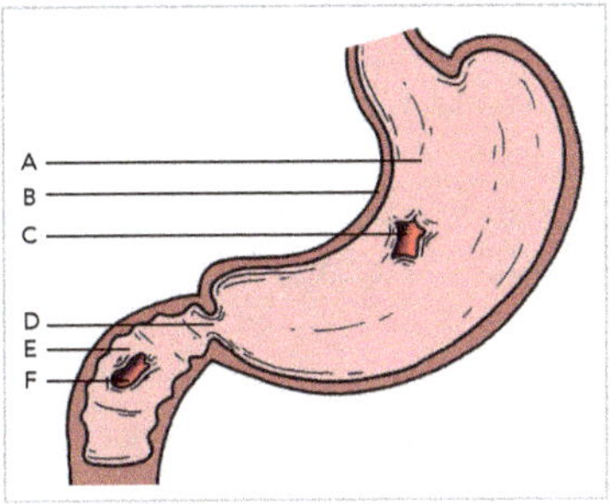

Figure 48 // Peptic ulcer: locations
A: Stomach **B:** Stomach wall **C:** Ventricular ulcer **D:** Pylorus **E:** Duodenum **F:** Duodenal ulcer

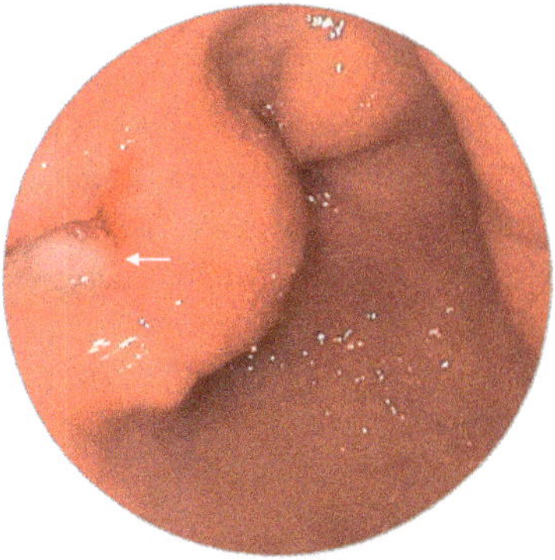

Figure 49 // Gastroscopy: ventricular ulcer

Hypergastrinemia is fasting serum gastrin >200 pg/mL, classified as appropriate (low acid) or inappropriate (normal/high acid). Zollinger-Ellison syndrome (ZES) often shows gastrin >1000 pg/mL, low gastric pH, and recurrent ulcers with diarrhoea. Diagnosis involves confirming low pH with elevated gastrin or using a secretin test if levels are less marked.

See section *Management of upper GI haemorrhage* for ulcer-related bleeding.

Gastric antral vascular ectasia (GAVE)

D GAVE, also called watermelon stomach, is characterised by capillary malformations in the gastric antrum that often lead to chronic blood loss and iron deficiency anaemia.

E Affects up to 14% of patients with liver cirrhosis, yet the link between GAVE and portal hypertension is uncertain

Ae Unknown

R Advanced age (++), ♀, associated with chronic kidney disease (+), liver cirrhosis, connective tissue disease (e.g. systemic sclerosis), DM, obesity, anticoagulants

Hx Symptoms consistent with iron deficiency anaemia or GI blood loss (including melaena)

PE Rectal exam may reveal melaena

Dx
- Upper endoscopy: parallel red antral folds representing ecstatic and sacculated vessels, resembling a watermelon (see Figure 50)
- Biopsy in selected cases for confirmation of diagnosis: dilated mucosal capillaries with fibrin thrombi, fibromuscular hyperplasia in lamina propria, spindle cell proliferation

Tx Iron supplements for iron deficiency anaemia, blood transfusion as needed, consider somatostatin analogues or thalidomide

Endoscopic treatment: upper endoscopy with coagulation of the capillary malformations, rubber band ligation, or RF ablation

P 62% of patients become transfusion-dependent

! Acute severe bleeding is rare, partial gastric resection may be considered for severe bleeding if endoscopic treatment proves ineffective

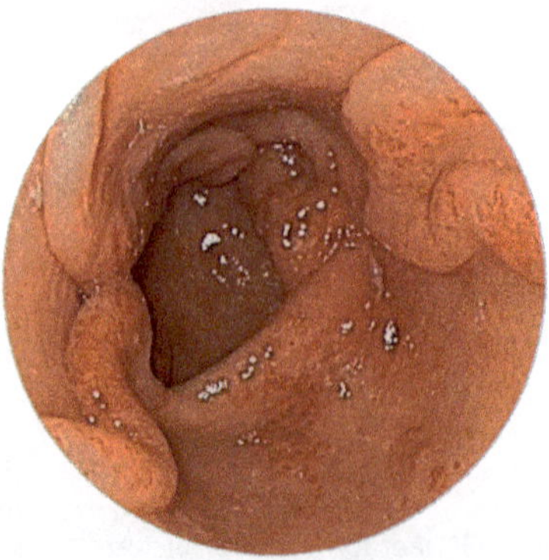

Figure 50 // Gastroscopy: erythematous antral folds, consistent with watermelon stomach

Small intestine

Small intestinal bacterial overgrowth (SIBO)

D SIBO is a disorder of the small intestine characterised by excessive bacterial colonisation, causing gastrointestinal symptoms. It is a controversial condition and a difficult diagnosis to make.

E Unclear, incidence increases with age

Ae Mechanisms such as gastric acid secretion, bile acids, pancreatic enzymes, intestinal motility, incl. a properly functioning ileocecal valve, and the immune system contribute to the maintenance of normal intestinal flora. Bacterial overgrowth can occur when one or more of these mechanisms malfunction: bacterial growth ↑, bacterial clearance ↓ (particularly *E. coli* and *Klebsiella*) → retrograde translocation of colon flora to small intestine.

R Advanced age, functional GI disorders/disorders of gut-brain interaction (e.g. IBS, functional dyspepsia), motility disorder (e.g. secondary to DM, systemic sclerosis, medication (opiates)), anatomic abnormalities esp. after surgery (adhesions, strictures, blind loop, status after ileocaecal resection or short bowel in general), chronic pancreatitis, immune deficiencies, coeliac disease, Crohn's disease

Hx Asymptomatic ⊕, bloating ⊕, flatulence ⊕, nausea, abdominal pain, abdominal cramps, diarrhoea, steatorrhoea ⊖, weight ↓

PE Not contributing

Dx
- Hydrogen breath testing (glucose hydrogen breath test)
- Small bowel aspirate (invasive procedure)
- Labs: to rule out malabsorption (e.g. pernicious anaemia)
- Optional: upper endoscopy to rule out other causes or predisposing conditions, MRI of small intestine to rule out anatomic abnormalities

Tx Treat underlying cause

ABx (e.g. rifaximin), consider vitamin and mineral supplements

P 40% have persistent symptoms after ABx. Recurrences are also frequent. Consider AB rotation.

! Limited data available to guide treatment decisions

Coeliac disease

D Coeliac disease is an IgA-mediated chronic autoimmune disorder of the small intestine caused by an autoimmune reaction triggered by the intake of gluten (see Figure 51).

E Prevalence 1%, more common in northern Europe

Ae
- Gliadin (gluten component) deamination by tissue transglutaminase → T-lymphocyte activation via HLA-DQ2-positive or DQ8-positive MHC II class molecules → production of pro-inflammatory cytokines and autoantibodies → enterocyte damage → villous atrophy
- Gliadin → IL-15 secretion by enterocytes ↑ → lymphocyte activation → enterocyte apoptosis → villous atrophy

R Genetic predisposition (positive HLA-DQ2 and/or HLA-DQ8 genes), ♀, positive FHx (screening recommended in asymptomatic first-degree relatives of patients with confirmed coeliac disease), DM type I, thyroid disorders, Down syndrome, Turner syndrome

Hx
- Asymptomatic ⊕, often undiagnosed: some symptoms are too mild to be experienced as complaints
- Diarrhoea ⊕⊕, steatorrhoea ⊕, abdominal pain ⊕, bloating, flatulence, appetite ↓
- Extraintestinal symptoms: general malaise, fatigue, symptoms consistent with anaemia, weight ↓ (but can also present in overweight people), dermatitis herpetiformis, delayed puberty, infertility, amenorrhoea, delayed menarche, depressive feelings, osteopenia/osteoporosis
- Childhood age: failure to thrive, possibly steatorrhoea/diarrhoea, abdominal cramps, abdominal bloating

PE Bulging abdomen, weight ↓, skin rash (dermatitis herpetiformis)

Dx
- Labs: anti-transglutaminase (TGA-IgA) ↑ (>10x normal) and anti-endomysium (EMA-IgA) ↑ (with gluten-rich diet), check for IgA deficiency, Hb ↓, vitamin and mineral deficiencies (vitamin B12, vitamin D, Ca, iron status, folic acid), TSH, consider ALT ↑ and AST ↑, HLA testing (second-line testing)
- Upper endoscopy with biopsy (≥5 duodenal biopsies): characteristic villous atrophy, intraepithelial lymphocytosis, crypt hyperplasia (Marsh classification)

Tx
Dietary recommendations: lifelong gluten-free diet, vitamin and mineral supplementation as needed

Age >50: treatment for osteoporosis/osteopenia if indicated by DEXA scan

P
- Gluten-free diet → symptoms disappear within weeks/months, and small intestine enteropathy disappears in 6-24 mo
- Risk of oesophageal and duodenal carcinoma and/or enteropathy-associated T-cell lymphoma ↑ or refractory coeliac disease

! Besides coeliac disease, there are many other causes of villous atrophy, e.g. other autoimmune disorders (e.g. Crohn's disease), drug-associated (esp. angiotensin receptor blockers), malignancy-related, infectious, ischaemic

In incidental diagnoses of iron deficiency anaemia, coeliac disease should always be considered as a possible cause.

Malabsorption symptoms include chronic diarrhoea, fatigue, weight ↓, vitamin deficiency, anaemia (iron deficiency or vitamin B12 deficiency), hypocalcaemia, and osteoporosis.

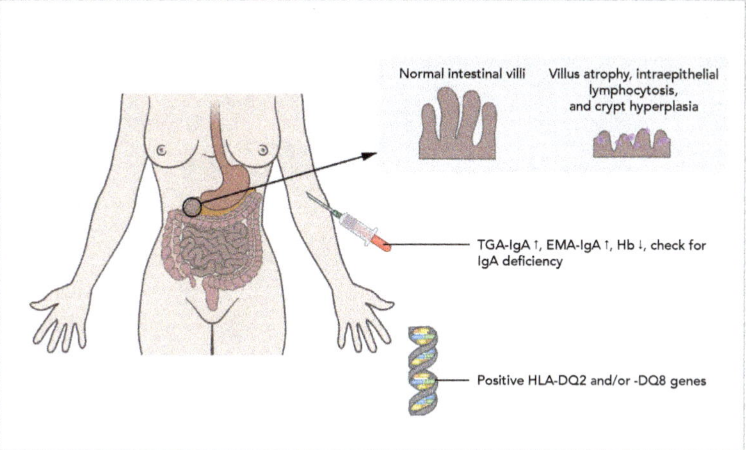

Figure 51 // Coeliac disease

Ileus

D Ileus is a motility disorder resulting in delayed passage of enteric contents. It is a clinical diagnosis with two subtypes: adynamic/paralytic ileus and mechanical obstruction (see Table 42 and Figure 52). Occurs more commonly in the small intestine (80%) than in the large intestine (20%).

SHAVING
Causes of an ileus include **s**trictures, **h**ernia, **a**dhesions, **v**olvulus, **i**ntussusception/IBD, **n**eoplasms, and **g**allstones.

<table>
<tr><th></th><th>ADYNAMIC ILEUS</th><th>MECHANICAL OBSTRUCTION</th></tr>
<tr><td>D</td><td>Ileus secondary to paralysis of the intestinal wall musculature.</td><td>Ileus secondary to obstruction of the intestinal lumen.</td></tr>
<tr><td>E</td><td colspan="2">Small intestine (80%) > colon (20%)</td></tr>
<tr><td>Ae</td><td>• Paralysis of intestinal wall musculature → peristalsis ↓
• Mostly secondary to disease</td><td>Mechanical obstruction of intestinal lumen → accumulation of intestinal contents proximally and collapsed intestinal lumen distal to obstruction → peristalsis ↑</td></tr>
<tr><td>R</td><td>Abdominal or retroperitoneal surgery ⊕, medication (e.g. anticholinergics, opiates, tricyclic antidepressants), sedentary lifestyle, peritonitis (e.g. infectious, carcinomatous), pancreatitis, arterial stenosis (perfusion ↓), electrolyte imbalances (e.g. K^+ ↓)</td><td>• Intraluminal: intussusception, volvulus, gallstones (gallstone ileus), faecal impaction, undigested food (phytobezoars), meconium, obstructive tumours (mainly in colon)
• Intramural: Crohn's disease, stricture due to radiotherapy, adenocarcinoma
• Extramural: abdominal surgery → postoperative adhesions ⊕, causing adhesive small bowel obstruction, incarcerated hernia</td></tr>
<tr><td>Hx</td><td colspan="2">Cramping abdominal pain (persistent, continuous pain in intestinal ischaemia), nausea, vomiting, failure to pass stools and flatus, distended abdomen, fever, if complicated by perforation and/or strangulation: signs of septic shock (BP ↓, heart rate ↑, clammy and pale skin)</td></tr>
<tr><td rowspan="2">PE</td><td colspan="2">Distended abdomen, hyperresonant percussion (tympany), absent liver muffling in the case of perforation, rectal digital exam reveals an empty ampulla, possibly signs of dehydration (heart rate ↑, BP ↓, turgor ↓)</td></tr>
<tr><td>Auscultation: peristalsis ↓ (absent bowel sounds for 4 min)</td><td>Auscultation: peristalsis ↑ (high-pitched, tinkling bowel sounds)</td></tr>
<tr><td rowspan="2">Dx</td><td colspan="2">• Lab: detection of dehydration (Na^+ ↓/↑, K^+ ↓, Cl^- ↓, pH ↑), WBC ↑, CRP ↑, lactate ↑ (in ischaemia), arterial blood gas (metabolic alkalosis due to vomiting)
• In principle, the abdominal X-ray is no longer used as a diagnostic tool</td></tr>
<tr><td>Abdominal contrast CT: diffuse dilation of all intestinal loops, no lead point, but diffuse paralysis due to gradual dilation of intestinal lumen, small bowel faeces sign</td><td>Abdominal contrast CT: lead point at obstruction site (e.g. strand, rotation, space-occupying lesion (SOL)), dilated bowel lumen starts from the lead point onwards, small bowel faeces sign</td></tr>
<tr><td rowspan="2">Tx</td><td colspan="2">Supportive, NPO, gastric drainage tube
IV fluids and electrolytes, consider TPN (not in the acute phase, but in prolonged ileus)</td></tr>
<tr><td>Consider prokinetics, if possible discontinue medication with negative effect on motility (e.g. opiates)
Surgery is only indicated for treatment of underlying cause and in case of complications</td><td>• Depending on underlying cause
• Endoscopic intervention (if no signs of strangulation or perforation), stool evacuation (for faecal impaction)
• Indications for emergency laparotomy: strangulation, necrosis, perforation</td></tr>
</table>

Table 42A // Types of ileus

	ADYNAMIC ILEUS	MECHANICAL OBSTRUCTION
P	• Failure to treat ileus in a timely manner can result in potentially fatal intestinal perforation • Ileus has a good prognosis if the underlying cause can be treated • 20-30% of patients with mechanical ileus undergo surgical intervention	
!	• DDx: chronic intestinal pseudo-obstruction (CIPO, mostly affecting the colon instead of the small intestine) • Complications ⊖: intestinal ischaemia, perforation	• Complications ⊖: bowel ischaemia, perforation, peritonitis • A prolonged mechanical ileus often develops into paralytic ileus

Table 42B // Types of ileus

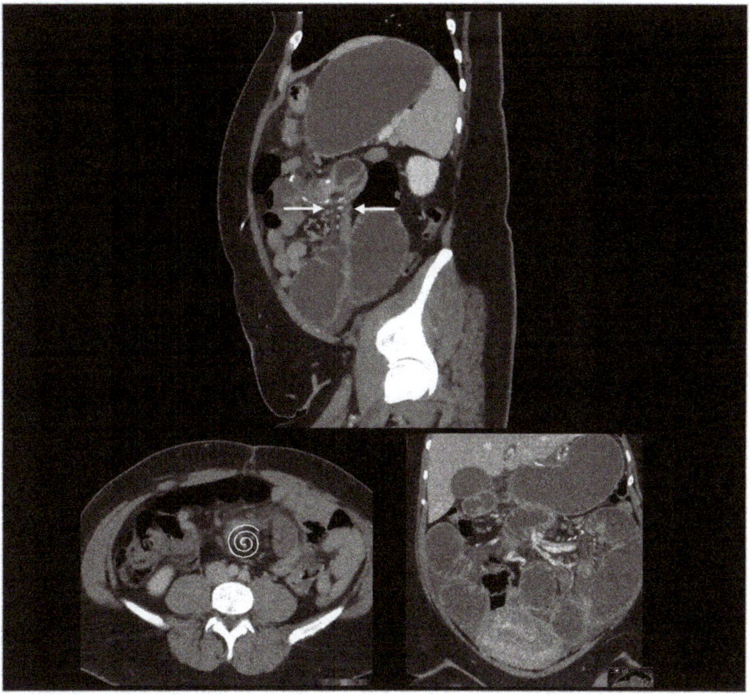

Figure 52 // Abdominal contrast CT: internal herniation after gastric bypass surgery with intestinal loops protruding through Petersen's space (white arrows). The herniation has caused mechanical obstruction (dilated intestinal loops) and the whirlpool sign is visible on axial slices.

The **'small bowel faeces sign'** is a radiological finding resembling solid faeces in the small intestinal lumen and is a sign of slow/obstructed passage.

Lactose intolerance

D Lactose intolerance is a condition characterised by the absence or low levels of the small intestinal enzyme lactase, preventing the intestines from absorbing lactose.

E Varying prevalence worldwide, with higher rates in South America, Africa, and Asia compared to North America, Europe, and Oceania

Ae
- Primary (acquired ⊕ or congenital ⊖): lactase deficiency → lactose absorption ↓ → intestinal lactose levels ↑ → bacterial fermentation → gas formation and osmotic diarrhoea
- Secondary: coeliac disease, GI infection, giardiasis, tropical sprue, bacterial overgrowth, candidiasis

R Advanced age, prematurity, ethnicity (African, Asian descent), small intestine disorders

Hx Symptoms occur 0.5-2h after significant lactose intake: stomach cramps, bloating, nausea, vomiting, diarrhoea (sometimes frothy, yellow, and acidic), flatus

PE Not contributing

Dx
- Elimination/provocation test, lactose hydrogen breath test (specificity > sensitivity), lactose tolerance test (glucose monitoring in plasma), consider genetic testing
- Biopsy of small intestine in case of suspicion of underlying primary aetiology, e.g. celiac disease (rarely used, and only in secondary lactose intolerance)
- Stool analysis (not specific for lactose intolerance): osmotic gap ↑, pH ↓

Tx Dietary recommendations: elimination diet

Lactase supplements prior to lactose intake, consider supplementation of calcium and vitamin D

P May be reversible by treating secondary causes

I Isolated lactose intolerance does not cause malabsorption or weight loss. Endoscopic evaluation and/or diagnostic imaging is recommended in patients with severe symptoms and/or alarm symptoms to rule out other causes (e.g. IBD).

> Food allergies produce symptoms by activating the immune system (IgE). A food intolerance is a reaction to food in which the immune system is not activated.

Meckel's diverticulum

D Meckel's diverticulum is a congenital bulge, usually located in the middle to distal region of the ileum (see Figure 53). In >50% of cases, the diverticulum contains ectopic gastric mucosa and/or pancreatic tissue in addition to intestinal mucosa.

E Prevalence 2%, often chance finding, if symptomatic: 80% of patients develop symptoms before age 15

Ae Both a persistent vitelline duct (or omphalomesenteric duct) and partially patent vetelline duct (90%) can lead to a Meckel's diverticulum

R ♂:♀ 2:1, malformation of umbilicus, GI tract, nervous system, or cardiovascular system

Hx
- Asymptomatic (++)
- Ectopic (gastric) mucosal bleeding: melaena, bright red rectal blood loss
- Inflammation and obstruction of the lumen of Meckel's diverticulum (Meckel's diverticulitis): resembles appendicitis
- Intestinal obstruction due to volvulus or invagination: resembles mechanical ileus

PE No specific abnormalities

Dx
- CTA and CTV in case of active bleeding: detect branch of superior mesenteric artery to Meckel's diverticulum and possibly coiling
- Meckel's scan: to detect ectopic mucosa
- Balloon-assisted endoscopy

Tx Surgical resection of Meckel diverticulum

P A Meckel's diverticulum is a possible lead point for intussusception

I Risk of complications (bleeding, inflammation, obstruction) ↑ if age <50, length >2 cm, or in the presence of ectopic tissue

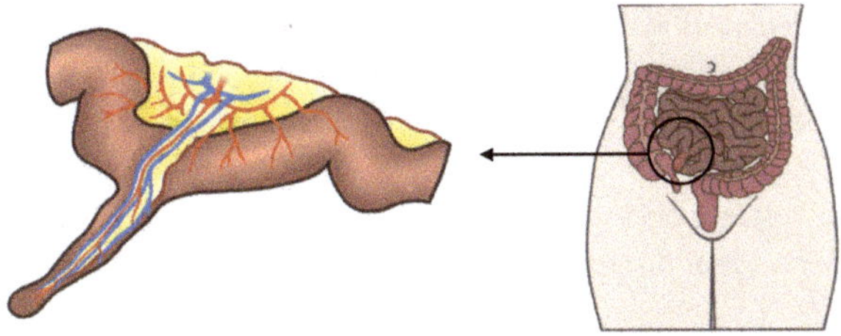

Figure 53 // Meckel's diverticulum

Refeeding syndrome

D Refeeding syndrome is a set of metabolic changes and electrolyte disturbances that occur after restarting enteral or parenteral nutrition following a period of prolonged low food intake or nutrient loss.

E Unknown due to lack of uniform definition

Ae See Figure 54

R
- Minimal or no food intake (including drinking, tube feeding, and/or parenteral nutrition) for ≥10d, esp. combined with pre-existing malnourishment and underlying disease (e.g. malignancies, HIV, malabsorption, alcohol use disorder)
- BMI <16 kg/m^2 and unintentional weight loss >15% in last 3-6 mo
- Alcohol, advanced age, anorexia nervosa
- Low serum P, K^+, and Mg^{2+} levels prior to restarting nutrition

Hx
- Gastrointestinal: nausea, vomiting
- Circulatory: heart failure
- Respiratory: dyspnoea, respiratory insufficiency
- Neurological: confusion, seizures, Wernicke-Korsakoff syndrome
- Extremities: muscle pain, muscle weakness, tremor

PE Tachypnoea, muscle weakness, oedema, signs of Wernicke encephalopathy

Dx
- Labs: electrolytes (Ca^{2+}, K^+, Mg^{2+}, Na^+, P) ↓, glucose intolerance, thiamine deficiency, lactate acidosis
- Reduced organ function (heart, kidney, lung) and fluid overload/dehydration
- ECG: to rule out cardiac arrhythmias

Tx Slow, tapered restart of feeding, monitor fluid balance, monitor weight, labs for electrolytes (Ca^{2+}, K^+, Mg^{2+}, Na^+, P), creatinine, glucose, and albumin before start of feeding, monitor electrolytes daily in the first 72h, glucose curve, consult dietician

Before starting the refeed schedule, administer IV thiamine with multivitamins and electrolyte supplementation if indicated

P Reintroducing food too rapidly can result in cardiac arrhythmias and impaired organ function and may be fatal

! Possible complications: heart failure, cardiac arrhythmias, respiratory insufficiency, muscular disorders, convulsions, delirium, kidney failure

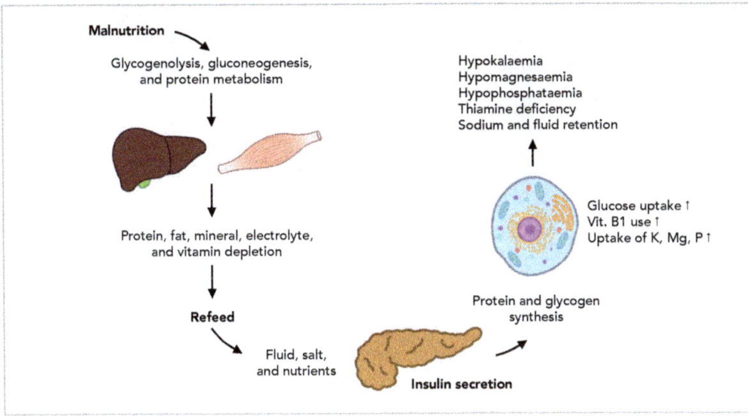

Figure 54 // Refeeding syndrome

Short bowel syndrome

D Short bowel syndrome is a combination of symptoms caused by malabsorption due to a lack of functional small intestine (approx. <2m), which can cause malnutrition despite a normal diet.

E Estimated 0.3:100,000 per year

Ae Insufficient residual functional small intestine → absorptive capacity ↓ → protein, vitamin, and mineral deficiency (including vitamin B12, Mg^{2+}, K^{+}, zinc, and iron)

R Resection of the small intestine (e.g. in Crohn's disease, tumours, necrotising enterocolitis (NEC) in infancy, or congenital malformation), volvulus complicated by necrosis, mesenteric ischaemia complicated by necrosis, radiation enteritis

Hx Weight ↓ (++), fatigue, malaise, abdominal cramps, bloating, flatus, diarrhoea, steatorrhoea

PE No specific abnormalities, weight ↓, muscle mass ↓, signs of vitamin and mineral deficiencies

Dx
- Length of small intestine <2m (surgical reports), check whether large intestine is in situ
- Labs and stool analysis: detect deficiencies

Tx Dietary recommendations: small meals spread throughout the day, specific recommendations dependent on excised intestine, stenoses, motility disorders, etc.

- Supplementation for deficiencies, intestinal motility inhibitors, Somatropin (recombinant growth hormone for SBS treatment)
- TPN, switch to enteral nutrition if possible and eventually to oral nutrition

P Prognosis depends on the length of the small intestine and aetiology, complications, and degree of intestinal adaptation

I
- Beware of gallstones, kidney stones (calcium oxalate), renal dysfunction (oxalate nephropathy), and D-lactic acidosis (neurological symptoms following carbohydrate consumption)
- Oral nutrition is usually possible if at least 30-50 cm of the small intestine remains after resection (excluding duodenum), provided the large intestine is in situ

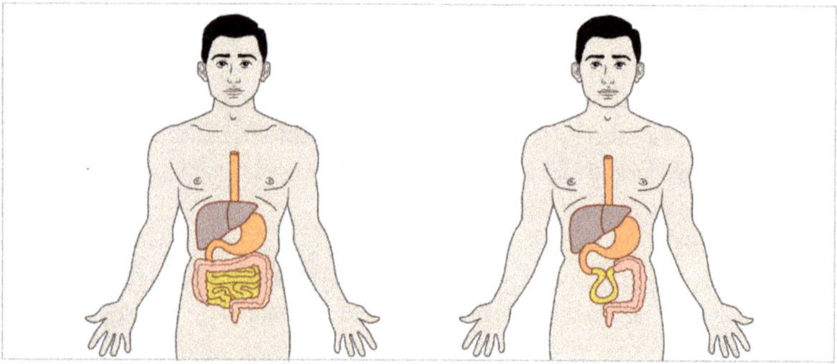

Figure 55 // Short bowel syndrome

Colon

Diverticular disease

	DIVERTICULOSIS	DIVERTICULITIS
D	Diverticulosis is the presence of multiple diverticula. Diverticula are sac-like protrusions of the colonic wall and occur when the mucosa, submucosa, and serosa bulge out through the muscle wall of the colon (see Figure 56). This is often an incidental finding.	Diverticulitis is inflammation of one or more diverticula (see Figure 56).

Table 43A // Diverticular disease

	DIVERTICULOSIS	DIVERTICULITIS
E	• Prevalence 5% age <40, 20-60% age >40, 70% age >80 • In Western Europe and North America, diverticula are mainly found in the sigmoid (90%), in patients of Asian descent mainly in the ascending colon (75%)	• Incidence ±180:100,000 • 4-15% of patients with diverticulosis develop diverticulitis
Ae	Intraluminal pressure ↑, strength of collagen fibres in colon wall ↓	Unknown, possibly faecal stasis or faecolith entrapment in a diverticulum → bacterial overgrowth → diverticulitis
R	Advanced age, low-fibre diet, constipation, lack of exercise, obesity, positive FHx, smoking	
	N/A	Use of corticosteroids, opiates, and NSAIDs
Hx	Asymptomatic (++), mild non-specific symptoms	Fever, LLQ pain (+), abdominal cramps, nausea, vomiting, possible changes in bowel habits (constipation, sometimes alternating with diarrhoea)
PE	Not contributing	T ↑, possible signs of peritoneal irritation, LLQ tenderness
Dx	Only perform colonoscopy in case of persistent symptoms to rule out colon carcinoma: visibility of intestinal wall bulges/ diverticula (see image 57)	• Labs: WBC ↑, CRP ↑ • Abdominal ultrasound in case of suspected uncomplicated diverticulitis: diverticulosis with peridiverticular fat stranding, bowel wall thickening • Abdominal contrast CT: if ultrasound is inconclusive or to detect possible complications (perforation, abscess) • Consider colonoscopy in patients with complicated diverticulitis, persistent symptoms, or alarm symptoms
Tx	Lifestyle recommendations: exercise, high-fibre diet, plenty of fluids, stop smoking Laxatives, fibre supplements	Depends on Hinchey stage (see Table 44) and clinical presentation No preventive medication is available for recurrent diverticulitis, avoid regular use of NSAIDs
P	• 4-15% develop diverticulitis • 5-15% develop diverticular bleeding (see Figure 58)	• 25% have complicated diverticulitis • 20% have recurring episodes <10y
!	Possible complications: diverticulitis, diverticular bleeding	Possible complications: abscess, fistula formation, obstruction, peritonitis, sepsis

Table 43B // Diverticular disease

STAGE	DEFINITION	TREATMENT
0	Mild clinical diverticulitis	Wait-and-see: liquid diet, analgesics as needed. Indications for ABx in uncomplicated diverticulitis: immunocompromised patients, refractory symptoms or vomiting, CRP >140 or WBC >15, fluid collection, or longer segment of inflammation
Ia	Limited pericolic inflammatory process/ inflammatory infiltrate	
Ib	Limited pericolic (mesenteric) abscess	Cannot be drained: IV fluids, analgesics, and ABx
II	Pelvic, intra-abdominal, or retroperitoneal abscess	Abscess size allows for drainage (≥4 cm): percutaneous drainage and ABx
III	Generalised purulent peritonitis (perforated abscess)	• For Hinchey III: consider laparoscopic peritoneal lavage (no consensus) • NPO, IV fluids, Hartmann procedure (sigmoid resection with anastomosis or terminal colostomy)
IV	Faecal peritonitis	

Table 44 // Hinchey classification and corresponding treatment options

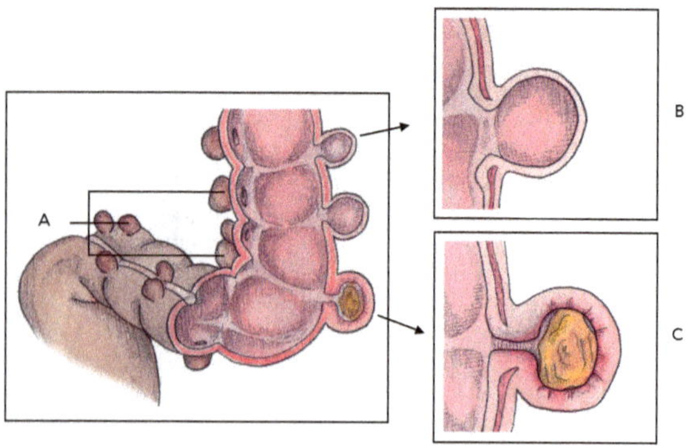

Figure 56 // Diverticulosis and diverticulitis
A: Diverticula **B:** Diverticulum **C:** Diverticulitis (inflamed diverticulum)

Patients with colonic diverticulosis can develop segmental colitis associated with diverticulosis (SCAD), most commonly located in the sigmoid colon. Clinical features include chronic diarrhoea, abdominal pain primarily in the left lower quadrant, and intermittent rectal blood loss. The endoscopic and histological features of SCAD can range from mild inflammatory changes to chronic active inflammation that resembles IBD.

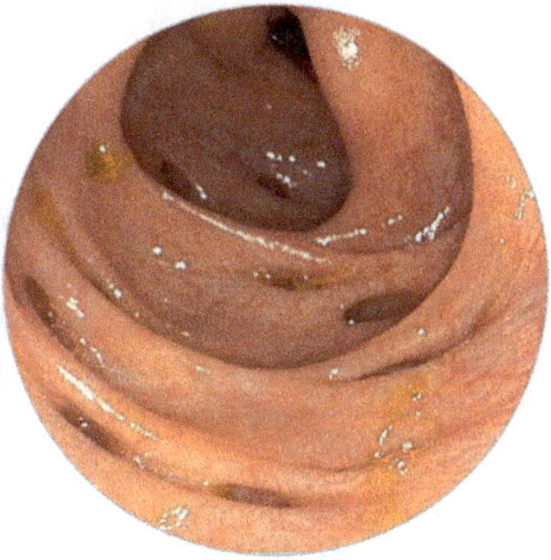

Figure 57 // Colonoscopy: diverticulosis

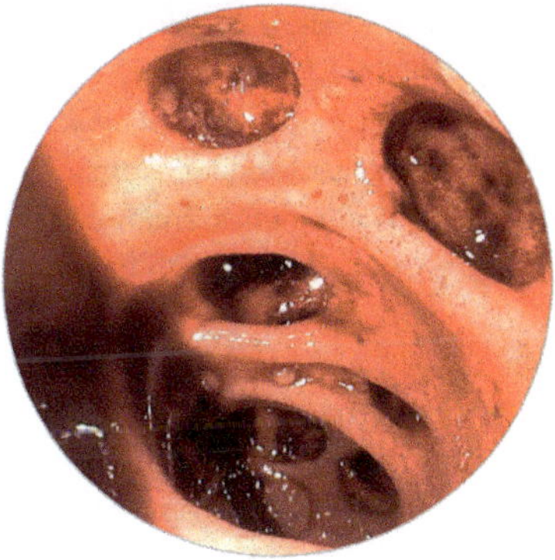

Figure 58 // Colonoscopy: aspect of colon following diverticular bleeding

Infectious colitis/gastroenteritis

D Inflammation of the intestinal mucosa due to bacterial, viral, or parasitic infection.

E Frequent, endemic. Epidemiology is highly dependent on pathogen and geographical location. Bacterial colitis accounts for half of all cases of acute diarrhoea. Campylobacter bacteria are the number 1 cause worldwide of infectious colitis, with a prevalence of 25-30:100,000.

Ae
- Bacteria: *Escherichia coli, Salmonella enterica, Shigella, Yersinia, Campylobacter, Clostridium difficile, Mycobacterium tuberculosis, Vibrio, Entamoeba histolytica, Listeria monocytogenes*
- Viruses: rotavirus, norovirus, cytomegalovirus, adenovirus
- Parasites: *Entamoeba histolytica, Giardia lamblia, Cryptosporidium parvum, Cyclospora cayetanensis, Strongyloides stercolaris*
- Sexually transmitted infections (STIs; esp. in HIV positive patients): *Neisseria gonorrhoeae, Chlamydia trachomatis, Herpes simplex, Treponema pallidum* (syphilis)

R Poor hygiene, contaminated drinking water or food, use of immunosuppressants, living or working in a health facility or day-care centre, recent AB use, travel to area with poor sanitation, receptive anal intercourse

Hx Fever, chills, nausea, vomiting, abdominal pain, abdominal cramps, bloating, bloody and/or watery diarrhoea, muscle pain, headache

PE T ↑, signs of dehydration, abdominal tenderness, high-pitched bowel sounds

Dx
- Stool culture/PCR: to detect possible pathogens

- Labs (if signs of dehydration): renal function ↓, electrolyte abnormalities, WBC ↑, CRP ↑

Tx Self-limiting ⊕, oral rehydration

- IV fluids, oral rehydration therapy (ORT)
- Anti-emetics, antimotility treatment (e.g. loperamide (contraindication: bloody stool with fever))
- AB for severe symptoms (e.g. persistent bloody diarrhoea or sepsis), specific pathogens, give to immunocompromised individuals at early stage

P Good prognosis

! Hx, PE, labs, and calprotectin do not always provide enough information to distinguish between IBD and infectious colitis. Always rule out infectious causes before diagnosing a patient with IBD.

Norovirus is the most common viral cause of infectious enteritis, *Campylobacter jejuni* is the most common bacterial cause. Travellers' diarrhoea is usually caused by *E. coli* species. In-hospital infectious enteritis is most commonly caused by *C. difficile*.

Irritable bowel syndrome (IBS)

	IBS WITH PREDOMINANT DIARRHOEA (IBS-D)	IBS WITH PREDOMINANT CONSTIPATION (IBS-C)	IBS WITH MIXED BOWEL HABITS (IBS-M)
D	IBS is a disorder of gut-brain interaction (DGBI) and comprises chronic abdominal pain and changed stool habits without an apparent physical cause. The diagnosis is made using the ROME IV criteria.		
E	Prevalence 4%		
Ae	• Multifactorial: intestinal permeability ↑, immune activation, mechanisms of gut-brain interaction, microbiome, motility • Visceral hypersensitivity, bowel motility disorders, psychological factors		
R	Young age, previous gastroenteritis, anxiety disorders, mood disorders, genetic factors, ♀		
Hx	Bloating, tenesmus, flatulence, bowel movements provide relief, headache, fatigue		
	>25% of bowel movements with Bristol stool types 6 or 7 and <25% of bowel movements with Bristol stool types 1 or 2	>25% of bowel movements with Bristol types 1 or 2, and <25% of bowel movements with Bristol stool types 6 or 7	Mixed: >25% of bowel movements with Bristol stool types 1 or 2, and >25% of bowel movements with Bristol stool types 6 or 7

Table 45A // Irritable bowel syndrome

	IBS WITH PREDOMINANT DIARRHOEA (IBS-D)	IBS WITH PREDOMINANT CONSTIPATION (IBS-C)	IBS WITH MIXED BOWEL HABITS (IBS-M)
PE	To rule out alternative diagnoses. Consider rectal exam to assess pelvic floor function.		
Dx	• Clinical diagnosis: ROME IV criteria • Labs to rule out other causes: CRP =, anti-tTG =. Other tests upon indication (e.g. Hb and TSH). • Faeces: calprotectin and cultures/PCR for diarrhoea • Colonoscopy if indicated (e.g. alarm symptoms or age of onset >50)		
Tx	Education, reassurance, dietary recommendations (e.g. low FODMAP, soluble fibre supplements (e.g. psyllium)), lifestyle modifications (exercise, sleep, stress reduction) Cognitive behavioural therapy, hypnotherapy, diaphragmatic breathing exercises, pelvic floor therapy • Symptomatic (e.g. pain, faecal incontinence) • Recommendations for pharmacological therapy vary between guidelines • Predominantly in IBS-D and IBS-C: analgesics, antispasmodics (peppermint oil), neuromodulators (e.g. tricyclic antidepressants (TCA), selective serotonin reuptake inhibitors (SSRI), gabapentinoids) • Predominantly in IBS-D: psyllium, antidiarrheals (e.g. loperamide), ABx in USA/ Canada (only rifaximin) • Predominantly in IBS-C: laxatives (bulk-forming, osmotic, stimulant), secretagogues (e.g. linaclotide). See Figure 59 for an example of step-up treatment.		
P	IBS has a chronic clinical course. It is more common in conjunction with chronic fatigue syndrome, fibromyalgia, and interstitial cystitis.		
!	Patients with e.g. endometriosis or IBD may be wrongly diagnosed with IBS because of the overlapping pattern of symptoms		

Table 45B // Irritable bowel syndrome

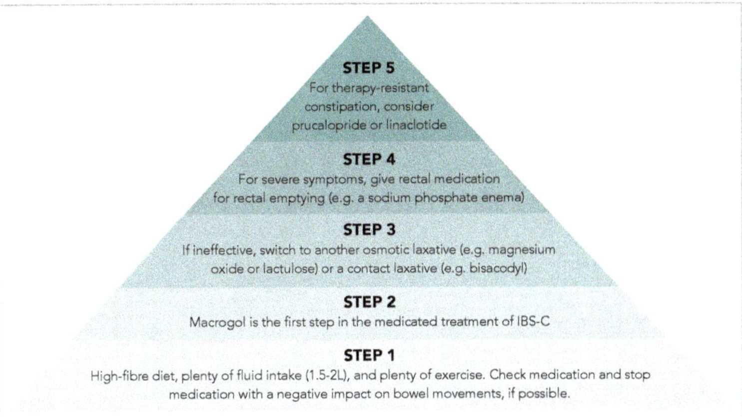

Figure 59 // Example step-up treatment for IBS-C

ROME IV criteria for irritable bowel syndrome

1. Recurrent abdominal pain (A), at least 1 d/wk of abdominal pain in the past 3 months, with onset of symptoms at least six months before diagnosis
2. ≥2 of the following criteria:
   - Related to defecation (B)
   - Associated with a change in frequency of stool (C)
   - Associated with a change in appearance of stool (D)

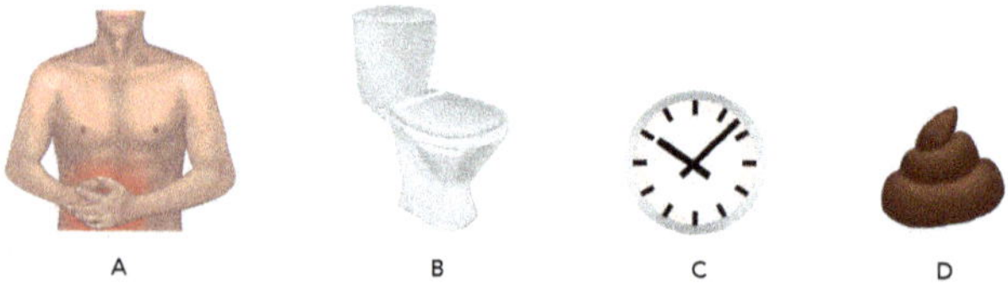

TYPE		DESCRIPTION
1	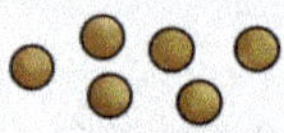	Separate hard lumps, like nuts (difficult to pass)
2	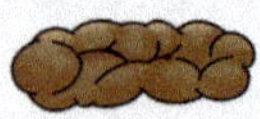	Sausage-shaped but lumpy
3	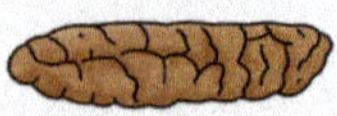	Like a sausage but with cracks on its surface
4	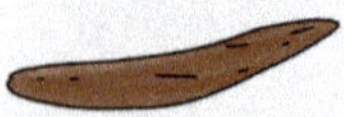	Like a sausage or snake, smooth and soft
5	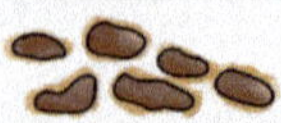	Soft blobs with clear-cut edges (easy to pass)
6	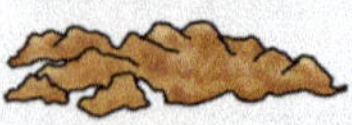	Fluffy pieces with ragged edges, a mushy stool
7	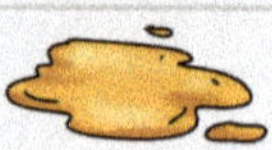	Watery, no solid pieces (entirely liquid)

Table 46 // Bristol Stool Form scale

Patients who present with any of the following symptoms must at least be evaluated for alternative diagnoses that might coexist with IBS:

- Blood in stool
- (Unexplained) iron deficiency anaemia
- Unintentional weight loss
- Palpable abdominal mass or lymphadenopathy on physical examination
- Onset of symptoms age >50 or family history of colon cancer and have not had age-appropriate colon cancer screening
- Sudden or acute onset of changes in bowel habits

Follow the 4 C's for further diagnostics: **C**RP, **c**oeliac serology, **c**alprotectin, and **c**olonoscopy in patients aged >50 or patients with alarm symptoms. Other diagnostics may be more appropriate for other DDx.

See section *Treatment // Pharmacotherapy* for an overview of pharmacological treatment options.

Polyps

	HYPERPLASTIC POLYP	SESSILE SERRATED POLYP	ADENOMATOUS POLYP
D	A polyp is an abnormal growth of a mucous membrane in the GI tract. Polyps vary greatly in both size and shape and are most common in the colon.		
	Most common non-neoplastic colon polyp	May show morphological signs of dysplasia	Most common dysplastic colon polyp
E	Incidence: 25-30% age >50		
Ae	Hereditary predisposition (see Table 48 on polyposis syndromes)		
R	Advanced age, ♂, positive family history, IBD, alcohol, smoking, obesity		
Hx	• Asymptomatic (++) • Large, distal, or neoplastic polyps: blood in stool, change in bowel habits, obstructive symptoms, positive FIT		
PE	Rectal exam to distinguish between other possible causes of rectal blood loss: palpable mass		

Table 47A // Polyps

	HYPERPLASTIC POLYP	SESSILE SERRATED POLYP	ADENOMATOUS POLYP
Dx	Colonoscopy: more common in rectosigmoid region, glassy	Colonoscopy: more common in proximal colon, flat with cloud-like appearance, indistinctive border, irregular shape (WASP classification). Their flat appearance makes detection during colonoscopy challenging.	• Colonoscopy: convex (sessile), flat, or stalked (see Figures 60, 61, and 62) • Histology: adenomatous with varying degrees of dysplasia
Tx	Polypectomy: • Endoscopic loop/snare polypectomy (with (hot) or without (cold) coagulation) • Endoscopic mucosal resection (EMR) for large polyps (>2 cm) • Endoscopic full thickness resection (eFTR) for complex polyps, complete removal of all layers • Endoscopic submucosal dissection (ESD) for suspected superficial malignant polyp (T1 carcinoma)		
P	Most polyps are benign, but can develop into colon carcinoma over time		
	Hyperplastic polyps do not appear to increase the risk of colorectal carcinoma	Dysplasia is common in sessile serrated lesions and it is important to track their size and number	Surveillance may be indicated, and diagnostics may be needed for suspected hereditary disease (see Hereditary colorectal cancer syndromes)
!	Pathologist assesses polyps to identify adenomatous features, degree of dysplasia, and/or adenocarcinoma		

Table 47B // Polyps

Hereditary colorectal cancer syndromes

	FAMILIAL ADENOMATOUS POLYPOSIS (FAP)	MUTYH-ASSOCIATED POLYPOSIS (MAP)
D	Hereditary disorder in which hundreds to thousands of adenomatous polyps develop in the colon and rectum. Risk of malignant transformation increases with age.	Hereditary disorder with a greatly increased risk of adenomatous polyps (dozens to hundreds per patient).
E	1% of colon cancer patients	0.7-1% of colon cancer patients
Ae	Hereditary mutation in APC gene (autosomal dominant), in 25-30% the mutation occurs spontaneously	Hereditary mutation in MUTYH gene (autosomal recessive)

Table 48A // Hereditary colon cancer syndromes

Over the past years, several countries have adopted colonoscopy surveillance programmes and/or national screening programmes for detection of neoplastic polyps or colorectal cancer. There is great variation between countries regarding surveillance programmes and cut-off age.

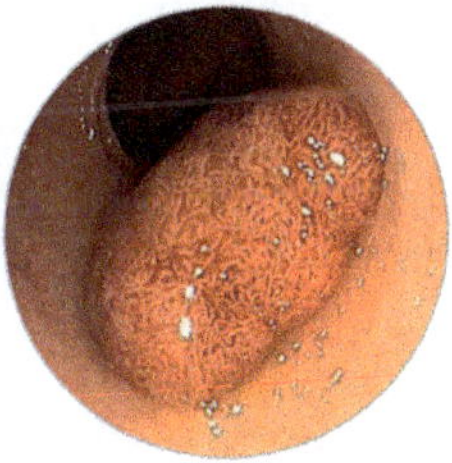

Figure 60 // Colonoscopy: sessile adenomatous polyp in the colon

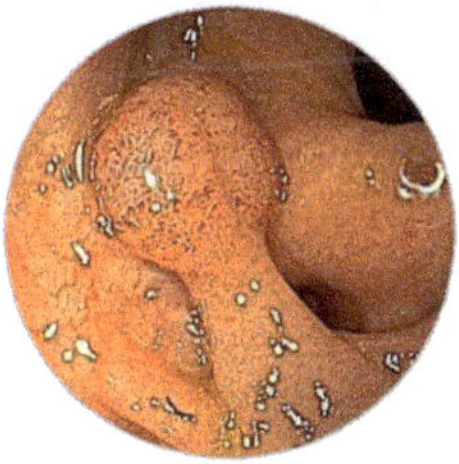

Figure 61 // Colonoscopy: pedunculated adenomatous polyp in the colon

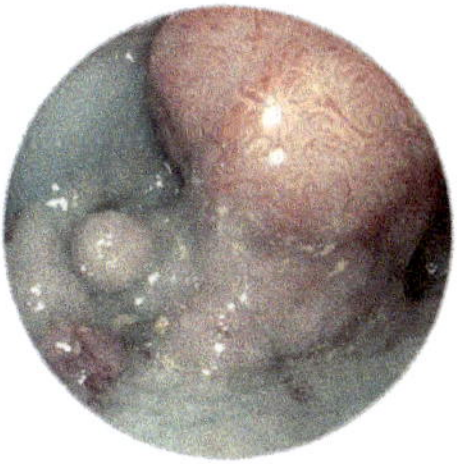

Figure 62 // Colonoscopy: flat elevated adenomatous polyp in the colon measuring about 30 mm after it is detected (e.g. with blue dye and adrenaline), which makes it clearly detectable

LYNCH (HNPCC)	PEUTZ-JEGHERS	SERRATED POLYPOSIS SYNDROME (SPS)
Hereditary disorder with increased risk of developing carcinomas in various organs, including colon carcinoma.	Hereditary disorder in which polyps (hamartomas) develop mainly in the small intestine.	Disorder with greatly increased risk of serrated polyps, typically proximal to the sigmoid.
Most common hereditary colorectal cancer syndrome, 2-3% of colon cancer patients	Incidence of 0.3-4:100,000	Unknown prevalence, extremely rare
Hereditary mutation in mismatch repair genes (MLH1, MSH2, MSH6, PMS2, and EPCAM) (autosomal dominant)	Hereditary mutation in the STK11 gene (autosomal dominant)	Pattern of inheritance unknown, mostly sporadic patients

<table>
<tr><th></th><th>FAMILIAL ADENOMATOUS POLYPOSIS (FAP)</th><th>MUTYH-ASSOCIATED POLYPOSIS (MAP)</th></tr>
<tr><td>R</td><td colspan="2">Hereditary predisposition</td></tr>
<tr><td>Hx</td><td colspan="2">Positive FHx for colorectal carcinoma at age <50, blood or mucus in stool, changed bowel habits, tenesmus, unexplained weight loss</td></tr>
<tr><td rowspan="2">PE</td><td colspan="2">Rectal exam (if contributing)</td></tr>
<tr><td colspan="2">N/A</td></tr>
<tr><td>Dx</td><td>• Colonoscopy: hundreds/thousands of adenomas in colon and rectum (see Figure 63)
• Upper endoscopy: gastric and duodenal adenomas, usually accompanied by fundic gland polyps in stomach
• DNA testing: APC mutation</td><td>• Colonoscopy: 10-100+ adenomas in colon and rectum
• Upper endoscopy: adenomas in duodenum
• DNA testing: MUTYH mutation</td></tr>
<tr><td>Tx</td><td>• From age 10-12, every 0,5-2y check-up colonoscopy
• Endoscopic surveillance of rectum/pouch every 6 mo/2y, removing all polyps >5 mm
• From age 25, biannual to 5-yearly upper endoscopy
Preventive proctocolectomy or colectomy: at young adult age (preferably age >18) based on number/size of polyps and degree of dysplasia. Severe rectal polyposis: proctocolectomy with ileoanal pouch. Mild rectal polyposis: total or subtotal colectomy with ileorectal or ileosigmoidal anastomosis.</td><td>• From age 18, every 2y check-up colonoscopy
• From age 35, biannual to 5-yearly upper endoscopy
Polypectomy for polyps >5 mm</td></tr>
<tr><td>P</td><td>Untreated (without preventive colectomy) 100% risk of colorectal carcinoma at age 35-45. A diagnosis of colorectal cancer has the same prognosis as non-hereditary colon carcinoma.</td><td>Numerous/large polyps or high-grade dysplasia that render check-ups ineffective are indications for colectomy</td></tr>
<tr><td>!</td><td>Increased risk of desmoid tumours, thyroid cancer, and epidermoid cysts</td><td>Possible increased risk of bladder and ovarian cancer</td></tr>
</table>

Table 48B // Hereditary colon cancer syndromes

LYNCH (HNPCC)	PEUTZ-JEGHERS	SERRATED POLYPOSIS SYNDROME (SPS)
Hereditary predisposition		Smoking
Positive FHx for colorectal carcinoma at age <50, blood or mucus in stool, changed bowel habits, tenesmus, unexplained weight loss	Dermal and mucosal pigmentation, polyps in the small intestine (obstipation or obstruction), anaemia when polyps bleed, invagination	Multiple family members with colorectal carcinoma or multiple types of polyps without polyposis syndromes
	Rectal exam (if contributing)	
N/A	Characteristic pigmentation (particularly on the inside of the lips)	N/A
• Colonoscopy: no more polyps than in normal population, polyps may be flatter • DNA testing: Lynch genes	• Colonoscopy: polyps in colon • Upper endoscopy: polyps in stomach, small intestine • MRI and/or video capsule endoscopy: assess small intestine	Colonoscopy: ≥5 histologically confirmed serrated lesions of which at least two >10 mm; or at any number of serrated polyps proximal to the sigmoid in patients with a first-degree relative with SPS; or >20 serrated polyps, of any size, scattered in the colon
From age 25, every 2y check-up colonoscopy with polypectomy as needed	From age 10, every 1-2y check-up with paediatrician. From age 25 colonoscopy every 2-5y. Surgical intervention only needed in case of invagination or ileus	Surveillance every 1-2y, depending on number of polyps • Consider surgical resection (e.g. subtotal colectomy) only if endoscopic polypectomies are impossible • Remove all adenomas and serrated polyps >3 mm
Average age at colorectal carcinoma diagnosis: • MLH1 mutation: 41-47y • MSH2 mutation: 44-46y • MSH6 mutation: 50-54y	Treatment is usually unnecessary because polyps grow slowly, and malignant development is rare. The average age of malignant development is 42.	There are no genetic tests for SPS, and the diagnosis is often missed, increasing the risk of missing colorectal carcinoma
Increased risk of uterine cancer and slightly increased risk of gastric, small intestine, pancreatic, urinary tract, and ovarian cancer	Increased risk of polyps in the nose, bladder, and gallbladder	Studies show that a large number of patients with SPS (68%) have polyps in the appendix, which is not specifically found in other polyposis syndromes

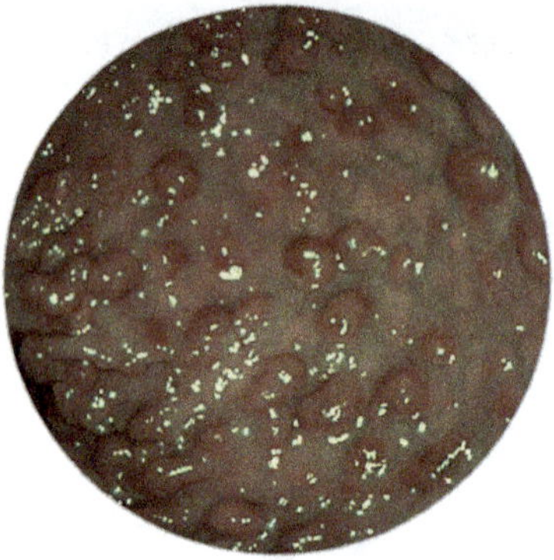

Figure 63 // Narrow band imaging (NBI) colonoscopy: tens of adenomatous polyps in familial adenomatous polyposis (FAP)

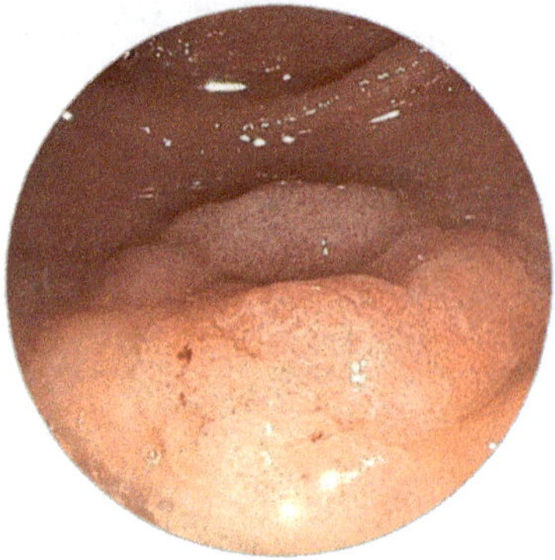

Figure 64 // Colonoscopy: sessile serrated polyp in serrated polyposis syndrome (SPS)

Sigmoid volvulus

D A sigmoid volvulus occurs when the sigmoid colon wraps around its own mesentery (see Figure 65), potentially causing ischaemia and necrosis.

E Prevalence 8:100,000, incidence 2:100,000 adults

Ae Strangulation of branches of the inferior mesenteric artery → ischaemia → necrosis

R Long and mobile sigmoid colon (dolicho-sigmoid) ⊕, chronic constipation, long-term bedridden, use of psychopharmaceuticals, neuroleptics, previous abdominal surgery

Hx Sudden attacks of severe abdominal pain (mostly not until perfusion defects or ischaemia), nausea, vomiting, abdominal distention, absence of stools, loss of appetite, reduced oral intake

PE Bulging abdomen, high-pitched bowel sounds, tenderness

Dx
- Abdominal X-ray: distended colon, coffee bean sign (see Figure 65)
- Abdominal contrast CT: visible torsion (see Figure 65), distended proximal colon, identification of possible complications (ischaemia, perforation)
- Labs if indicated: electrolytes, lactate, Hb, CRP, WBC, renal function

Tx
- Sigmoidoscopy (toffee sign, see Figure 65): endoscopic decompression and detorsion of affected segment to normal position and rectal tube for at least 24h (often falls out earlier)
- Suspected severe ischaemia/necrosis: Surgery consultation (consider sigmoid resection)

P
- Elective sigmoid resection should be considered for recurrent sigmoid volvulus
- Recurrence rate after colonoscopic decompression and subsequent conservative treatment is 45-71%

I Watch out for intestinal perforation, temporary or permanent colostomy if a large part of the colon is damaged

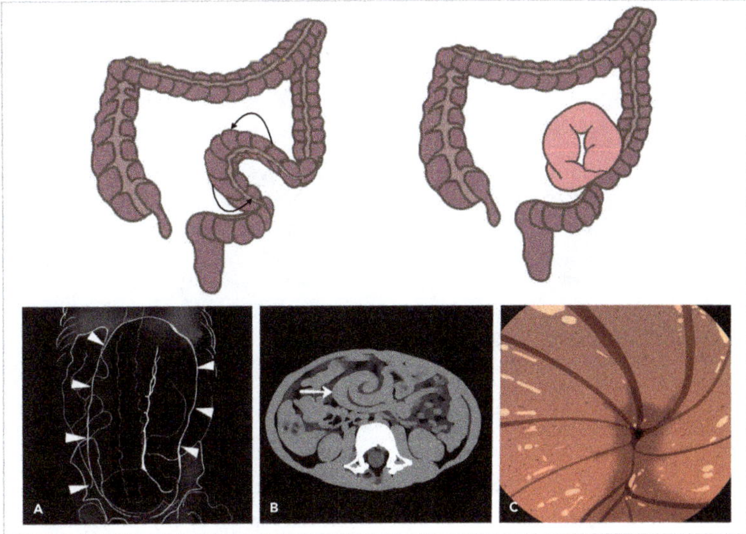

Figure 65 // Sigmoid volvulus
A: Coffee bean sign on abdominal X-ray, **B:** Rotation on CT, and **C:** Toffee sign during colonoscopy

Toxic megacolon

D Toxic megacolon is characterised by acute, extreme, and non-obstructive segmental or total dilation of the colon and is a serious complication of IBD and sometimes of infectious colitis (pseudomembranous colitis due to *C. difficile*, *Shigella* spp.) (see Table 49).

E 1-5% of patients with IBD, 1% of patients admitted with *C. difficile*

Ae Inflammation ↑ → nitric oxide production ↑, paralysis of smooth muscle tissue → colon dilation

R Ulcerative colitis (++), pseudomembranous colitis due to *C. difficile* (+), Crohn's disease, Cytomegalovirus (leading cause in HIV patients)

Hx Fever, general malaise, abdominal pain (+), bloody diarrhoea

PE T ↑, signs of shock, abdominal distention

Dx Abdominal contrast CT: colon dilatation to ≥6 cm, loss of haustration, pericolic fat stranding, pseudopolyps may protrude into the intestinal lumen due to intestinal wall ulcerations

Tx Parenteral nutrition, rehydration, consider corticosteroids (contraindicated in infectious colitis), consider biological in IBD patients, ABx

Subtotal colectomy

P Mortality 7.9-10%

! Beware of perforation → peritonitis → septic shock. Colon perforation increases mortality 3-5 fold. A colonoscopy is contraindicated due to the risk of perforation.

Diagnostic criteria for toxic megacolon:

1. Radiographic evidence of colonic dilatation ≥6 cm
2. Any 3 of the following: **a)** fever, **b)** tachycardia, **c)** leukocytosis, **d)** anaemia
3. Any of the following: **a)** hypotension, **b)** hypovolemia, **c)** altered mental status, **d)** electrolyte disorders

Chronic bowel diseases

Inflammatory bowel disease (IBD)

D IBDs are chronic diseases of the gastrointestinal tract affecting the mucosa and have an unpredictable clinical course. The diseases are characterised by quiet periods (remission) and flare-ups (exacerbation). Treatment goals are clinical remission (no symptoms), biochemical remission (low faecal calprotectin and CRP), endoscopic remission (no inflammation on colonoscopy/imaging), and a normal quality of life. IBD usually manifests between age 15-35, followed by a second peak between age 55-70. The two main entities are Crohn's disease and ulcerative colitis. When no distinction can be made between these two diseases, they are referred to as 'inflammatory bowel disease unclassified' (IBD-U). See Table 49 and Figure 67.

The typical patient with inflammatory bowel disease is a young adult who presents to their doctor with diarrhoea (possibly nocturnal), bloody stool, and abdominal pain. Patients may also present with microcytic anaemia and unintentional weight loss.

<table>
<tr><th></th><th>CROHN'S DISEASE</th><th>ULCERATIVE COLITIS</th></tr>
<tr><td>D</td><td>Bowel inflammation can occur from mouth to anus, affecting all layers of the intestinal wall. Affected areas are often scattered throughout the GI tract (see Figure 69). The rectum is often spared.</td><td>Bowel inflammation is limited to the colon, with the rectum always affected and inflammation extending further toward the caecum (see Figure 70).</td></tr>
<tr><td>E</td><td>Prevalence 500:100,000</td><td>Prevalence 50-150:100,000</td></tr>
<tr><td>Ae</td><td colspan="2">Unknown, possibly combination of genetic factors, environmental factors, diet, bacterial flora, and autoimmunity</td></tr>
<tr><td rowspan="2">R</td><td colspan="2">Positive family history, other autoimmune diseases (e.g. psoriasis, spondylarthritis)</td></tr>
<tr><td>Smoking</td><td>Smoking cessation</td></tr>
<tr><td rowspan="2">Hx</td><td colspan="2">Abdominal pain, general malaise, fever, fatigue, weight loss</td></tr>
<tr><td>Chronic diarrhoea (possibly bloody), mouth ulcers, perianal disorders such as fistulas and abscesses, malabsorption (skin turgor ↓, hair loss, oedema, muscle loss)</td><td>Chronic diarrhoea with blood and mucus (sometimes up to 30 x/d), urgency, incontinence</td></tr>
<tr><td rowspan="2">PE</td><td colspan="2">T ↑, abdominal tenderness, weight loss, extraintestinal manifestations: uveitis, arthritis, pyoderma gangrenosum, erythema nodosum (esp. in Crohn's disease)</td></tr>
<tr><td>Aphthous ulcers in the mouth, perianal disorders (fissure, abscess, fistula, skin tags: perianal Crohn's disease)</td><td>Rectal exam: sometimes blood on the glove</td></tr>
<tr><td rowspan="2">Dx</td><td colspan="2">• Labs: Hb ↓ (microcytic or normocytic), platelets ↑, albumin ↓, BSE ↑, WBC ↑, CRP ↑
• Faeces: calprotectin ↑↑ for disease monitoring, stool culture to rule out infection</td></tr>
<tr><td>• Colonoscopy: ulcers, cobblestones, alternating unaffected tissue (skip lesions), stenosis, pseudopolyps. In case of clinical suspicion with normal endoscopy, a video capsule endoscopy should be considered to rule out small bowel involvement. In patients with upper GI symptoms, upper endoscopy is recommended.
• Biopsy: granuloma formation, all layers intestinal wall affected, chronic inflammation
• Intestinal ultrasound: bowel wall thickening, hyperaemia, decreased motility
• Abdominal contrast CT or MRI: stenosis, fistula, abscess</td><td>• Colonoscopy or sigmoidoscopy: erythematous and oedematous mucosa, pseudopolyps, haemorrhages, ulcers, lesions starting immediately after the anorectal junction and continuing proximally
• Biopsy: chronically active inflammation, only mucosa and submucosa affected
• Intestinal ultrasound if inflammation reaches beyond the rectum: bowel wall thickening, hyperaemia, decreased motility
• Abdominal X-ray: only in acute severe ulcerative colitis to rule out toxic megacolon
• Abdominal contrast CT to rule out complications: perforation, abscess</td></tr>
</table>

Table 49A // Inflammatory bowel diseases

	CROHN'S DISEASE	ULCERATIVE COLITIS
Tx	Lifestyle changes: smoking cessation (esp. in Crohn's disease), dietary modifications. Relative contraindication to NSAIDs. No curative medication available. See Pharmacology for an overview of IBD medications, see Figure 68 for the step-up and top-down methods to treat IBD. Clinical and biochemical response to treatment should be assessed <12 wk after initiation of therapy, endoscopic evaluation can be considered 3–9 months after starting treatment to assess mucosal healing.	
	Surgery: ileocaecal resection, segmental resection, stricturoplasty, abscess drainage, fistula surgery, colectomy, ostomy. Stenosis: consider endoscopic balloon dilation.	Surgery: proctocolectomy, ostomy, ileal pouch-anal anastomosis
!	• In acute abdomen, consider a complicated course: toxic megacolon, perforation, or intra-abdominal abscess • Increased risk of colorectal carcinoma for which surveillance may be indicated, 8y after onset of disease, thereafter every 1, 3, or 5y • Psychosocial component and impact on quality of life: fatigue, irritable bowel, depression • Risk of primary sclerosing cholangitis ↑ (esp. in ulcerative colitis) • Recommend pneumococcal vaccine and yearly influenza vaccine, living vaccines should be avoided in patients treated with immunosuppressive therapy	

Table 49B // Inflammatory bowel diseases

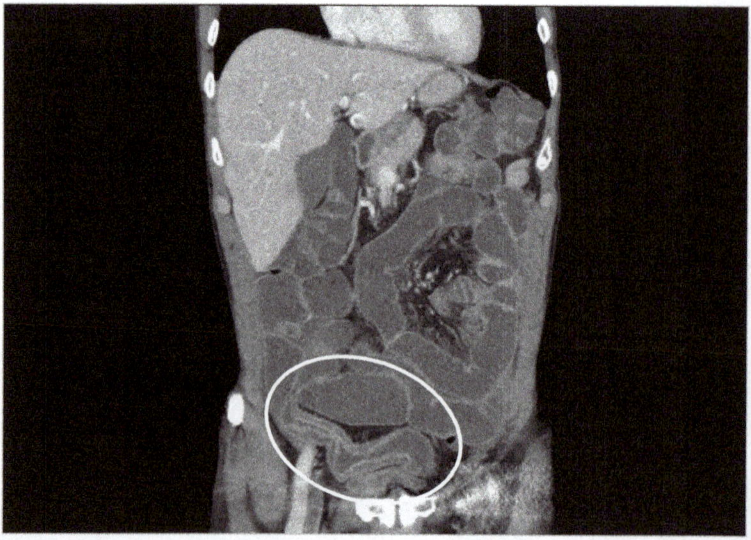

Figure 66 // Abdominal CT: terminal ileitis in Crohn's disease with dilated small intestine lumen

Inflammatory bowel disease is often abbreviated as IBD and should not be confused with irritable bowel syndrome (IBS).

Patients hospitalised with an IBD exacerbation are given prophylactic LMWHs to prevent venous thrombosis and embolisms. Nutrition is very important for patients hospitalised with an exacerbation. Consult a dietitian and start tube feeding at an early stage. Esp. in paediatric patients with IBD, exclusive enteral nutrition may have a therapeutic effect as well. Promptly consult a surgeon.

Acute severe ulcerative colitis (ASUC) is a serious complication that affects 20-25% of patients with ulcerative colitis; it is characterised by an increase in bloody stools and signs of systemic inflammation. The standard treatment for ASUC consists of intravenous corticosteroids. Infliximab or cyclosporine is added in patients with steroid-refractory ASUC. The Travis criteria can be used to identify patients who are at high risk of needing a colectomy during an episode of ASUC (see Appendix 2).

Step-up and top-down treatment:

- Step-up method: start with locally acting agents with mild adverse effects (aminosalicylates such as mesalazine for ulcerative colitis, topical corticosteroids like a budesonide enema). If ineffective, opt for a systemic corticosteroid, immunomodulator (e.g. thiopurine), and/or biological/small molecule.
- Top-down method: the most potent agents (biologicals or small molecules) are used first
- Accelerated use method: accelerated treatment option with most potent agents for IBD patients with large/deep ulcers, young patients, recurrence after bowel resection, extensive involvement of the proximal small intestine (Crohn's disease), or presence of symptomatic fistula (Crohn's disease). Surgical intervention is usually needed if medicated treatment fails.

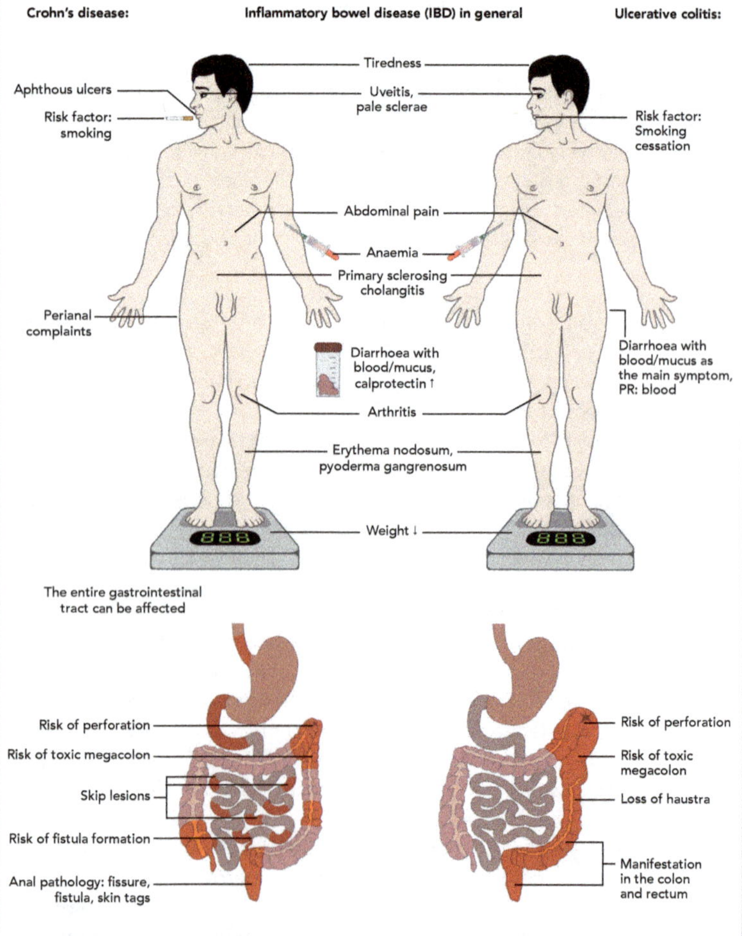

Figure 67 // Overview of the differences and similarities between Crohn's disease and ulcerative colitis

Medicated treatment for IBD consists of two phases: remission induction and maintenance treatment. See sections *Treatment* and *Pharmacological treatment* for an overview of medications used to treat IBD.

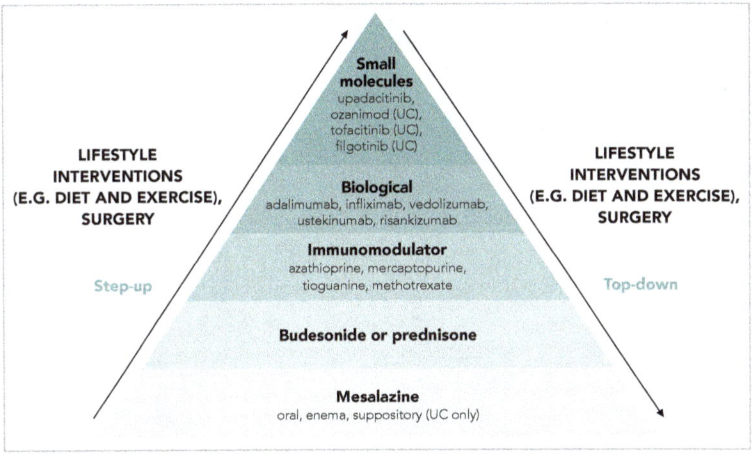

Figure 68 // Pyramid diagram of the step-up and top-down IBD therapies

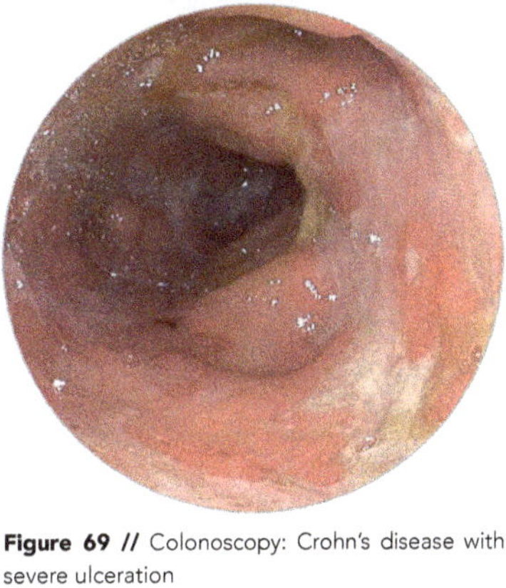

Figure 69 // Colonoscopy: Crohn's disease with severe ulceration

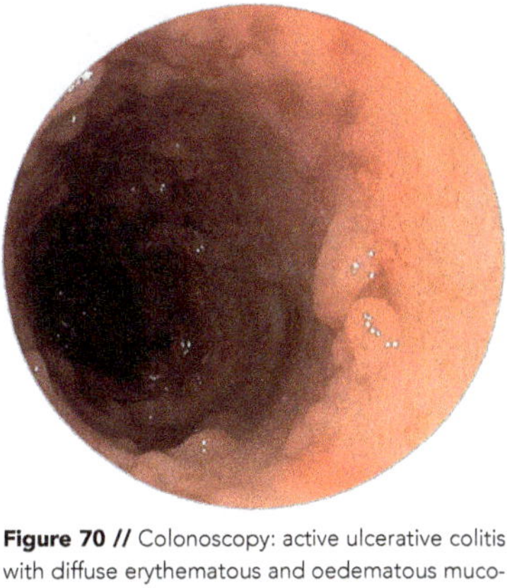

Figure 70 // Colonoscopy: active ulcerative colitis with diffuse erythematous and oedematous mucosa, ulceration, and extensive pseudopolyps

Proctitis

	IBD	STI	RADIATION PROCTITIS
D	Proctitis is inflammation of the mucous membrane lining the rectum and/or rectosigmoid (see Figure 71).		
E	30% of patients with IBD have proctitis	25% of men with an STI develop proctitis	10-20% of patients undergoing small-pelvis radiotherapy

Table 50A // Proctitis and its various causes

	IBD	STI	RADIATION PROCTITIS
Ae	Unknown, possibly combination of genetic factors, environmental factors, diet, bacterial flora, and autoimmune		
R	Ulcerative colitis (++), Crohn's disease, known IBD (+)	STIs (e.g. gonorrhoea, chlamydia), multiple sexual partners, sex work, receptive and unprotected anorectal sex	After small-pelvis radiotherapy, causing progressive epithelial atrophy and fibrosis → chronic mucosal ischaemia (prostate carcinoma (+)), combination of radiotherapy with chemotherapy, increasing with number of treatments
Hx	Rectal mucus or blood loss, anorectal pain		
	Bloody diarrhoea, increased urgency, faecal incontinence	Itching, constipation, receptive anorectal sex	Bloody diarrhoea, urgency ↑, abdominal or pelvic pain, tenesmus
PE	Rectal exam: painful, blood		
	No specific abnormalities	Inspect perianal region (ulcers, anal warts)	No specific abnormalities
Dx	Colonoscopy with biopsies: consistent with IBD, negative CMV PCR	Rectal swab	Endoscopy (colonoscopy or sigmoidoscopy): oedema, erythematous mucosa, telangiectasias (cause of blood loss), ulceration
Tx	Mesalazine or corticosteroid (suppository or enema)	ABx: e.g. ceftriaxone + doxycycline/azitromycine	Sucralfate enema (little evidence) Endoscopic therapy (e.g. coagulation) or hyperbaric oxygen therapy
P	Recurring problem	Good when treated with AB	Clinically challenging problem: some patients do not respond to any treatment option

Table 50B // Proctitis and its various causes

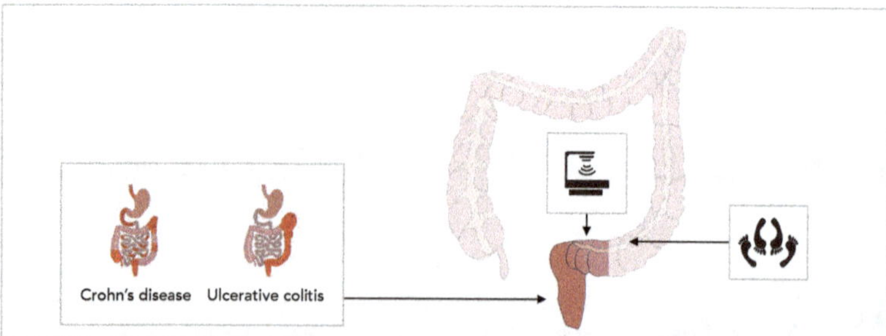

Figure 71 // Proctitis: possible causes

Anus and rectum

Anal fissure

D An anal fissure is a superficial lesion of the anodermis, usually in the posterior midline of the anal canal (see Figure 72). Laterally located fissures may indicate an underlying medical condition (e.g. infectious, immunosuppressive disorder, malignancy).

E Unknown, mostly affects infants and middle-aged patients

Ae Straining → superficial damage to the anodermis (acute fissure) → pain → internal sphincter tone ↑ → compression of the terminal branches of the inferior rectal artery → anodermal perfusion ↓ → healing ↓ → chronic fissure (6-8 wk) (vicious circle)

R Local trauma (e.g.constipation, vaginal delivery, anal intercourse, diarrhoea, Crohn's disease, granulomatous diseases (TBC, sarcoidosis), infectious diseases (HIV, syphilis), malignancy)

Hx Sharp pain during and after defaecation (<2h), bright red rectal bleeding, hard stools

PE Chronic fissures with a skin tag or sentinel pile, almost always in posterior midline, rectal exam will be extremely painful and should be avoided

Dx
- Clinical diagnosis. Additional diagnostics may be required when an underlying medical cause is suspected.
- Biopsy in all longstanding fissures: rule out malignancy

Tx Lifestyle recommendations: adequate intake of fluids, high-fibre diet, warm sitz baths

- Laxatives for constipation, local anaesthesia (lidocaine), local (i.e. intra-anal) nitrate ointment or calcium antagonist (diltiazem: internal sphincter tone ↓ → anodermal perfusion ↑)
- Botox injection (internal sphincter tone ↓ → anodermal perfusion ↑)
- Chemical denervation (injection of Botulinum A toxin): chemically paralyses the internal sphincter, which lowers the resting anal pressure and increases blood flow

Lateral internal sphincterotomy, fissurectomy with V-Y advancement flap

P Risk of developing chronic fissure ↑

! Beware of faecal incontinence after lateral internal sphincterotomy

The typical patient with anal fissure presents with severe pain during and after defaecation, in the absence of nocturnal pain. Bright red blood may be visible on toilet paper after wiping.

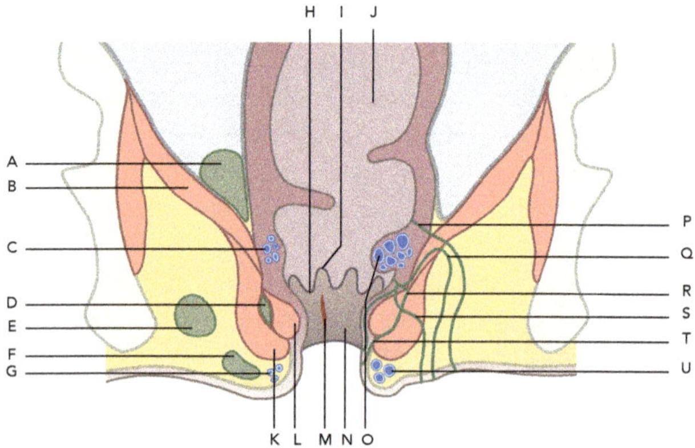

Figure 72 // Perianal pathology

A: Supralevator abscess **B:** Levator ani muscle **C:** Internal venous plexus **D:** Intersphincteric abscess **E:** Ischio-anal abscess **F:** Perianal abscess **G:** External venous plexus **H:** Crypt of Morgagni **I:** Dentate line **J:** Rectum **K:** External anal sphincter **L:** Internal anal sphincter **M:** Anal fissure **N:** Anal canal **O:** Internal haemorrhoid **P:** Extrasphincteric fistula **Q:** Suprasphincteric fistula **R:** Intersphincteric fistula **S:** Trans-sphincteric fistula **T:** Subcutaneous fistula **U:** External haemorrhoid

Haemorrhoids

D Haemorrhoids, or piles, are symptomatic prolapses of engorged tissue of the superior haemorrhoidal plexus (internal haemorrhoids) or inferior haemorrhoidal plexus (external haemorrhoids). External haemorrhoids (caudal to dentate line) are covered by anodermis (squamous epithelium of the anus), and only thrombosed haemorrhoids are symptomatic. Internal haemorrhoids (cephalad to dentate line) are covered by mucosa and are classified by the degree of prolapse (see Table 51 and Figure 73).

E Unknown

Ae Degeneration of supporting tissue → engorged tissue of the superior haemorrhoidal plexus prolapses → entrapment → venous drainage ↓ → congestion and oedema formation → pain → internal sphincter tone ↑ → congestion ↑ → pain ↑ (vicious circle)

R Intra-abdominal pressure ↑ (obesity, constipation, COPD, pregnancy/vaginal delivery, ascites, pelvic mass), middle age (45-65), sedentary lifestyle

Hx Bright red rectal bleeding (often on toilet paper), prolapse sensation, soiling (accidental loss of fluids/faeces through the anus), itching, pain (with thrombosis)

PE Protruding haemorrhoids (on straining), rectal exam: to rule out rectal tumour, only thrombosed haemorrhoids are palpable

Dx
- Proctoscopy: to rule out rectal tumour and to detect and treat haemorrhoids. Haemorrhoids are typically paired and located in the right posterior, right anterior, and left lateral locations.
- Colonoscopy to rule out malignancy in patients above a certain age (mostly >40-50y, cut-off varies between guidelines) presenting with rectal bleeding or other alarm symptoms

Tx Lifestyle recommendations: adequate intake of fluids, high-fibre diet, exercise, warm sitz baths

Laxatives for constipation, local anaesthetics and short-term corticosteroids for itching

- In patients with grade III and grade IV hemorrhoids and those with persistent symptoms despite conservative and office-based procedures
- Grade I-II: rubber band ligation (RBL), sclerotherapy, infrared coagulation
- Grade III: RBL, if ineffective see grade IV
- Grade IV: haemorrhoidectomy/haemorrhoidopexy

P High recurrence rate, risk of soiling and incontinence after haemorrhoidectomy

! DDx: rectal prolapse

CLASSIFICATION	FEATURES
Grade I	Does not prolapse when intra-abdominal pressure ↑, only visible on proctoscopy
Grade II	Prolapses when intra-abdominal pressure ↑, reduces spontaneously
Grade III	Prolapses spontaneously and/or when intra-abdominal pressure ↑, does not reduce spontaneously and must be manually reduced
Grade IV	Prolapses continuously, cannot be reduced manually, risk of strangulation

Table 51 // Classification of internal haemorrhoids

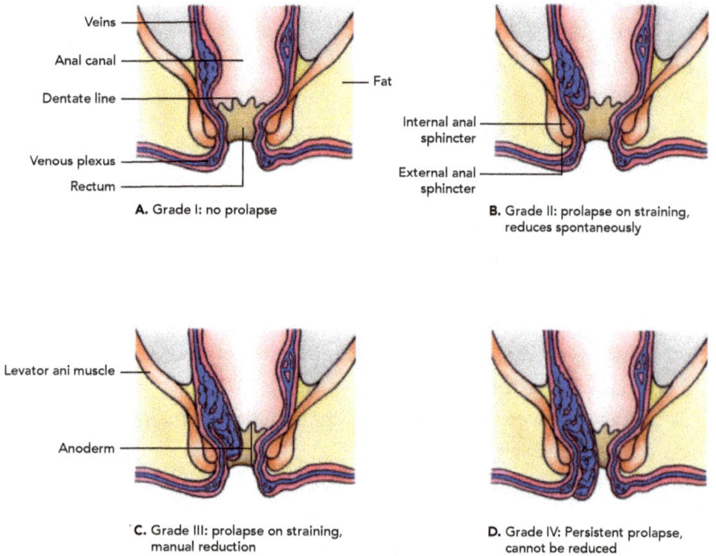

Figure 73 // Haemorrhoid classification
A: Grade I **B:** Grade II **C:** Grade III **D:** Grade IV

Perianal fistula

D A perianal fistula is a tunnel between the anal canal and the perianal skin, most often formed after a perianal abscess ruptures or is drained (see Figure 72).

E Incidence ♂ 12:100,000 per year, ♀ 5:100,000 per year

Ae Perianal abscess → drainage following path of least resistance → perianal fistula. Perianal fistulas can also occur without a previous perianal abscess.

R Perianal abscess ⊕, Crohn's disease ⊕, ♂, radiotherapy, obstetric injury, infectious diseases (HIV/TBC), malignancy, rectal foreign body

Hx Pain ⊕, intermittent perianal discharge, itching, faecal incontinence, lumps

PE External opening, internal fistula may be palpable during rectal exam, anal discharge (pus and/or blood)

Dx
- Local exam under anaesthesia
- MRI scan (fistula protocol): visualise tract and position relative to sphincters for surgical planning
- Endoanal or transperianal ultrasound performed by an experienced operator can be an alternative to MRI

Tx Depends on classification

- Simple fistula (low transsphincteric fistula, intersphincteric fistula, superficial fistula): fistulotomy (opening the fistula)
- Complex fistula (high transphincteric fistula, suprasphincteric fistula, extrasphincteric fistula, >1 fistula tract, recurrent fistulas, fistulas associated with infectious diseases (HIV/TBC) and Crohn's disease, anterior fistula in women, faecal incontinence present, or a history of regional radiation, obstetric trauma, or prior anorectal surgery): seton and ABx, dependent on localisation of fistula followed by ligation of intersphincteric fistula tract (LIFT), mucosal advancement flap, or proctectomy
- Refractory fistulas: consider stem cell therapy and hyperbaric oxygen therapy as alternative treatment options

P High recurrence rate, 30-50% faecal incontinence after surgical treatment

Risk factors for perianal fistula: **FRIENDS**

- **F**oreign body
- **R**adiation
- **I**nfection
- **E**pithelialisation
- **N**eoplasm
- **D**istal obstruction
- **S**teroid use

Hepatology

Acute liver failure

D Acute liver failure is characterised by elevated transaminases, impaired liver function (jaundice and INR >1.5), and hepatic encephalopathy in patients without pre-existing liver disease.

E Rare, high mortality

Ae R Hx PE Dx Tx See *Management of acute liver failure*

P 80% survival rate after liver transplantation, 55% without liver transplantation.

Hyperacute liver failure carries a lower risk of mortality than acute/subacute liver failure, but a higher risk of cerebral oedema.

I Possible complications: circulatory disorders (arrhythmias, hypotension), respiratory insufficiency, renal insufficiency (hepatorenal syndrome), pancreatitis, sepsis (multi-organ failure), cerebral oedema

In case of suspected drug-induced acute liver failure, notify the corresponding agency if available in your country:

EudraVigilance | FDA | Lareb

For a comprehensive roadmap for patients with acute liver failure, see *Management of acute liver failure.*

Autoimmune biliary diseases

	PRIMARY BILIARY CHOLANGITIS (PBC)	PRIMARY SCLEROSING CHOLANGITIS (PSC)
D	Progressive, immunologically mediated destruction of small intrahepatic bile ducts (see Figure 81).	Progressive, fibro-inflammatory disease of intrahepatic and/or extrahepatic bile ducts characterized by strictures and dilatations.
E	Rare, incidence 1.1:100,000 per year, ♂:♀ 1:9	Rare, incidence 0.5:100,000 per year, ♂:♀ 2:1
Ae	Immune-mediated liver disease, exact aetiology unknown	
R	Possible presence of concomitant autoimmune hepatitis features (AIH-PBC variant syndrome and AIH-PSC variant syndrome)	
	Peak age 40-60, 75% age >50, comorbidities: autoimmune diseases (e.g. Sjögren's syndrome, sicca syndrome, Raynaud's syndrome, thyroid disorders, coeliac disease, rheumatoid arthritis)	Peak age 40, comorbidity 50-80%: IBD (particularly ulcerative colitis)

Table 52A // Autoimmune biliary diseases

<table>
<tr><th></th><th>PRIMARY BILIARY CHOLANGITIS (PBC)</th><th>PRIMARY SCLEROSING CHOLANGITIS (PSC)</th></tr>
<tr><td rowspan="2">Hx</td><td colspan="2">Asymptomatic (+) in early stages, malaise, pruritus, jaundice</td></tr>
<tr><td>Fatigue (++)</td><td>RUQ pain, fatigue (−)</td></tr>
<tr><td rowspan="2">PE</td><td colspan="2">Non-specific symptoms (50%), as disease progresses:
jaundice, scratch marks, stigmata of liver cirrhosis</td></tr>
<tr><td>Skin lesions (e.g. xanthelasmata, dry skin, hyperpigmentation (25-50%))</td><td>Possible signs of IBD</td></tr>
<tr><td rowspan="2">Dx</td><td colspan="2">Labs: ALP ↑, GGT ↑, bilirubin =/↑, AST and ALT slightly ↑, labs may be consistent with
liver cirrhosis (platelets ↓, INR ↑, albumin ↓), see Diagram 10</td></tr>
<tr><td>• Labs: cholesterol ↑, IgG ↑, IgM ↑, AMA + (95%), ANA + (70%) (PBC-specific: anti-sp100, anti-gp210), centromere antibodies
• Liver biopsy: cholangitis of the interlobular and septal bile ducts, bile duct loss, granulomas</td><td>• Labs: ANA +/ANCA +, IgM ↑ (40-50%) (but not disease-specific), IgG4 if indicated
• MRCP: bile duct strictures and dilatations (string of pearls sign)
• Liver biopsy: little added value, yet diagnosis of small-duct PSC and AIH-PSC variant syndrome (5-10%) can only be made based on histology. Small duct can evolve into a large duct (−).</td></tr>
<tr><td>Tx</td><td>Surveillance of disease progression (elastography), osteoporosis (DEXA scan), HCC (in case of liver cirrhosis)
• First line: UDCA 13 mg/kg, consider treating osteoporosis and symptomatic treatment of itching (bezafibrate or rifampicin)
• Second line: add PPAR agonists (bezafibrate off-label, elafibranor, seladelpar), FXR agonists (obeticholic acid)
Liver transplantation</td><td>No treatment available (ursodeoxycholic acid (UDCA) at doses of 15-20 mg/kg/d improves liver tests and surrogate markers for prognosis, but beware: high doses of 28-30 mg/kg/d should not be given)
Yearly surveillance for IBD/colorectal carcinoma (colonoscopy) and gallbladder carcinoma (ultrasound/MRI), disease progression (elastography), osteoporosis (DEXA scan), HCC (in case of liver cirrhosis)
• ERCP in cases of severe stenosis (endoscopic balloon dilatation, stent placement)
• Liver transplantation</td></tr>
<tr><td>P</td><td>• Strongly improved with UDCA treatment, particularly in responders
• GLOBE score, Paris II score</td><td>Mayo risk score, median survival without liver transplantation: 13- 21y, worse prognosis if patient is symptomatic at time of diagnosis</td></tr>
<tr><td rowspan="2">!</td><td colspan="2">Possible complications: liver cirrhosis and its sequels,
HCC (in patients with liver cirrhosis), osteoporosis, vitamin deficiencies (A, D, E, K)</td></tr>
<tr><td>Patients should be evaluated for the development of disease progression</td><td>Beware of secondary bacterial cholangitis, colorectal carcinoma, cholangiocarcinoma, gallbladder carcinoma, strictures, peristomal varices (25% of patients that undergo proctocolectomy with ileostomy)</td></tr>
</table>

Table 52B // Autoimmune biliary diseases

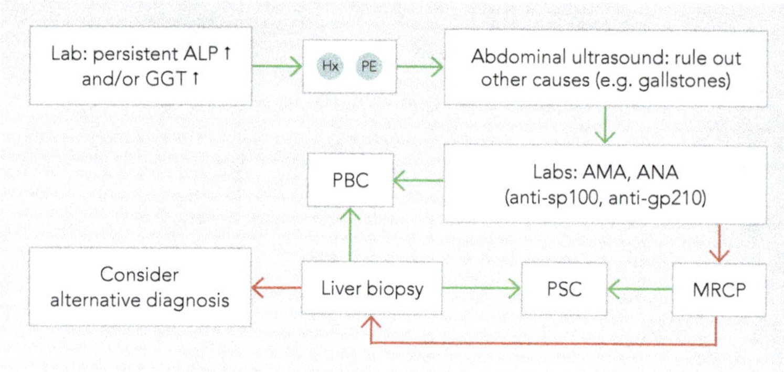

Diagram 10 // Dx in autoimmune biliary diseases

Autoimmune hepatitis (AIH)

D Autoimmune hepatitis is a progressive, chronic inflammatory liver disease characterised by autoimmune-mediated liver damage.

E Rare, European prevalence 17-23:100,000

Ae Idiopathic, autoimmune-mediated liver disease, likely involving the adaptive immune system, genetic factors, and extrinsic triggers such as drugs or infection

R ♀ (++), possible overlap with PBC or PSC, comorbidity: other autoimmune diseases (e.g. Graves' disease, rheumatoid arthritis, ulcerative colitis), peak age 40-75

Hx Highly heterogeneous presentation with nonspecific symptoms: asymptomatic (++), fatigue, malaise, appetite ↓, RUQ pain, joint pain, amenorrhoea

PE Highly heterogeneous presentation: liver cirrhosis (30% at first presentation), if liver cirrhosis: stigmata

Dx
- Labs: IgG ↑, AST ↑, ALT ↑, autoantibodies (ANA +, SMA +, LKM1 +, SLA +), possible: bilirubin ↑, ALP ↑, GGT ↑, labs may be consistent with liver cirrhosis, rule out viral hepatitis
- Liver biopsy (clinical standard for diagnosing AIH): interface hepatitis, portal lymphoplasmacytic hepatitis, lobular hepatitis, absence of histological features suggestive of other liver conditions

Tx Frequent lab testing to check for flare of activity, even if patient is stable
- Corticosteroids (prednisone 0.5-1.0 mg/kg) and immunosuppressants (first-line: azathioprine or mycophenolate mofetil as maintenance treatment, second-line: e.g. 6-mercaptopurine, third-line: e.g. tacrolimus)

- Liver transplantation for very severe and progressive liver disease despite treatment

P
- Vast majority of patients need lifelong treatment
- Timely diagnosis of the disease is crucial, as untreated AIH has a low 10-year survival rate

> Use the simplified criteria for diagnosing AIH.
> Scan the QR code.

Benign liver abnormalities

Liver abscess

D A liver abscess is an encapsulated collection of pus in the liver caused by bacteria (usually polymicrobial), parasites, or fungi. It can also develop after ischaemia or surgical trauma.

E Most common intra-abdominal abscess, incidence 2.3:100,000, ♀>♂, highest incidence in Asia

Ae Route of dissemination depends on the organism: intestines and bile ducts (*Escherichia coli, Klebsiella pneumoniae*, enterococci), hematogenous dissemination (streptococci, staphylococci). Less common pathogens: *Entamoeba histolytica*, fungi.

R DM, hepatobiliary disease, liver transplantation, poor dental hygiene

Hx Malaise, fever, chills, jaundice, nausea, vomiting, RUQ pain, appetite ↓, weight loss. Travel history (Africa, India, Central and South America for amoebiasis), recent surgery (abdominal or other), or dental treatment.

PE T ↑, jaundice, hepatomegaly, abdominal tenderness, rebound tenderness, possibly hypotension, and tachycardia in patients with sepsis

Dx
- Labs: abnormal liver test results (ALT ↑, AST ↑, ALP ↑, GGT ↑), elevated inflammation parameters (CRP ↑, WBC ↑), albumin ↓, blood cultures
- Abdominal ultrasound: variable appearance (hyper- to hypoechoic), often poorly demarcated, possibly gas bubbles
- Abdominal contrast CT (see Figure 74): collection with hypodense centre (fluid-filled) and peripheral enhancement, oedema of the surrounding liver parenchyma (double target sign)

- Aspiration or drainage sample analysis: microbiology (pathogen and antibiogram) and pathology (if malignancy in DDx)

Tx Broad-spectrum IV ABx (after taking cultures), usually for several weeks

Ultrasound or CT-guided drainage if possible, with drain placement. Flush the abscess over the drains frequently, check location of drain and collected volume when production declines or new fever spike occurs.

P Mortality 2-12%, higher with surgical drainage, underlying malignancy, or anaerobic infection

I Watch out for underlying colorectal malignancy or IBD in *Klebsiella pneumoniae* or *Streptococcus milleri*, watch out for pylephlebitis (rare) in portal vein thrombosis

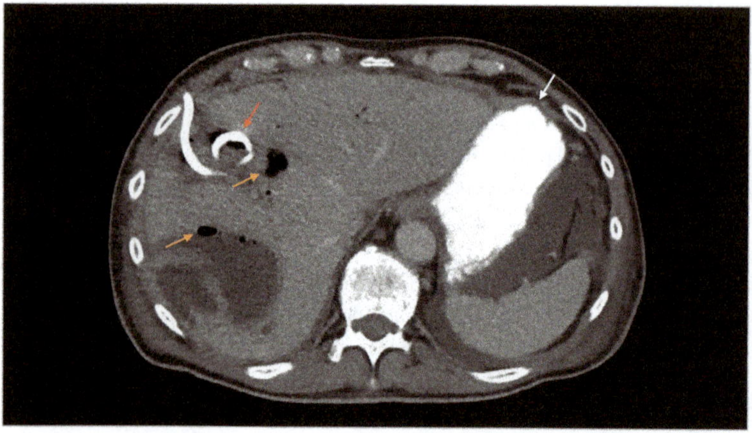

Figure 74 // Abdominal contrast CT and oral contrast in stomach (white arrow): liver abscess with air bubbles (orange arrows) and pigtail drain in the ventrally located abscess (red arrow). Note oral contrast is not indicated to visualise liver abscesses.

Hepatic adenoma

D A hepatic adenoma is a benign tumour of the liver consisting of densely packed, normally differentiated hepatocytes, without sinusoids or portal fields.

E Incidence 3-4:100,000 per year

Ae Oral contraceptives, pregnancy (oestrogen levels ↑ → adenoma)

R ♀, contraceptives, pregnancy, androgens, anabolic steroids, obesity

Hx Asymptomatic (<5 cm) ⊕, RUQ pain (>5 cm)

PE RUQ tenderness

Dx Liver contrast MRI (pref. with liver-specific contrast agent e.g. Primovist®): lesion with variable T1 characteristics, slightly hyperintense signal on T2 sequences, early arterial enhancement, and isointense to hypointense (in liver-specific contrast agent) on delayed images

Tx Stop hormonal medication

Indication for surgical resection/embolisation of hepatic artery: adenoma >5 cm (♀: wait for regression after discontinuing hormonal medication)

P Unknown, risk of malignant transformation ↑, risk of spontaneous rupture and bleeding ↑

! Adenoma rupture → life-threatening intraperitoneal haemorrhage

---

Hepatic cyst

D A hepatic cyst is a cavity filled with serous fluid that is lined with bile duct epithelium, and which is usually not connected to the intrahepatic bile ducts. Liver cysts vary in size from one to several centimetres and are usually an incidental finding. Patients with ten or more liver cysts are classified as polycystic liver disease.

E Most common benign hepatic abnormality alongside hepatic haemangiomas, prevalence 5-18%

Ae Congenital defect of the intrahepatic bile ducts, in which a dilated embryonic bile duct unconnected to the intrahepatic bile ducts forms a hepatic cyst

R ♂:♀ 1:1.5

Hx Asymptomatic ⊕, symptomatic in case of large or multiple hepatic cysts: mechanical symptoms in the upper abdomen (e.g. nausea, vomiting, heartburn, bloating)

PE Nonspecific, possibly palpable swelling and hepatomegaly

Dx Ultrasound, contrast CT, or MRI: hepatic cysts, inhomogeneous content in case of haemorrhagic component, assessment of wall thickening, septation, and/or nodular enhancement as possible signs of infection or malignancy

Tx Asymptomatic: wait-and-see

Somatostatin analogues for multiple small cysts scattered throughout the liver

- Symptomatic (choice of treatment depends on phenotype):
- Ultrasound-guided aspiration with sclerotherapy for large, superficial cysts
- Deroofing for multiple large ventral and caudal cysts

- Resection if several liver segments are severely affected and other segments are cyst-free
- Liver transplantation for very severe and disabling polycystic liver disease (e.g. severe malnutrition due to liver volume ↑)

P Mostly no effect on liver function

! Watch out for mucinous cystic neoplasms of the liver (♀), hepatic cyst infections (esp. for Echinococcus), and spontaneous haemorrhages, which may show different characteristics on imaging

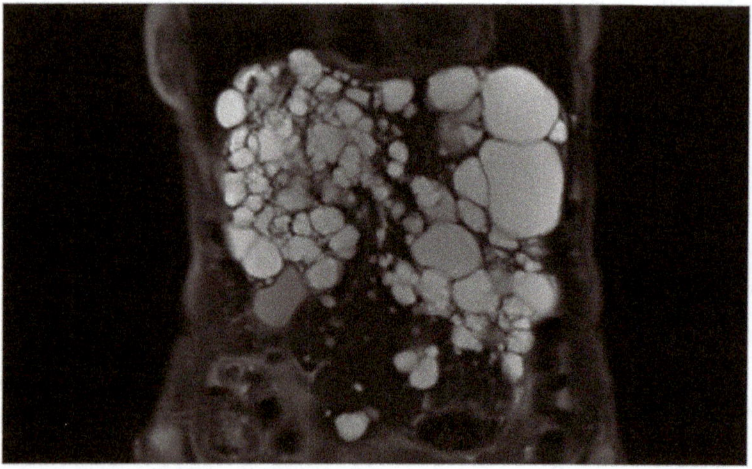

Figure 75 // Abdominal MRI T2-weighted images with fat suppression: multiple hepatic cysts (hyperintense). The liver is enlarged due to the space-occupying cysts.

Hepatic haemangioma

D A hepatic haemangioma is a benign, highly vascularised lesion, usually under five centimetres, arising from proliferation of endothelial cells.

E Most common benign liver abnormality, prevalence 10-20%, ±20% have multiple haemangiomas, usually an incidental finding

Ae Not fully known, may arise from congenital vascular malformations

R Oestrogen (e.g. pregnancy, oral contraceptives)

Hx Asymptomatic ⊕, nonspecific symptoms in hepatic haemangiomas >5 cm (giant haemangiomas) due to mechanical effect: epigastric pain, nausea, vomiting

PE No added value

Dx
- Ultrasound: often hyperechoic lesion, but can be variable
- Contrast MRI following liver protocol if ultrasound is inconclusive: nodular peripheral enhancement in arterial phase with enhancement comparable to liver parenchyma in portal venous phase

Tx Asymptomatic: wait-and-see

Symptomatic: surgical resection

P Complications are rare

! Consumptive coagulopathy (Kasabach-Merritt syndrome) with giant haemangioma (platelets ↓, fibrinogen ↓, fibrin degradation products ↑, erythrocyte fragmentation)

Haemochromatosis

D Haemochromatosis (iron overload) is characterised by uncontrolled intestinal iron absorption and the inability to mobilise absorbed iron in cells (decreased activity of iron homeostasis mechanisms). It occurs mainly in the liver, but can also affect the heart and pancreas, leading to organ damage. There is a hereditary and a secondary variant (see Figure 76).

E 10% of Northern European population carries the HFE gene, 0.5-1.5% is homozygous for C282Y mutation, His63Asp mutation ⊖. Onset in middle age (♂ age >40, ♀ age >50).

Ae Mutation in the HFE gene (C282Y) → hepcidin synthesis ↓ → excessive uptake from enterocytes and macrophages → circulating iron levels ↑ → accumulation in multiple organs (liver, pancreas, heart, testes, joints) → production of oxygen free radicals ↑ → organ damage

Hx
- Often nonspecific, depending on the organ affected, see Figure 76
- Asymptomatic (++), fatigue (++), muscle and joint pain, positive FHx

PE Hyperpigmentation (++), stigmata of liver cirrhosis, leg oedema

Dx
- Lab: ferritin ↑, iron ↑, transferrin ↑, transferrin saturation ↑ (>45%), total iron-binding capacity ↓
- DNA diagnostics: HFE gene mutations
- MRI with contrast according to liver protocol with iron quantification: serves to determine liver iron levels in patients with negative DNA diagnostics and persistently elevated ferritin without an alternative explanation
- Liver biopsy: needed to estimate degree of liver damage, not to set diagnosis

- Elastography: used to assess fibrosis stage, low liver stiffness measurement rules out advanced fibrosis
- Liver elastography: used for assessment of fibrosis stage, low liver stiffness measurement rules out advanced fibrosis

Tx Lifestyle recommendations: limit alcohol consumption, avoid obesity, avoid red meat, and foods high in vitamin C

- Start treatment in C282Y homozygous patients with transferrin saturation >45% with increased ferritin/AST/ALT. When transferrin saturation >45% with normal ferritin, AST and ALT, or in heterozygous patients, further evaluation is required before initiation of treatment.
- Iron chelation treatment (e.g. deferoxamine (iron bond ↑ → secretion ↑)), hepatitis B vaccination

Phlebotomy (guided by ferritin and transferrin saturation, this blood can also be donated if several criteria are satisfied), erythrocytapheresis

P Lifelong treatment is indicated to prevent organ damage

I Risk of liver fibrosis and cirrhosis ↑ with ferritin >1000 μg/L (see Figure 76)

Hepatitis

Viral hepatitis

	HEPATITIS A (HAV)	HEPATITIS B (HBV)
D	Hepatitis is an acute or chronic inflammation of the liver, causing liver cell damage and potentially leading to serious and irreversible damage.	
E	Worldwide, 1 in 3 individuals is infected with viral hepatitis, high prevalence in China, India, Indonesia, Nigeria, Pakistan, Ethiopia, Bangladesh, Vietnam, the Philippines, and Russia	
Ae	• Viral replication in hepatocytes → immune response • Acute (<6 mo): transient form with full recovery • Chronic (>6 mo): persistent with ongoing hepatitis, fibrosis, and risk of liver cirrhosis and HCC	
R	Faecal-oral transmission, 2-6 wk incubation period. Childhood, endemic areas (South America, Africa, Asia), poor hygiene, contaminated food and water.	Haematogenous transmission, 1-6 mo incubation period. Occurs worldwide, IV drug use, contact with contaminated body fluids through damaged skin and healthy mucous membranes, unprotected sexual intercourse. Babies born to hepatitis B carrier mothers.
Hx	30% of children and 70% of adults are symptomatic	10% of children and 40% of adults are symptomatic

Table 53A // Types of viral hepatitis

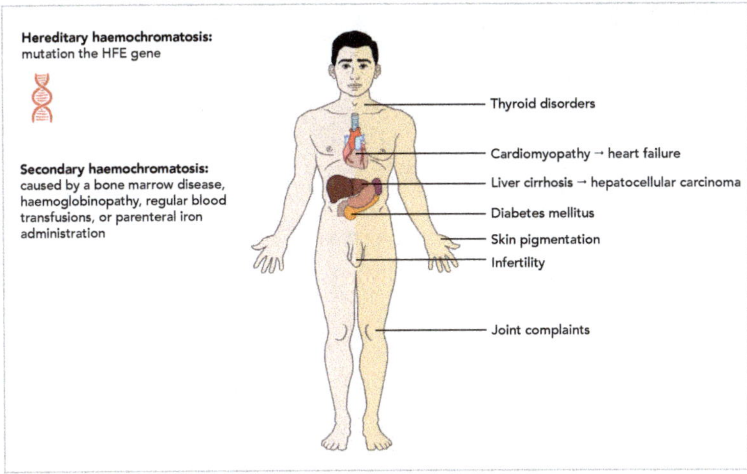

Figure 76 // Causes, symptoms, and complications of haemochromatosis

HEPATITIS C (HCV)	HEPATITIS D (HDV)
Hepatitis is an acute or chronic inflammation of the liver, causing liver cell damage and potentially leading to serious and irreversible damage.	
Worldwide, 1 in 3 individuals is infected with viral hepatitis, high prevalence in China, India, Indonesia, Nigeria, Pakistan, Ethiopia, Bangladesh, Vietnam, the Philippines, and Russia	
• Viral replication in hepatocytes → immune response • Acute (<6 mo): transient form with full recovery • Chronic (>6 mo): persistent with ongoing hepatitis, fibrosis, and risk of liver cirrhosis and HCC	
Haematogenous transmission, 15-150d incubation period. Seen worldwide but is esp. common in endemic areas, IV drug use, iatrogenic spread caused by unsterile procedures or blood products, anal sex.	Haematogenous transmission, 1-2 mo incubation time. Only in combination with hepatitis B infection.
30-50% symptomatic	Rarely symptomatic

<table>
<tr><th></th><th>HEPATITIS A (HAV)</th><th>HEPATITIS B (HBV)</th></tr>
<tr><td>Hx</td><td colspan="2">Symptoms include general malaise, fever, abdominal pain, nausea, jaundice, dark urine, light stools, itching, appetite ↓, fatigue</td></tr>
<tr><td>PE</td><td colspan="2">Liver cirrhosis: stigmata of liver cirrhosis</td></tr>
<tr><td rowspan="2">Dx</td><td colspan="2">• Labs: AST ↑ and ALT ↑ (liver cell destruction), labs may be consistent with liver cirrhosis; in case of cholestasis: bilirubin ↑, ALP ↑, GGT ↑, urobilin (urine) ↓
• Abdominal ultrasound or elastography: in suspected liver cirrhosis</td></tr>
<tr><td>Anti-HAV IgM and IgG</td><td>HBs antigen (HBsAg), HBe antigen (HBeAg), HBV DNA. If indicated: anti-HBs (antibody titre for vaccination, lifelong protection at >10 IU/L), anti-HBc (chronic or cleared infection), see Figure 77 for clinical course.</td></tr>
<tr><td rowspan="2">Tx</td><td colspan="2">Preventive: active/passive immunisation</td></tr>
<tr><td>No curative treatment</td><td>For specific groups: nucleoside/nucleotide analogues, possibly experimental new drugs</td></tr>
<tr><td>P</td><td>Self-limiting, no chronic form, 10% recurrence rate</td><td>• Chronic form: 90% of newborns, 25-30% of children aged <5, <5% of adults
• 95% self-limiting in adults</td></tr>
</table>

Table 53B // Types of viral hepatitis

	HEPATITIS E (HEV)
D	Hepatitis is an acute or chronic inflammation of the liver, causing liver cell destruction and potentially leading to serious and irreversible damage.
E	20,000,000 per year, most common in Southeast Asia
Ae	• Viral replication in hepatocytes → immune response • Acute (<6 mo): transient form with full recovery • Chronic (>6 mo): persistent with ongoing hepatitis, fibrosis, and risk of liver cirrhosis
R	Faecal-oral transmission, 2-8 wk incubation period
Hx	• Asymptomatic • Symptoms include general malaise, fever, abdominal pain, nausea, jaundice, dark urine, light stools, itching, appetite ↓, fatigue

Table 53C // Types of viral hepatitis

HEPATITIS C (HCV)	HEPATITIS D (HDV)
Symptoms include general malaise, fever, abdominal pain, nausea, jaundice, dark urine, light stools, itching, appetite ↓, fatigue	
Liver cirrhosis: stigmata of liver cirrhosis	
• Labs: AST ↑ and ALT ↑ (liver cell destruction), labs may be consistent with liver cirrhosis; in case of cholestasis: bilirubin ↑, ALP ↑, GGT ↑, urobilin (urine) ↓ • Abdominal ultrasound or elastography: in suspected liver cirrhosis	
Anti-HCV, HCV-RNA	Anti-HDV, HDV-RNA
• No immunisation • Direct-acting antiviral (DAA) therapy	• No specific HDV immunisation • HBV immunisation confers immunity to HDV • Only with symptoms/abnormal liver function: interferon • Treatment of HBV, no specific treatment of HDV
• 80% have chronic form • Sustained virological response after 8-12 wk of treatment: >95% • Antibodies don't confer immunity	• With co-infection, 5% have chronic form, with superinfection 90% • Fastest progression to liver cirrhosis, HCC, and mortality

CYTOMEGALOVIRUS (CMV)	EPSTEIN-BARR VIRUS (EBV)
Hepatitis is an acute or chronic inflammation of the liver, causing liver cell destruction and potentially leading to serious and irreversible damage.	
45-95% of fertile women worldwide have antibodies	90% of adults worldwide have antibodies
• Viral replication in hepatocytes → immune response • Acute (<6 mo): transient form with full recovery • Chronic (>6 mo): persistent with ongoing hepatitis, fibrosis, and risk of liver cirrhosis	
Faecal-oral and haematogenous transmission, 1-3 mo incubation period. Peaks at infant, toddler and adolescent age, close contact with young children.	Transmission via saliva, 32-40 d incubation period. Peak age <5, adolescents and young adults.
Asymptomatic (++), sore throat, fever, lymphadenopathy, jaundice (−)	• Asymptomatic (++) • Symptoms depend on age: sore throat, fever, and lymphadenopathy common in young adults, jaundice and signs of hepatitis more common in elderly patients

	HEPATITIS E (HEV)
PE	Jaundice, RUQ pain
Dx	• Labs: AST ↑ and ALT ↑ (liver cell destruction), labs may be consistent with liver cirrhosis; in case of cholestasis: bilirubin ↑, ALP ↑, GGT ↑, urobilin (urine) ↓ • Abdominal ultrasound or elastography: in suspected liver cirrhosis Anti-HEV IgM and IgG, HEV RNA
Tx	• No curative treatment • Severe acute hepatitis, acute-on-chronic liver failure, immunocompromised patients, or chronic hepatitis: ribavirin • No vaccine
P	Generally self-limiting, 50-60% of immunocompromised patients have chronic form

Table 53D // Types of viral hepatitis

EBV: VCA is short for viral capsid antigen and EBNA is the nuclear antigen of EBV. Testing for antibodies to these antigens makes it possible to distinguish between acute EBV infection (IgM-VCA and IgG-VCA positive, Ig-EBNA negative) and a transmitted infection (IgM-VCA negative, IgG-VCA positive, Ig-EBNA positive). IgG-VCA and Ig-EBNA remain detectable for life.

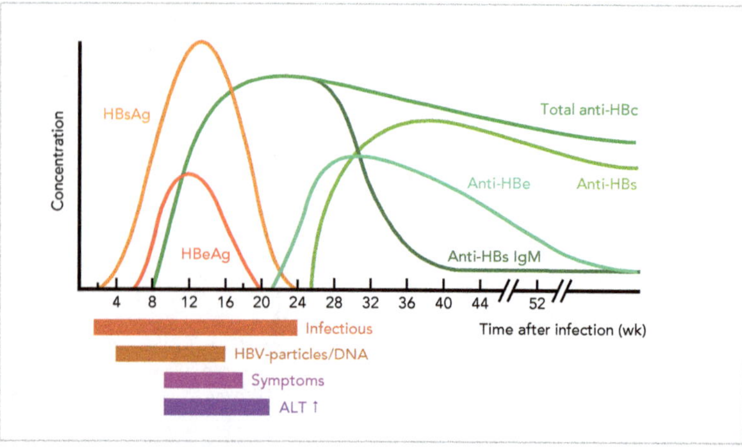

Figure 77 // Hepatitis B serology

CYTOMEGALOVIRUS (CMV)	EPSTEIN-BARR VIRUS (EBV)
T ↑, lymphadenopathy, pharyngitis, exanthema, RUQ pain ⊖, jaundice ⊖	• Adolescents: T ↑, lymphadenopathy, pharyngitis, exanthema • Elderly: RUQ pain, jaundice
• Labs: AST ↑ and ALT ↑ (liver cell destruction), labs may be consistent with liver cirrhosis; in case of cholestasis: bilirubin ↑, ALP ↑, GGT ↑, urobilin (urine) ↓ • Abdominal ultrasound or elastography: in suspected liver cirrhosis	
Anti-CMV IgM and IgG, CMV-DNA	IgM-VCA, IgG-VCA, Ig-EBNA, anti-EBV-EA, or PCR virus detection
For immunocompromised patients: e.g. ganciclovir, valganciclovir	
Generally self-limiting	

Alcoholic hepatitis

D Alcoholic hepatitis is a clinical syndrome characterised by onset of jaundice within three months with possible other signs of decompensated liver disease (e.g. ascites) in patients with long-term excessive alcohol consumption.

E Incidence 20% of heavy alcohol users

Ae 90% of heavy alcohol users develop steatosis, which can be associated with hepatitis. Alcoholic hepatitis is a more severe, inflammatory form of liver damage: Kupffer cell activation (hepatic macrophages) → hepatocyte swelling, neutrophilic infiltration, and formation of Mallory-Denk bodies.

R Alcohol consumption >100 g/d (= 6-7 units), age 40-50, possible genetic predisposition, malnourishment, obesity, environmental factors (e.g. low socioeconomic status, unemployment, stress). Alcoholic hepatitis can also develop after heavy alcohol consumption for a short period.

Hx Jaundice ⊕, fever, general malaise, RUQ pain, vomiting, appetite ↓, weight ↓, symptoms consistent with decompensated liver disease

PE Jaundice, T ↑, poor personal hygiene, hepatomegaly, weight ↓ (malnourishment), proximal muscle atrophy and poor grip strength, possible signs of decompensated liver disease, GCS in case of altered consciousness

Dx
- Labs: bilirubin ↑ (total bilirubin >50 µmol/L, essential for diagnosis), AST and ALT ↑ (both usually 50-400 IU/L, AST:ALT ratio ≥1.5), GGT ↑ (> 100 IU/L), ALP ↑, macrocytic anaemia, WBC ↑ (esp. neutrophils), CRP ↑, ferritin ↑, tri-

glycerides ↑, labs may be consistent with liver cirrhosis

- Abdominal ultrasound: rule out other causes of cholestasis (e.g. obstructing gallstones or intrahepatic lesions) and check hepatic vein patency
- Rule out viral hepatitis by serological testing
- When in doubt: liver biopsy

Tx
- Lifestyle recommendations: stop alcohol use immediately (monitor for alcohol withdrawal syndrome, see *Alcohol-related conditions*), high-protein, high-calorie diet (possibly by feeding tube)
- Consult with transplantation centre at first presentation
- Vitamin supplementation (vitamin B-complex, vitamin C, vitamin B1 (thiamine) and vitamin K if necessary)
- Consider corticosteroids for patients with a MELD score ≥18 or a Maddrey score ≥32, evaluate the effect of corticosteroids >1 wk using Lille score, in responders continue corticosteroids for 4 wk, if not consider liver transplantation
- Consider N-acetylcysteine in cases of severe alcoholic hepatitis

P One-month mortality up to 50% in cases of severe alcoholic hepatitis. Many patients with alcoholic hepatitis also have diagnosed/undiagnosed liver cirrhosis.

> Patients may have stopped consuming alcohol for days to weeks prior to the onset of alcoholic hepatitis symptoms, so always make sure by taking a thorough alcohol use history.

> If AST >400 IU/L, rule out DILI.

> See *www.mdcalc.com* for how to calculate the Maddrey, Lille, and MELD scores. Scan the QR code.

Drug-induced liver injury (DILI)

<table>
<tr><th colspan="6">DRUG-INDUCED LIVER INJURY (DILI)</th></tr>
<tr><td>D</td><td colspan="5">Liver damage (usually acute hepatitis) secondary to prescription or non-prescription medication.</td></tr>
<tr><td>E</td><td colspan="5">1-19:100,000, most common cause acute liver failure, 10% of acute hepatitis is caused by DILI</td></tr>
<tr><td rowspan="6">Ae</td><td>Direct</td><td colspan="3">Idiosyncratic</td><td>Indirect</td></tr>
<tr><td rowspan="3">• Directly hepatotoxic medication
• Dose-dependent
• Predictable
• Occurs soon after use</td><td colspan="3">• Non-intrinsically hepatotoxic medication
• Unpredictable
• Can occur immediately or up to months after use
• Immune-mediated form usually develops sooner (weeks) than metabolic form (months)</td><td rowspan="3">• Effect of the drug produces liver damage
• Unpredictable
• Occurs weeks to months after use</td></tr>
<tr><td>Immune-mediated</td><td>Metabolic</td><td>Auto-immune</td></tr>
<tr><td>• Allergic
• Can cause Stevens-Johnson syndrome or toxic epidermal necrolysis in severe cases</td><td>Probably caused by abnormal metabolism due to genetic factors</td><td>Body responds to reactive metabolites formed by hepatic metabolism as foreign substances</td></tr>
<tr><td colspan="5">Examples</td></tr>
<tr><td>Paracetamol</td><td>Penicillin</td><td>Amiodarone</td><td>Nitrofurantoin</td><td>Tamoxifen</td></tr>
<tr><td>R</td><td colspan="5">Excessive alcohol use, medication interactions, certain genetic polymorphisms of CYP enzymes (hepatic metabolism), and HLA antigens</td></tr>
<tr><td>Hx</td><td colspan="5">• Detailed medication history (OTC medicines, natural remedies (mushrooms, herbs, teas, alternative medicines), dietary supplements, drug use)
• Asymptomatic ⊕, RUQ pain, nausea, vomiting, features associated with cholestasis (jaundice, clay-coloured stools, dark urine, itching)
• Immune-mediated: skin rash, fever, joint pain, lymphadenopathy</td></tr>
<tr><td>PE</td><td colspan="5">Hepatomegaly, if disease progresses to liver cirrhosis: stigmata of liver cirrhosis, possible signs of decompensated liver disease</td></tr>
<tr><td>Dx</td><td colspan="5">• Lab:
- Hepatocellular DILI → ALT ↑ (normally 3x ULN), ALT:ALP ≥5
- Cholestatic DILI → ALP ↑ (normally 2x ULN), ALT:ALP ≤2
- Mix of the above (ALP:ALT = 2:5)
- Rule out other causes: viral hepatitis, autoimmune hepatitis, Wilson's disease, Budd-Chiari syndrome, ischaemic liver injury
• When in doubt: liver biopsy (histological findings differ according to mechanism of DILI and are therefore not diagnostic but rather helpful in ruling out other causes of liver injury)</td></tr>
<tr><td>Tx</td><td colspan="5">Discontinue medication, record contraindication in hospital system and specify reason
• N-acetylcysteine for paracetamol intoxication (start immediately, do not wait for labs, and even if serum paracetamol concentration is low).
• Corticosteroids for autoimmune idiosyncratic DILI</td></tr>
</table>

Table 54A // Drug-induced liver injury (DILI)

DRUG-INDUCED LIVER INJURY (DILI)	
P	• Patients usually recover after medication is discontinued • In some cases, patients may even recover despite continued exposure (adaptation) • In severe cases, the liver does not recover after medication is discontinued, causing acute liver failure and necessitating liver transplantation • Prognostic factors for poor outcomes: jaundice with ALT ↑ (normally 3x the ULN), acute liver failure due to antiepileptic drugs in children, acute liver failure due to paracetamol, pre-existing hepatic pathology, African American descent • Cholestatic liver damage has a better prognosis than hepatocellular liver damage

Table 54B // Drug-induced liver injury (DILI)

Visit 'LiverTox' for a list of hepatotoxic prescription and nonprescription medications and dietary supplements. Scan the QR code.

Liver cirrhosis

D Liver cirrhosis is a late stage of progressive liver fibrosis and is characterised by changes in liver structure (fibrosis bridges and regenerative nodules), resulting in impaired liver function (see Figure 78). Decompensated liver cirrhosis is a complication of liver cirrhosis. Possible complications include variceal haemorrhage, ascites, spontaneous bacterial peritonitis, hepatic encephalopathy, hepatocellular carcinoma, hepatorenal syndrome, and hepatopulmonary syndrome.

E
- Prevalence 100:100,000
- Every year, ±5-11% of patients with liver cirrhosis develop decompensated cirrhosis

Ae Many causes of liver disease can result in liver cirrhosis due to e.g. chronic inflammation or cholestasis. Most common causes: viral hepatitis (hepatitis B, C), alcoholic liver disease, haemochromatosis, MASLD. Other causes: autoimmune hepatitis, PBC, PSC, cystic fibrosis, haemochromatosis, Wilson's disease, alpha-1 antitrypsin deficiency, medication, veno-occlusive disease (Budd-Chiari syndrome), cardiac cirrhosis.

R Risk factors for decompensated liver cirrhosis: haemorrhage, infection, alcohol consumption, hepatotoxic medication, dehydration (e.g. due to diuretics), constipation, obesity

Hx
- Asymptomatic, nonspecific symptoms: general malaise, fatigue, weight ↓, appetite ↓, possible muscle cramps, anovulation (♀), hypogonadism (♂)

- Advanced liver cirrhosis or decompensated liver cirrhosis: jaundice, itching, signs of possible complications (e.g. variceal haemorrhage, ascites, hepatic encephalopathy)

PE
- General: BP ↓, muscle weakness, sluggishness
- Inspection: jaundice, spider naevi, palmar erythema, gynaecomastia (♂), testicular atrophy (♂), caput medusae, oedema, asterixis (flapping tremor)
- Palpation: liver feels firm and bumpy, hepatomegaly, splenomegaly ⊖
- Advanced liver cirrhosis or decompensated liver cirrhosis: including hepatic foetor, hepatic encephalopathy, jaundice, ascites

Dx
- Labs: platelets ↓, INR ↑, albumin ↓, Na^+ ↓, total protein ↓, AST =/slightly ↑, ALT =/slightly ↑, bilirubin =/↑, ALP =/↑ (2-3x ULN is normal), GGT =/↑, later: Hb ↓, WBC ↓, creatinine ↑
- Abdominal ultrasound: nodular thickening of liver capsule, inhomogeneous liver parenchyma, portal venous flow ↓, spleen size, also used for HCC screening
- Elastography: stage of fibrosis (see Diagnostics)
- Abdominal contrast CT: liver volume ↓ and change in liver segment volume ratios (hypertrophic caudate lobe), heterogeneous enhancement of liver parenchyma, nodular aspect of liver surface, ascites, splenomegaly, possibly recanalisation of the umbilical vein, and paraoesophageal varices
- Liver biopsy: fibrous margins, nodular rounding of the liver parenchyma, large sections of connective tissue, absence of normal portal triads
- In decompensated liver cirrhosis: rule out eliciting factor for decompensation (see R), investigate specific complications (see below)

Tx
- Treatment goal: treating the underlying liver disease (aetiological analysis) and preventing further damage (e.g. portal hypertension or HCC), screening for complications (HCC, oesophageal varices)
- In decompensated liver cirrhosis: pursue liver recompensation, depending on complications
- Stop alcohol use, stop hepatotoxic drugs
- Prophylaxis of oesophageal varices: non-selective beta blockers
- Vaccinations for HAV and HBV to prevent further liver injury

Liver transplantation

P Chance of progression to chronic liver disease, risk of HCC ↑ (1:3 lifetime prevalence of developing HCC), high mortality, measured by Child-Pugh classification and MELD score (see Appendix 2)

I Watch out for primary HCC, decompensated liver cirrhosis, oesophageal varices

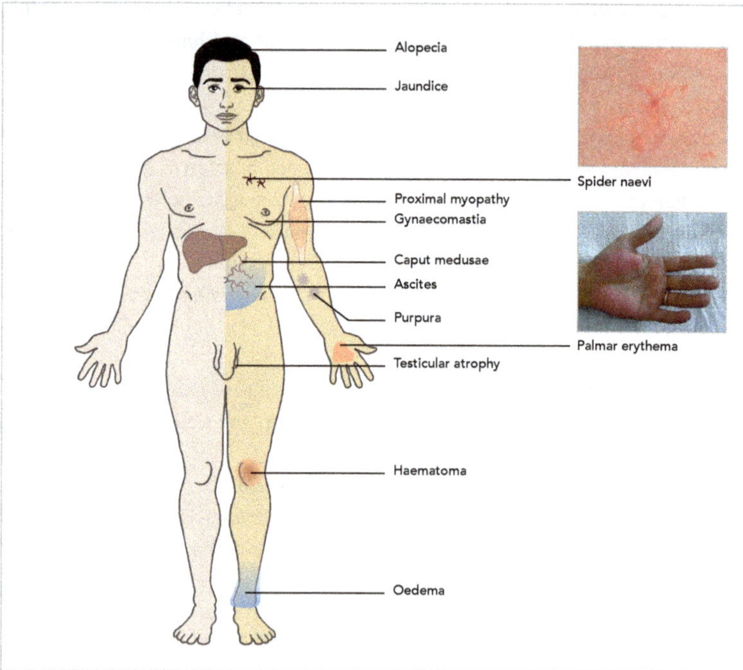

Figure 78 // Stigmata of liver cirrhosis

Liver cirrhosis complicated by ascites

D Ascites is the pathological accumulation of fluid in the abdominal cavity resulting from e.g. portal hypertension in liver cirrhosis.

E 50% of patients with liver cirrhosis develop ascites <10y

Ae In liver cirrhosis (hepatic, 85%): portal hypertension (>8 mmHg) → splanchnic vasodilation → RAAS activation → Na^+ and H_2O retention → oncotic pressure ↓ → fluid shift in peritoneal cavity → ascites

R Hepatic cirrhosis with portal hypertension, alcohol use disorder

Hx Increased abdominal girth (see Figure 78), weight ↑, abdominal discomfort (occasionally pain), feeling full, early satiety, shortness of breath, feeling of decreased mobility, ankle oedema

PE
- Inspection: increased abdominal girth, dilated flanks, flat navel
- Percussion: shifting dullness
- Palpation: undulation

Dx • Abdominal ultrasound: presence and semi-quantification of ascites
• Diagnostic paracentesis: analyse ascites to rule out spontaneous bacterial peritonitis (SBP), malignancy, albumin level (transudate/exudate; see the Appendix 1, Paracentesis)

Tx Lifestyle recommendations: stop alcohol use, low-sodium diet

Diuretics (monotherapy spironolactone or combination therapy spironolactone with furosemide, 100:40 mg)

Large volumes of ascites leading to mechanical distress (dyspnoea, reduced mobility due to abdominal girth) are an indication for therapeutic drainage (first rule out SBP, beware of potential coagulation disorder); with >5L ascites, therapeutic paracentesis with IV albumin according to local protocol

P 5-year mortality 36-43%

Hepatic encephalopathy

D Hepatic encephalopathy is a reversible neuropsychiatric syndrome caused by metabolic changes in cases of advanced liver dysfunction.

E 30-40% of patients with cirrhosis will experience hepatic encephalopathy at least once

Ae Hepatic cell damage (acute/chronic) → liver insufficiency, portosystemic collateral circulation and eliciting factor (haemorrhage, sedatives, infection) → degradation of toxic substances ↓ → ammonia (NH_3) ↑ → excessive conversion to glutamate ↑ → GABA activity ↑, cerebral oedema, oxidative stress, changes in blood-brain barrier → coma

R Combination of severe liver failure, extent of portosystemic shunting (TIPS), and triggers (GI haemorrhage ⊕, infections, constipation, dehydration, medication)

Hx PE Depends on severity (West Haven criteria, see Table 55), possible jaundice, stigmata of liver cirrhosis

Dx Labs: NH_3^+ ↑ (only if indicated, clinical diagnosis), EEG: slowing of background activity, triphasic waves and rule out non-convulsive seizures

Tx Symptomatic treatment, ICU admission (preventive intubation if encephalopathy progresses to coma), treat triggers/precipitating factors, avoid morphine and sedatives

Lactulose (oral and/or rectal, depending on grade) → ammonia absorption ↓, consider adding rifaximin in case of recurring episodes

Liver transplantation

GRADE	MENTAL STATUS
0	No confusion
1	Slight confusion, euphoria/anxiety, concentration ↓, changes in sleeping habits, irritability
2	Lethargy/apathy, disorientation to time and place, personality changes, inappropriate behaviour, apraxia, tremor
3	Somnolence, responsive to stimuli, confusion, disorientation to time and place, bizarre behaviour, speech disorder
4	Coma

Table 55 // West Haven criteria for grading hepatic encephalopathy

Patients with hepatic encephalopathy are prescribed lactulose to inhibit intestinal ammonia production and uptake. Lactulose lowers pH in the small intestine, resulting in reduced ammonia production by gut bacteria. Its laxative effect shortens the time for ammonia absorption. Keep the minimum dose of lactulose to obtain 2 evacuations/day, reduce in case of diarrhoea.

Hepatorenal syndrome (HRS)

	HRS TYPE 1	HRS TYPE 2
D	Hepatorenal syndrome (HRS) is characterised by renal insufficiency in patients with liver cirrhosis and ascites, having ruled out other causes of renal insufficiency. This makes HRS a diagnosis of exclusion. See Appendix 3 for the diagnostic and therapeutic pathway.	
	HRS type 1 is now defined as HRS-AKI: absolute increase in serum creatinine ≥0.3 mg/dl within 48h or increase in serum creatinine >1.5 times baseline level; or urinary output <0.5 ml/kg/h for 6h	HRS type 2 is now defined as HRS-CKD: eGFR <60 ml/min/1.73 m^2 for ≥3 mo in the absence of other (structural) causes
E	Incidence: 10% of patients hospitalised with liver cirrhosis and ascites	
Ae	Liver cirrhosis, portal hypertension → permeability of the intestinal mucosa ↑ → barrier function ↓ → chronic inflammation → plasma levels of inflammatory mediators and vasodilators ↑ → systemic vasodilation → systemic vascular resistance ↓, hypotension → RAAS and sympathetic activation → renal vasoconstriction → eGFR ↓	
R	Hepatic cirrhosis (++), spontaneous bacterial peritonitis, GI haemorrhage, diuretics, NSAID	Liver cirrhosis (++), refractory ascites (++)

Table 56A // Hepatorenal syndrome

	HRS TYPE 1	HRS TYPE 2
Hx	General malaise, oliguria/anuria ⊕, fatigue, weight ↓, appetite ↓	
PE	BP ↓, stigmata of liver cirrhosis, signs of possible other complications of liver cirrhosis	
Dx	Labs: creatinine >133 µmol/L or >50% increase between baseline and 2 wk	Labs: creatinine >133 µmol/L
Tx	Terlipressin (vasoconstrictor, watch out for severe adverse effects (e.g. ischaemia)) + albumin Liver transplantation	
P	• Mortality without transplantation: 3-9 wk • Possibly reversible if spotted early and treated with vasoconstriction and albumin for volume expansion	2-year mortality without transplantation: 42-70%

Table 56B // Hepatorenal syndrome

Criteria for hepatorenal syndrome:

- Liver cirrhosis with ascites
- No shock
- No hypovolaemia (no improvement after 48h of fluid expansion with albumin and withdrawal of diuretics)
- No recent use of nephrotoxic drugs
- No renal or postrenal explanation for AKI

A patient with liver cirrhosis has **acute-on-chronic liver failure** (AoCLF) when an eliciting event leads to acute deterioration of liver function. The main difference between AoCLF and decompensated liver cirrhosis is the degree of reversibility, hence the prognosis. If spotted on time, liver function may be reversible in AoCLF, as opposed to decompensated liver cirrhosis, for which liver transplantation is the only curative treatment.

Spontaneous bacterial peritonitis (SBP)

D SBP is acute or subacute inflammation of the peritoneum with neutrophilic granulocytes in ascites, without another intra-abdominal inflammatory focus or malignancy.

E Incidence 7-30% patients hospitalised with liver cirrhosis and ascites

Ae Liver cirrhosis, portal hypertension → permeability of intestinal mucosa ↑ → barrier function ↓ → translocation of intestinal bacteria to abdominal cavity → infected ascitic fluid

R Hepatic cirrhosis ⊕⊕, GI haemorrhage ⊕, infection elsewhere, prior episodes of SBP

Hx Asymptomatic ⊕⊕, abdominal pain ⊕, fever ⊕ and chills, general malaise, vomiting, diarrhoea, ileus, unexplained clinical deterioration

PE Fragile, T ↑, ascites, abdominal tenderness, irritated abdomen ⊖

Dx
- Labs: eGFR ↓, CRP ↑, WBC ↑, blood cultures
- Immediate diagnostic paracentesis: leukocytes and differential count (neutrophil granulocytes >0.25 x 10^9/L/ >250/mm^3), ascites culture (most common are *Escherichia coli*, *Klebsiella pneumoniae*, and *Streptococcus pneumoniae*), albumin, cytology if indicated. For a comprehensive overview, see the Appendix 1 on Paracentesis.

Tx
- Stop diuretics and potentially nephrotoxic drugs, consider stopping beta blockers (in patients with hypotension, AKI, or hyponatremia), and PPI
- Supportive therapy as needed
- IV ABx (3rd-generation cephalosporin (e.g. ceftriaxone)), IV albumin (1.5 g/kg on day 1 of diagnosis and 1 g/kg on day 3 after diagnosis)
- Check levels of neutrophils in ascites after 24-72h to evaluate response to treatment and indication to modify ABx
- Patients who have had an episode of SBP need lifelong secondary prophylaxis: oral norfloxacin 1x/day 400 mg

P Hospital mortality 10-50%

! One-year risk of recurrence without prophylaxis is 70%, poor long-term prognosis (depending on stage of liver cirrhosis). Ascitic fluid cultures often have false-negative results; the diagnosis is based on the number of neutrophilic granulocytes.

> The most common cause of death in patients admitted with SBP is hepatorenal syndrome. Immediately administering IV albumin has a beneficial effect on mortality.

Variceal haemorrhage

See section *Oesophagus*.

Metabolic dysfunction-associated steatotic liver disease (MASLD)/Metabolic dysfunction-associated steatohepatitis (MASH; formerly NAFLD/NASH)

D MASLD is characterised by hepatic steatosis (>5%), with the presence of one or more cardiometabolic risk factors (see R) and no other identifiable cause of steatosis (such as alcohol use disorder), see Diagram 11. MASLD progresses to metabolic dysfunction-associated steatohepatitis (MASH) in case of present inflammation, which may lead to fibrosis. Also consider MASLD with increased alcohol intake (MetALD), alcohol associated liver disease (ALD), specific causes of steatotic liver disease (SLD), cryptogenic SLD (SLD without known aetiology and no cardiovascular risk factors present), or chronic liver disease, see Figure 79.

E Prevalence 30% worldwide (45% in Latin America, 30-35% in Middle East, North Africa, South Asia, and Southeast Asia, 25-30% in North America, East Asia, and Western Europe), 50-80% of DM type II patients.

Ae Exact pathways still not fully understood, most widely accepted theory is that insulin resistance plays a central role in the pathogenesis

R Obesity (++), DM (+), hypertension, hypercholesterolemia, hypertriglyceridemia, metabolic syndrome, most common in patients aged 40-50

Hx Asymptomatic (++), malaise (−), fatigue (−), pain right upper quadrant (−)

PE Hepatomegaly

Dx
- Lab: AST ↑ < ALT ↑ (2-5x ULN), ALP ↑ (2-3x ULN), GGT ↑, glucose ↑, mostly normal albumin and bilirubin, rule out viral/autoimmune hepatitis or haemochromatosis
- Elastography: staging of steatosis and fibrosis (see section *Diagnostics*)
- Liver biopsy (usually not necessary for diagnosis of MASLD, predominantly used for evaluation of disease activity and presence of fibrosis in MASH): steatosis, hepatocellular 'ballooning', lobular and/or portal inflammation

Tx
- Lifestyle recommendations: diet, stop alcohol use, weight reduction, physical exercise
- Resmetirom, vaccination HAV and HBV, optimisation of DM, hypertension, and/or hypercholesterolemia treatment
- Bariatric surgery, liver transplantation (after ≥6 mo alcohol abstinence)

P Steatosis initially reversible, 10-30% progression to MASH, 3-5% progression to cirrhosis

I
- Risk HCC ↑
- Expected to be the leading indication for liver transplantation globally by 2040

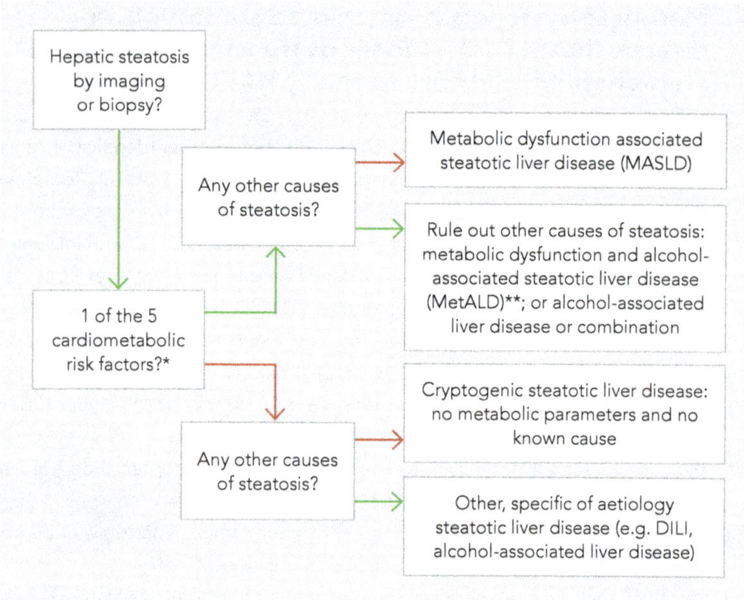

Diagram 11 // Diagnostic criteria for MASLD

*Obestity, DM type II, hypertension, dyslipidaemia, or hypertriglyceridaemia

**Consumption of high amounts of alcohol per week (♀ 140-350 g/wk, ♂ 210-420 g/wk)

The AST/ALT ratio is >1 in alcoholic liver disease and <1 in MASLD.

Noninvasive, prognostic serum markers are being developed to detect patients at high risk for developing fibrosis and cirrhosis. The FIB-4 Index comprised of AST, ALT, platelets, and age is being increasingly used in clinical practice.

MASLD can be regarded as the hepatic manifestation of metabolic syndrome. Cardiovascular morbidity and mortality is high in these patients, increasing with each disease stage. Drug therapies with varying metabolic mechanisms of action are currently under investigation for (fibrotic) MASLD, including GLP-1 agonists, glucagon agonists, FGF21 analogues, and pan-PPAR agonists.

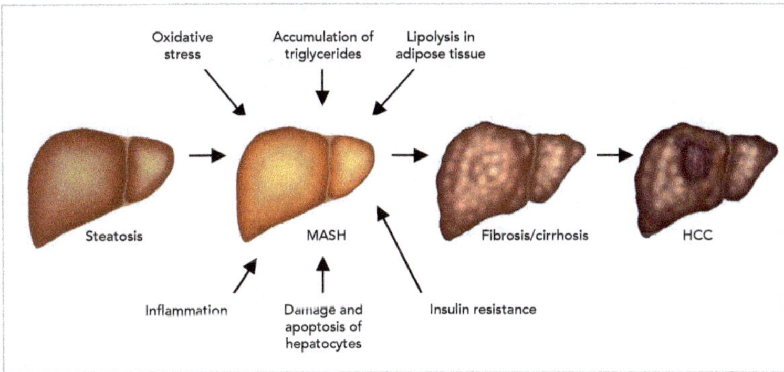

Figure 79 // MASH: pathophysiology

Portal hypertension

D Portal hypertension is a persistently elevated pressure in the portal vein. Portal vein pressure is determined by the portal blood volume flowing through the liver and the resistance of the portal vein.

E 80-90% of patients with liver cirrhosis have increased portal pressure

Ae
- Prehepatic: portal or splenic vein thrombosis, portal vein obstruction secondary to malignancy
- Intrahepatic (++): hepatic cirrhosis (++), schistosomiasis (+), sarcoidosis, hepatic fibrosis, hepatic vein thrombosis, nodular regenerative hyperplasia, hepatic metastases, PBC, medications (e.g. methotrexate, amiodarone), viral hepatitis
- Posthepatic: Budd-Chiari syndrome, constrictive pericarditis, right-sided congestive heart failure
- Left-sided: caused by necrotising pancreatitis or splenic vein obstruction secondary to pancreatic malignancy

Hx Asymptomatic (+), fatigue, weight ↓, appetite ↓, haemorrhoids, symptoms of complications, symptoms of underlying disease

PE Caput medusae, stigmata of liver cirrhosis, hepatosplenomegaly, signs of complications

Dx
- Aetiological analysis
- Labs: Hb ↓, platelets ↓, SAAG ≥11 g/L, signs of underlying cause
- Hepatic venous pressure gradient measurement ≥10 mmHg: clinically significant portal hypertension (CSPH); >12 mmHg is associated with complications (see !)

CONDITIONS

- Transient elastography: liver stiffness
- Upper endoscopy: congestive gastropathy, oesophagogastric varices
- Abdominal ultrasound: ascites, splenomegaly, hepatic nodules, portal flow <12 cm/sec, reflow in portal vein, portosystemic collateral pathways, portal vein diameter >13 mm, portal vein and superior mesenteric vein diameters do not vary with respiration, portal or superior mesenteric vein thrombosis

Tx Treat underlying cause and possible complications

Non-selective beta blockers (e.g. carvedilol)

Transjugular intrahepatic portosystemic shunt (TIPS)

P Depends on severity of portal hypertension and presence of complications

! Possible complications: variceal haemorrhage, ascites, SBP, hepatic encephalopathy, hepatorenal syndrome, hepatopulmonary syndrome

---

Wilson's disease

D Wilson's disease is an inherited disorder presenting with impaired excretion of copper via the bile canaliculi and accumulation of copper in tissues. The disease is characterised by a combination of hepatic, neurological, and psychiatric symptoms and is often diagnosed between ages 5-35.

E Live birth prevalence 3.3:100,000

Ae Autosomal recessive, ATP7B gene defects: ceruloplasmin (copper transporter protein) ↓ and copper excretion via bile ↓

Hx PE
- Hepatic: jaundice, ALF (hepatic encephalopathy and severe coagulopathy), RUQ pain, hepatosplenomegaly, liver cirrhosis stigmata, positive FHx (liver cirrhosis in infancy)
- Neurological: speech disorders (++), movement disorder, rigid dystonia, parkinsonism, frontotemporal dementia
- Psychiatric: cognitive decline, mood disorders (esp. depression), psychoses
- Other: Kayser-Fleischer rings (annular discolouration in the iris) (++), palpitations, joint pain, positive family history, self-limited hemolytic anaemia

Dx Labs (see Figure 80), ocular examination, 24-hour urinary copper excretion, brain MRI (if neurological symptoms), if uncertain: liver biopsy (hepatic copper concentration) and/or genetic testing (ATP7B mutation)

Tx Diet: low copper, consult dietician

D-penicillamine or trientine (copper: binding ↑ → excretion ↑, zinc: absorption ↓), for maintenance: zinc acetate (interferes with intestinal copper absorption)

P Proper treatment with good adherence leads to complete remission, discontinuation leads to progressive liver abnormalities and eventually lethal liver cirrhosis. In 5% of all cases, the disease presents with acute liver failure.

! Patients that present with acute liver failure may have hemolytic anemia (copper from necrotic hepatocytes → circulation → hemolysis) and kidney injury (from copper complexes)

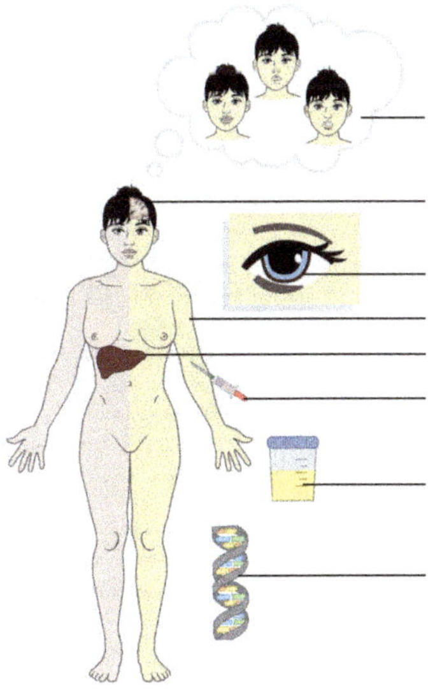

Figure 80 // Wilson's disease

Gallbladder and bile ducts

Cholelithiasis

	CHOLECYSTOLITHIASIS	CHOLEDOCHOLITHIASIS
D	Gallstone(s) located in the gallbladder.	Gallstone(s) located in common bile duct (CBD), see Figure 81.
E	Prevalence 15%, ♂:♀ 1:2	10-15% of people with gallstones develop symptomatic gallstone disease in <10y

Table 57A // Cholecystolithiasis and choledocholithiasis

	CHOLECYSTOLITHIASIS	CHOLEDOCHOLITHIASIS
Ae	Increased cholesterol levels (in populations with Western lifestyle cholesterol gallstones account for 90-95% of all gallstones), increased crystallisation tendency, decreased gallbladder motility, bile stasis (e.g. cystic fibrosis)	
R	♀, obesity, pregnancy, positive FHx, Western lifestyle, rapid weight loss (e.g. after bariatric surgery), oral contraceptives, liver cirrhosis	
Hx	Asymptomatic (++), episodic attacks of severe RUQ colic pain due to intermittent obstruction of the cystic duct (<6h), referred pain in back or right shoulder	Colic pain (urge to move) RUQ or epigastric region (>6h), referred pain in back or right shoulder, nausea, vomiting, jaundice with dark urine, clay-coloured stool
PE	Not contributing	Jaundice, RUQ tenderness
Dx	• Labs: normal liver enzymes, no cholestasis, no inflammation • Abdominal ultrasound: stones or sludge in gallbladder	Labs: AST ↑, ALT ↑, bilirubin ↑↑, ALP ↑↑, GGT ↑↑, sometimes lipase ↑ (beware of biliary pancreatitis) • Abdominal ultrasound (sensitivity 38-42%): dilated intrahepatic bile ducts (tram-track sign) and extrahepatic bile ducts, CBD >6 mm (if age <70 and no prior cholecystectomy), acoustic shadowing (stones) • MRCP (specificity >95%): dilated intrahepatic and extrahepatic bile ducts, gallstones in CBD • EUS (specificity >95%): dilated intrahepatic and extrahepatic bile ducts, stones and/or sludge in CBD
Tx	Analgesics for pain Laparoscopic cholecystectomy for recurrent biliary colic	Analgesics (preferably NSAIDs) • Gallstone extraction during ERCP with endoscopic sphincterotomy. Consider percutaneous bile duct drainage (PTC) in case of unsuccessful ERCP (possibly with rendezvous procedure). • Laparoscopic cholecystectomy recommended <2 wk after ERCP or PTC
P	5-year risk of biliary colic 10%	>95% of gallstones can be removed using ERCP
!	Possible complications: cholecystitis, choledocholithiasis (if small gallstones pass into the bile ducts), cholangitis, biliary pancreatitis	Possible complications: biliary pancreatitis, cholangitis

Table 57B // Cholecystolithiasis and choledocholithiasis

In cases of elevated liver tests in a cholestatic pattern and cholecystolithiasis without gallstones in the CBD, consider **Mirizzi syndrome.** This syndrome is a rare cause of cholestasis and jaundice. It occurs when the hepatic duct or CBD is compressed by a gallstone in the neck of the gallbladder or the cystic duct.

The risk factors of cholelithiasis are the **7 F's**: **f**at (BMI >30), **f**emale, **f**ertile (pregnancies), **f**orty (age >40), **f**air skin, **f**asting (also parenteral nutrition), positive **F**Hx.

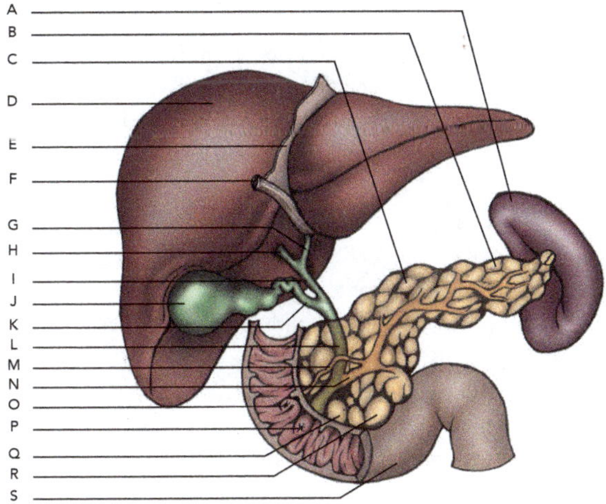

Figure 81 // The pancreas and surrounding structures
A: Spleen **B:** Pancreatic tail **C:** Pancreatic body **D:** Liver **E:** Falciform ligament **F:** Round ligament **G:** Left hepatic duct **H:** Right hepatic duct **I:** Common hepatic duct **J:** Gallbladder **K:** Cystic duct **L:** Common bile duct **M:** Accessory pancreatic duct **N:** Pancreatic duct **O:** Minor duodenal papilla **P:** Major duodenal papilla (papilla of Vater) **Q:** Pancreatic head **R:** Uncinate process of the pancreas **S:** Duodenum

Cholangitis

D Cholangitis is a bacterial infection of the biliary tract, sometimes accompanied by bile duct obstruction and subsequent cholestasis. The diagnosis is made using the Tokyo criteria (see Figure 82).

E ♂:♀ 1:1, up to 9% of patients with cholelithiasis

Ae Bile duct obstruction → bile stasis → bacteria ascending from duodenum → bacterial infection (most common: *E. coli, Klebsiella, Enterococcus, Pseudomonas, Enterobacter*)

R Obstruction by gallstones, bile duct stenosis (e.g. strictures secondary to primary sclerosing cholangitis or compression by tumours (pancreatic, ampullary, gallbladder, or duodenal)), bile duct anastomosis (hepaticojejunostomy), obstruction of biliary stent

Hx Charcot's triad (high specificity, low sensitivity): RUQ pain (80%), fever (chills) (80%), jaundice (60-70%)

PE
- T ↑, BP ↓, consciousness ↓, jaundice
- Features of sepsis may be present, depending on the severity of the condition

Dx
- Labs: bilirubin ↑, ALP ↑, GGT ↑, AST ↑, ALT ↑, CRP ↑, WBC ↑, blood cultures (before starting ABx). CA19-9 may be elevated in the setting of biliary obstruction. Recheck after resolution (cholangitis).
- Abdominal ultrasound: dilated intrahepatic bile ducts (tram-track sign), possible thickening of bile duct wall, possible cholelithiasis/choledocholithiasis
- MRCP: dilated bile ducts with thickening and contrast enhancement of bile duct wall, possible choledocholithiasis/obstruction/stenosis
- EUS: to detect gallstones or sludge and as a diagnostic tool for pancreatic obstructing lesions. This procedure has no place in the treatment of acute cholangitis.
- Abdominal contrast CT (pref. liver protocol): to rule out other pathology in inconclusive ultrasound, inhomogeneous enhancement of liver parenchyma on CTA, enhancement of biliary duct wall, possibly biliary dilation incl. CBD, stenosis, and location of the obstruction
- Tokyo criteria (see Figure 82)

Tx ABx (targeting gram-negative pathogens according to local protocol, e.g. piperacillin-tazobactam or ceftriaxon + metronidazol) and IV fluids in case of sepsis

Bile duct decompression during ERCP with papillotomy, balloon dilatation, gallstone extraction and/or biliary stent placement in case of stenosis. Consider percutaneous bile duct drainage by an interventional radiologist in case of unsuccessful ERCP or contraindications for ERCP.

P Mortality 11-30% (in cases of severe acute cholangitis)

I Possible complications: sepsis, multi-organ failure

Tokyo criteria for acute cholangitis (see Figure 82). Suspicion with I + II/III; diagnosis with I + II + III.
I: Systemic inflammation (T >38°C, chills, WBC <4 or >10, or CRP ≥10)
II: Cholestasis (jaundice or elevated cholestasis parameters and transaminases (ALP, GGT, ALT, AST >1.5x normal upper limit))
III: Imaging (dilated bile ducts (CBD >7 mm) or evidence of obstruction (e.g. gallstone, stent, stricture)

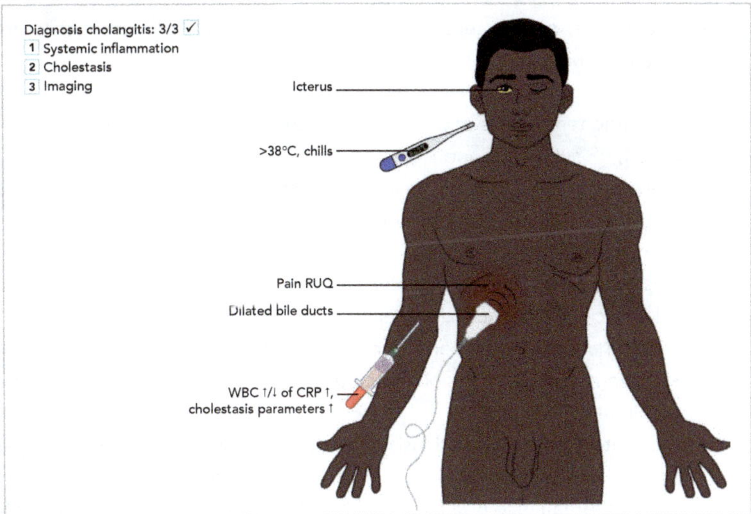

Figure 82 // Tokyo criteria for cholangitis

Pancreas

Acute pancreatitis

D Acute inflammation of the pancreas, diagnosed using the Atlanta criteria (see Figure 83). Subtypes of acute pancreatitis include interstitial oedematous (±80%) and necrotising pancreatitis (±20%, see Diagram 12).

E Incidence 5-56:100,000 and rising

Ae
- Proteolytic enzyme activation → pancreatic autodigestion → local inflammation, possible systemic inflammatory response syndrome (SIRS) with potential hypovolaemic shock due to redistribution
- Causes: cholelithiasis (++), alcohol use (++), trauma, medication (e.g. ACE inhibitors, statins, thiopurines), infections, metabolic (hypercalcaemia, hypertriglyceridaemia), post-ERCP, pancreatic carcinoma, anatomical variant (e.g. pancreas divisum (-)), autoimmune (-), idiopathic (+), ischaemia, cystic fibrosis

R Cholelithiasis (++), alcohol use disorder (++), obesity, genetic predisposition, DM type II

Hx
- Acute epigastric pain (radiating to back in 50% of patients), urge to move (colic), nausea, vomiting

- Alcohol use, patient recently started medication for pancreatitis, recent surgery/trauma, see (R)
- Eating/coughing/deep inspiration → pain ↑

(PE)
- Epigastric tenderness and/or rebound tenderness, T ↑/subfebrile, BP ↑/↓, pulse ↑, RR superficial and ↑
- Late onset signs: Cullen's sign (periumbilical ecchymosis) ⊖, Grey Turner's sign (ecchymosis or discoloration of the flank) ⊖

(Dx)
- Atlanta criteria (see Figure 83)
- Labs: lipase/amylase ↑ (>3x the upper limit of normal), CRP ↑, WBC ↑, possible: calcium ↑, triglycerides ↑, glucose ↑
- Abdominal ultrasound: perform at initial presentation given biliary aetiology is most common (i.e. obstructing gallstone, dilated bile ducts, cholecystolithiasis)
- EUS: detect choledocholithiasis, cholecystolithiasis, or intraductal sludge. Indicated if suspicion persists after negative abdominal ultrasound.
- MRCP: alternative to EUS for suspected choledocholithiasis in negative ultrasound. Rule out pancreas divisum.
- Abdominal contrast CT in acute phase only when in doubt about diagnosis. A CT can be performed >72h for suspected secondary complications of pancreatitis and to differentiate between oedematous or necrotising pancreatitis, but findings have no clinical consequences. Oedematous pancreatitis: normal enhancement of pancreatic tissue, diffuse parenchymal oedema, and mild peripancreatic fat infiltration. Necrotising pancreatitis: parenchymal oedema, peripancreatic fat infiltration, decreased parenchymal enhancement, non-enhancing necrotising regions, and fluid collections with/without wall enhancement.
- ECG: to rule out anterior myocardial infarction as cause of symptoms when in doubt

(Tx) Monitor fluid balance, optimise nutritional status (consult dietitian, enteral nutrition), monitor renal function

- Crystalloid (Ringer's lactate) IV guided by urine output, usually 3L/24h after a bolus with a target urine output of >0.5 ml/kg/h, analgesics, LMWH, consider anti-emetics, replete electrolytes as needed. No AB, only for infected necrosis (often only >2-4 wk).
- Pain management, e.g. NSAIDs and preferably only short-acting opioids
- ERCP in case of cholangitis <24h, elective in symptomatic choledocholithiasis

- Laparoscopic cholecystectomy for biliary pancreatitis, preferably <72h in patients with a mild (uncomplicated) clinical course (wait for at least 6 wk in patients with a more severe clinical course)
- Percutaneous/transgastric drainage of necrotic collections

Treatment of proven or suspected infected necrotising pancreatitis (minimally invasive step-up approach):

- ABx (broad-spectrum, e.g. meropenem)
- Drainage (transgastric endoscopic or retroperitoneal percutaneous drainage) of infected necrotising collection in case of walled-off necrosis (WON) optimally delayed up to >4 wk, followed by minimally invasive necrosectomy if necessary (endoscopic or video-assisted retroperitoneal debridement (VARD))

P
- Mild pancreatitis has low mortality: <5%
- CRP >150 mg/L within 48h → predictor of severe pancreatitis
- 15-20% of patients with acute pancreatitis develop necrotising pancreatitis → mortality ↑ (17%)
- Define severity of pancreatitis: Imrie score, BISAP score, APACHE score, and SIRS criteria

!
- Complications of acute pancreatitis (see Diagram 12)
- Watch out for cholangitis in case of a biliary cause

Although not yet routinely used, procalcitonin is the most sensitive lab test to detect pancreatic infection. Low serum values → strong negative predictor for infected necrosis.

GET SMASHID is a mnemonic for the most common causes of acute pancreatitis: **G**allstones, **E**thanol, **T**rauma, **S**teroids, **M**umps, **A**utoimmune, **S**corpion sting, **H**yperlipidaemia, **I**diopathic, **D**rugs.

Encapsulated pancreatic necrotising fluid collections are also known as walled-off necrosis. Drainage should preferably be delayed until encapsulation is complete, which often takes about 4 weeks.

Lipase has a higher specificity for pancreatitis than amylase.

Lipase (high sensitivity and specificity) rises within 4-8h from symptom onset and peaks after 24h. Return to baseline is seen after 8-14d. This is useful in patients with onset of symptoms over 24h. Lipase is more sensitive in alcohol-induced pancreatitis.

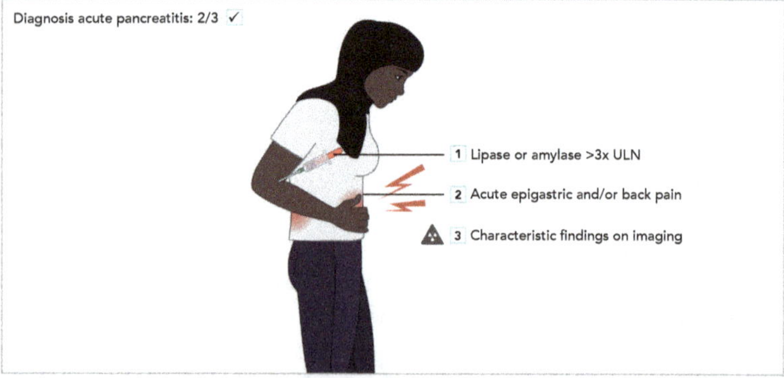

Figure 83 // Revised Atlanta Classification: pancreatitis diagnosis requires ≥2 criteria

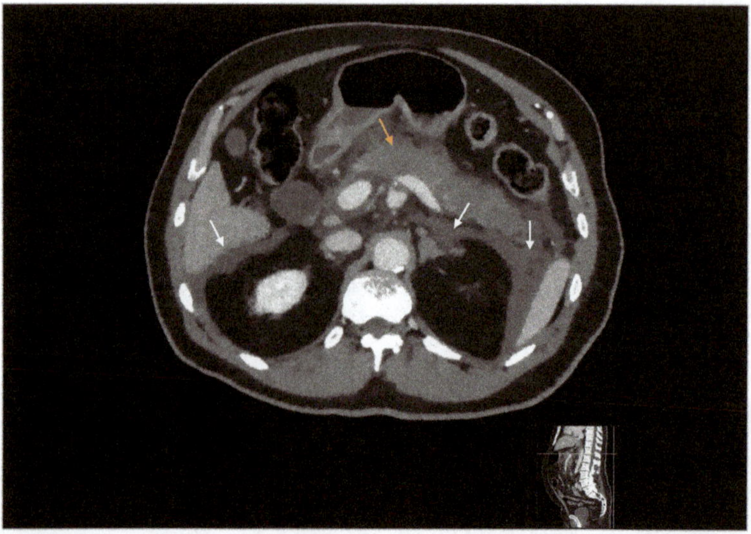

Figure 84 // Abdominal contrast CT: uncomplicated pancreatitis with oedematous swollen pancreas (orange arrow) and retroperitoneal free fluid (white arrows) No evidence of abscess formation (fluid collections are without peripheral enhancement).

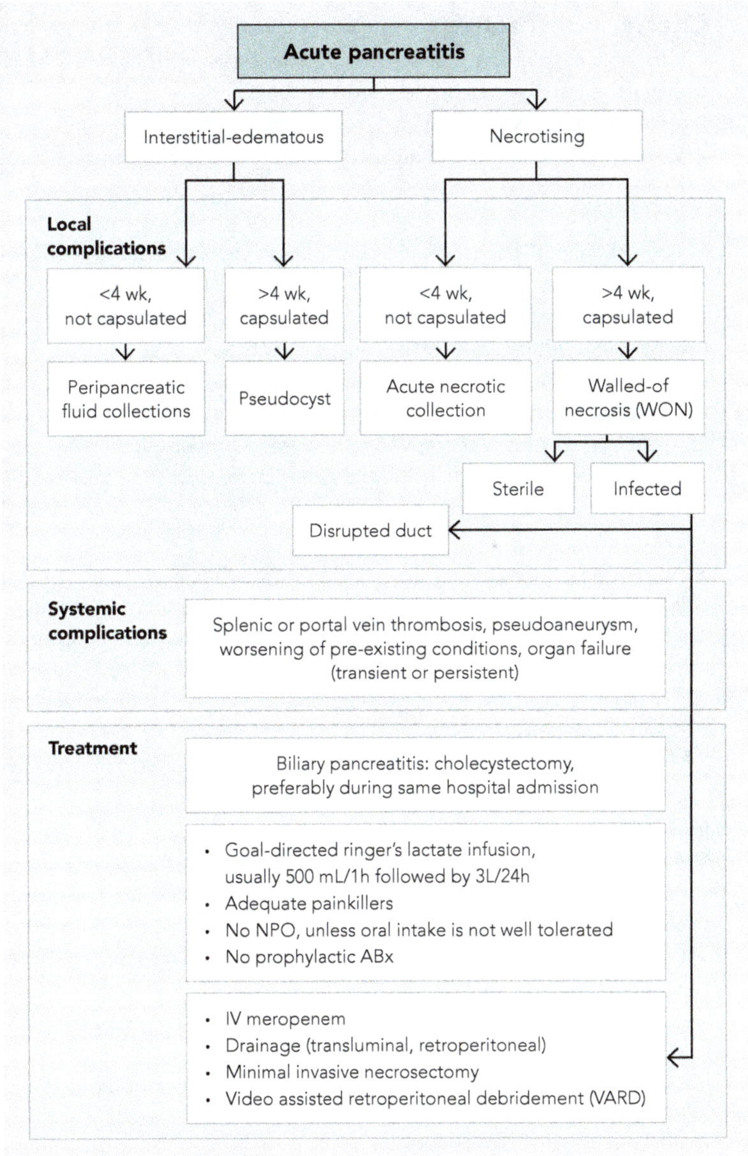

Diagram 12 // Subtypes of acute pancreatitis with corresponding complications

Chronic pancreatitis

D Chronic inflammation of the pancreas with fibrosis causing irreversible changes with impairment of exocrine and endocrine functions.

E Prevalence 25-75:100,000

Ae
- Fibrosis, duct stenosis/dilation, calcification → pressure in pancreatic duct or interstitial tissue ↑ → destruction of pancreatic tissue → pancreatic insufficiency
- Causes: alcohol ⊕⊕, pancreatic ductal obstruction/strictures ⊕, autoimmune pancreatitis ⊖, tropical pancreatitis (Southern India), idiopathic ⊕

R Alcohol use disorder ⊕⊕, smoking ⊕⊕, recurrent acute pancreatitis, genetic predisposition, systemic conditions (e.g. cystic fibrosis)

Hx Chronic epigastric pain, symptoms consistent with pancreatic enzyme insufficiency (e.g. steatorrhoea, malabsorption, weight loss), asymptomatic

PE Epigastric tenderness and/or rebound tenderness, underweight

Dx
- Labs: fasting glucose ↑, HbA1c ↑, possible: vitamin A, D, E, K ↓, AST ↑, ALT ↑, IgG4 ↑ (in case of autoimmune pancreatitis)
- Faecal elastase ↓
- Abdominal contrast CT/MRCP: parenchymal atrophy and/or calcifications, pseudocysts, strictures with prestenotic dilatation of the pancreatic duct

Tx
Lifestyle recommendations: stop smoking and drinking alcohol, optimise nutritional status

Analgesics, pancreatic enzyme replacement therapy, DM treatment, supplemental nutrition

Complications: consider surgery (e.g. pancreaticojejunostomy), splanchnic nerve block, ERCP (stent, extraction of small stones)

P Irreversible, acute exacerbations may occur

!
- Possible complications of chronic pancreatitis: e.g. endocrine/exocrine pancreatic insufficiency, pancreatic pseudocysts, pancreatic malignancy, splenic vein thrombosis
- Possible consequences for patient: weight loss, chronic pain syndrome, quality of life ↓
- Chronic pancreatitis may result in pancreatic ductal obstruction/strictures due to fibrosis → risk of recurrence ↑
- Perform DEXA scan in follow-up: risk of osteopenia/osteoporosis due to malabsorption

In **chronic pancreatitis**, serum amylase and lipase are often normal during flairs and therefore are not appropriate parameters. When analysing endocrine and exocrine pancreatic insufficiency, use functional parameters such as serum glucose and faecal elastase.

Pancreatic insufficiency

	ENDOCRINE PANCREATIC INSUFFICIENCY	**EXOCRINE PANCREATIC INSUFFICIENCY**
D	Inability of the pancreas to adequately produce and secrete insulin, resulting in impaired glucose regulation (DM). Pancreatic insufficiency-related DM is classified as DM type 3c.	Inability of the pancreas to adequately produce and secrete enzymes and bicarbonate, resulting in impaired absorption and digestion of nutrients, and fat-soluble vitamins (e.g. A, D, E, K).
E	Prevalence in patients with DM type 1 is 300:100,000	Unknown in the general population, prevalence in patients with chronic pancreatitis 30-85% (usually >5y of disease) and cystic fibrosis (CF) ±85%
Ae	• Primary: acute or chronic pancreatitis, pancreatic carcinoma (esp. pancreatic head adenocarcinoma), haemochromatosis, trauma • Secondary: pancreatectomy	
R	Recurrent pancreatitis, alcohol use disorder, hereditary factors (e.g. hereditary pancreatitis and CF), autoimmune disease	
Hx	Weight ↓, fatigue	
	Polyuria, polydipsia, malaise	• Abdominal pain, swollen abdomen, bloating, excessive flatulence, steatorrhoea, malnourishment • Malabsorption: skin turgor ↓, hair loss, oedema, muscle loss, concentration ↓
PE	BMI ↓, weight ↓	
Dx	Labs: fasting glucose ↑, HbA1c ↑	• Faecal elastase ↓ (<100 ug/g high sensitivity, 100-200 ug/g is indeterminate) • Faecal fat/24h ↑ • Secretin stimulation test +
Tx	Lifestyle recommendations: dietary changes, education, consider consulting Endocrinology Metformin, insulin	Lifestyle recommendations: stop smoking and drinking alcohol, optimise nutritional status Surveillance DEXA scan for osteopenia/osteoporosis Pancreatic enzyme replacement therapy (PERT)
P	Irreversible	

Table 58A // Endocrine and exocrine pancreatic insufficiency

	ENDOCRINE PANCREATIC INSUFFICIENCY	EXOCRINE PANCREATIC INSUFFICIENCY
P	Depends on patient-related factors and the underlying pancreatic condition causing DM type 3c	Outcomes of successful treatment with PERT include: • Steatorrhea and associated gastrointestinal symptoms ↓ • Gain of weight, muscle mass, and muscle function • Improvement in fat-soluble vitamin levels
!	High risk of hypoglycaemic episodes	Follow-up should include a DEXA scan at least every 1-2y, assessment of muscle mass and strength

Table 58B // Endocrine and exocrine pancreatic insufficiency

Intraductal papillary mucinous neoplasm (IPMN)

D A mucin-secreting premalignant or malignant cystic lesion in the pancreatic duct that usually grows slowly. A distinction is made between main-duct IPMN (MD-IPMN) and branch duct IPMN (BD-IPMN). A third, mixed-type IPMN (MT-IPMN) affects both the main duct and the side branches.

E Prevalence of pancreatic cysts is 2-45% and rises with age

Ae Unknown

R Age, DM, chronic pancreatitis

Hx Asymptomatic and incidental finding (++), abdominal pain, steatorrhoea, weight loss, new onset DM

PE Jaundice (−)

Dx
- Labs: CA 19-9 ↑ in invasive IPMN/malignancy, amylase ↑ → suggestive of connection with pancreatic duct (e.g. IPMN, pseudocyst)
- MRCP (1st choice in IPMN surveillance, see Figure 85): cyst with or without a nodule or solid mass, possibly dilated pancreatic duct, bunch of grapes, connection with pancreatic duct, monitor for worrisome features
- Abdominal contrast CT: cyst with/without a nodule or solid mass, possibly dilated pancreatic duct with atrophy of prestenotic pancreatic parenchyma
- EUS and aspiration cytology: CEA ↑ (nonspecific marker) suggestive of mucinous cystic neoplasm

Tx Surveillance depends on indication for surgery and comorbidity, see Table 59 for IPMN monitoring

Surgical resection (total pancreatectomy, pancreaticoduodenectomy, distal pancreatectomy, or central pancreatectomy in exceptional cases, depending on the location, see Table 60) if:
- ≥1 absolute indications for resection
- 1 relative indication for resection in healthy, fit patients

- 2 relative indications for resection in patients with significant comorbidities

P MD-IPMN has the highest malignancy potential

I Patients undergoing partial pancreatectomy require life-long check-ups for their residual pancreatic function (endocrine and exocrine insufficiency)

SURVEILLANCE STRATEGY	
No indication for surgery	MRI twice in one year after diagnosis, thereafter MRI annually, and clinical evaluation if unchanged
Indication for surgery and significant comorbidity	Biannual MRI, CA 19-9 serum, and clinical evaluation
After partial pancreatectomy due to IPMN	Depends on degree of dysplasia, usually identical to non-resected IPMN

Table 59 // IPMN monitoring

RELATIVE INDICATIONS FOR RESECTION	ABSOLUTE INDICATIONS FOR RESECTION
• Growth ≥5 mm/y • Elevated serum CA 19-9 • Dilated pancreatic duct 5-9.9 mm • Cyst diameter ≥40 mm • New DM • Acute pancreatitis (secondary to IPMN) • Enhancing nodule (<5 mm)	• Cytology: high-grade dysplasia • Solid mass • Jaundice • Enhancing nodule (≥5 mm) • Dilated pancreatic duct ≥10 mm

Table 60 // Relative and absolute indications for resection in IPMN

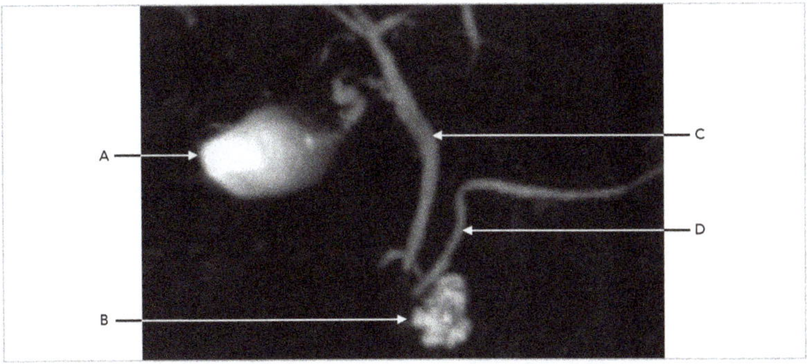

Figure 85 // MRI T2: side-branch IPMN in the pancreatic head. Note the contact of the cysts with the pancreatic duct

A: Gallbladder **B:** IPMN **C:** Common bile duct **D:** Pancreatic duct

Oncology

5% of cancer patients have a demonstrable genetic predisposition. Some types of cancer are clearly associated with e.g. smoking, alcohol consumption, UV radiation, advanced age, or previous radiotherapy, but the vast majority of cases have no clear cause.

As new, optimised, and more targeted cancer treatments are constantly being developed, it is very important to always consult the latest guidelines and local protocols. Treatment can consist of a combination of chemotherapy/radiotherapy/immunotherapy, and surgical/endoscopic resection and depends on e.g. TNM stage and performance status. This section describes general options only and does not address stage-specific choices.

Anal carcinoma

D Most anal carcinomas are squamous cell carcinomas (SCC) arising from the anal canal or perianal skin.

E Rare, incidence rising, ♀>♂

R HIV, HPV infection (types 16 and 18) ⊕, receptive anal intercourse, immunocompromised patients, smoking, history of vulvar or cervical carcinoma, genital warts

Hx Anal blood or mucus loss (45%), tenesmus, perianal itching, anorectal pain, STI (e.g. genital warts), weight ↓, appetite ↓, history of immunosuppressant use

PE Weight ↓, abnormal lesion in perianal area, palpable lymph nodes in groin, rectal exam: ulcer ⊕, palpable, hard, irregular swelling

Dx
- Biopsy: squamous cell carcinoma (SCC)
- Rectal MRI: evaluation of local and regional tumour spread, incl. lymph nodes
- Chest and abdominal contrast CT (with PET-CT as needed): staging
- Consider EUS: transmural spread when contemplating local resection

Tx
- Curative: 1st choice treatment is definitive chemoradiotherapy, local excision is often impossible
- Palliative: chemotherapy

P High risk of local recurrence, 5-year survival: stage T1N0 88%, stage T2N0 82%, stage T3N0 74%, stage T4N0 57%

(!) Some guidelines recommend screening for anal cancer in various groups such as chronically immunosuppressed patients

Colorectal carcinoma

<table>
<tr><th></th><th>COLON CARCINOMA</th><th>RECTAL CARCINOMA</th></tr>
<tr><td>D</td><td colspan="2">Colorectal cancer is one of the most common malignancies (♀: second, ♂: third). Adenocarcinomas are most common and 75% of tumours are located in the last 40 cm of the intestines (see Figures 86 and 87).</td></tr>
<tr><td>E</td><td colspan="2">• Incidence varies globally, highest in Australia, New Zealand, Europe, North America, lowest in Africa and South-Central Asia
• $^2/_3$ colon carcinoma, $^1/_3$ rectal carcinoma
• ♂>♀</td></tr>
<tr><td>R</td><td colspan="2">• Genetic predisposition (e.g. Lynch syndrome), familial adenomatous polyposis, IBD, PSC, positive FHx, history of colorectal carcinoma
• Environmental factors: obesity, physical inactivity, processed and red meat</td></tr>
<tr><td>Hx</td><td colspan="2">Changes in bowel habits (diarrhoea/obstipation) (++), blood and/or mucus in stool (+), tenesmus and/or painful defaecation (with rectal tumours), abdominal pain, abdominal mass, weight ↓, symptoms consistent with anaemia</td></tr>
<tr><td>PE</td><td>Obstructive tumours may produce signs of mechanical ileus, palpable abdominal mass, rectal exam: possible blood on glove</td><td>Rectal exam: palpable mass if tumour is located in the lower $^2/_3$ of rectum, blood on glove</td></tr>
<tr><td>Dx</td><td colspan="2">• Labs: iron deficiency anaemia, CEA ↑
• Colonoscopy with biopsies (see Figures 86 and 87)
• Chest and abdominal contrast CT: staging
• Rectal MRI for rectal carcinoma: location, invasion, locoregional lymph nodes
• Consider EUS for rectal carcinoma: differentiate between stage cT1 and cT2 (in treatment implications)</td></tr>
<tr><td rowspan="4">Tx</td><td colspan="2">Treatment depends on TNM stage, size, and location</td></tr>
<tr><td>Adjuvant chemotherapy (or neo-adjuvant for locally advanced cancer), research setting: neo-adjuvant immunotherapy in selected patients</td><td>Neo-adjuvant radiotherapy or chemoradiotherapy. In the absence of residual tumours following treatment, consider an expectative approach (preferably in a study context).</td></tr>
<tr><td colspan="2">Curative:</td></tr>
<tr><td>Surgical resection (open/laparoscopic): e.g. right or left hemicolectomy, transversectomy, sigmoid resection, low anterior resection (LAR)</td><td>Surgical resection (open/laparoscopic): e.g. transanal endoscopic microsurgery (TEM), abdominoperineal resection (APR), total mesorectal excision (TME)</td></tr>
</table>

Table 61A // Colorectal carcinoma

	COLON CARCINOMA	RECTAL CARCINOMA
	• For metastases confined to the liver: resection, radiofrequency or microwave ablation, liver transplantation (consult local protocols) • For metastases confined to the peritoneum (peritoneal cancer index (PCI) score <21): consider cytoreduction with HIPEC • Endoscopic submucosal dissection (ESD) (see Figure 88 or endoscopic full thickness resection (eFTR) for stage T1 • For obstructive tumours: temporary or permanent ostomy	
	Palliative:	
	Systemic therapy based on microsatellite instability (MSI) status, BRAF, and RAS mutation status Obstructive stoma: create decompressing ostomy, place endoscopic stent	
P	5-year survival: stage I 95%, stage II 88%, stage III 72%, stage IV 12%	5-year survival: stage I 95%, stage II 83%, stage III 75%, stage IV 14%
!	• MSI is associated with hereditary cancer (Lynch syndrome) • Mortality rates are higher in men	

Table 61B // Colorectal carcinoma

Nationwide screening programmes for colorectal carcinoma have been rolled out in Western Europe, USA, China, Japan, Thailand, Australia, New Zealand, Canada, Argentina, and Chile. Such programmes consist of FIT testing for occult blood in faecal samples. A positive test is an indication for diagnostics (colonoscopy).

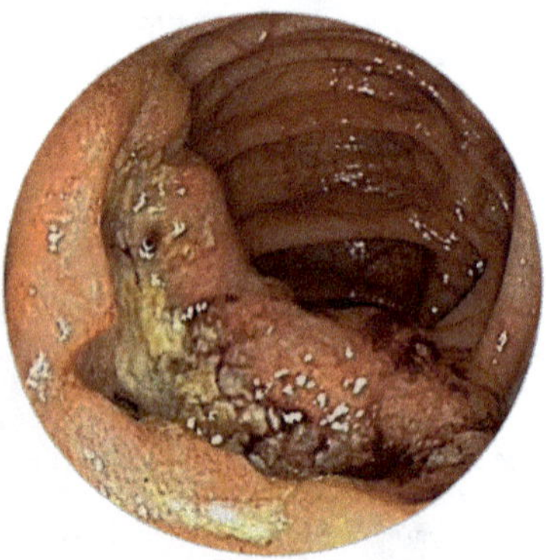

Figure 86 // Colonoscopy: colon carcinoma

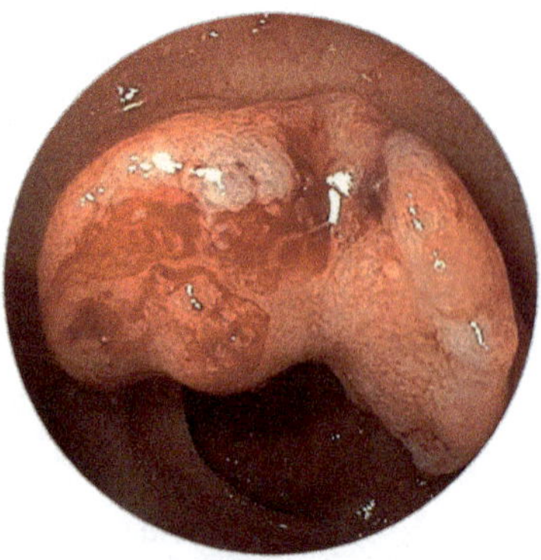

Figure 87 // Colonoscopy: rectal carcinoma

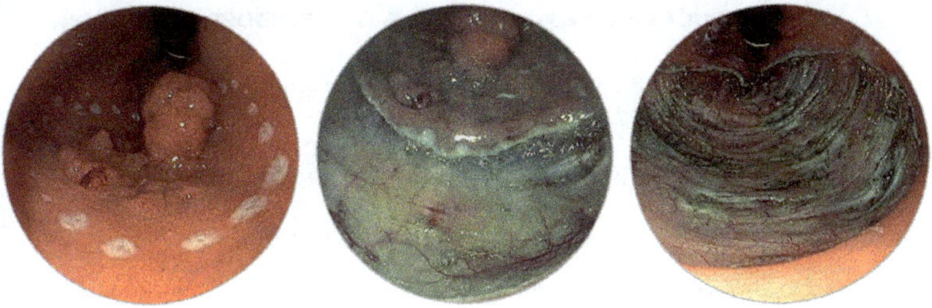

A B C

Figure 88 // Colonoscopy: image before **(A)**, during **(B)**, and after **(C)** endoscopic submucosal dissection (ESD) of a rectal carcinoma

> The typical patient with rectal carcinoma is aged >60 and has a positive family history of colon carcinoma with symptoms incl. weight loss, changes in bowel habits, and tenesmus.

Bile duct and gallbladder carcinoma

	BILE DUCT CARCINOMA	GALLBLADDER CARCINOMA
D	A bile duct carcinoma (cholangiocarcinoma (CCA)) is a malignant tumour arising from the epithelial cells of the bile ducts (intra/extrahepatic (perihilar and distal)). Perihilar cholangiocarcinoma is also known as Klatskin tumour.	More than 90% of gallbladder carcinomas are adenocarcinomas originating in the gallbladder and are associated with high mortality.
E	Rare, 5-10% intrahepatic cholangiocarcinomas, ♂>♀	Rare, incidence highest in India, Chile, and Eastern Europe, ♀>♂
R	Primary sclerosing cholangitis, bile duct cyst, hepatolithiasis, liver cirrhosis, hepatitis B and C, Lynch syndrome	Cholecystolithiasis (++), porcelain gallbladder (calcified gallbladder) (++), advanced age (75% age >70), gallbladder polyps, primary sclerosing cholangitis, Salmonella infection, obesity
Hx	• Only obstructive tumours are usually symptomatic • Weight ↓, appetite ↓, fever (beware of cholangitis), RUQ pain, possibly radiating to shoulder, signs of cholestasis in extrahepatic CCA (jaundice, itching, clay-coloured stools, dark urine)	Asymptomatic (++) or non-specific complaints, weight ↓, RUQ pain, jaundice (−), nausea (−), vomiting (−)
PE	Weight ↓, T ↑, jaundice (extrahepatic: 90%; intrahepatic: (−)), hepatomegaly	Weight ↓, jaundice (−), palpable gallbladder

Table 62A // Bile duct and gallbladder carcinoma

	BILE DUCT CARCINOMA	GALLBLADDER CARCINOMA
Dx	• Labs: bilirubin ↑, ALP ↑, GGT ↑, CA 19-9 ↑ • Abdominal ultrasound: dilated bile ducts, tumour • Chest and abdominal contrast CT: staging • ERCP with brush for PA, consider stent placement • Bismuth-Corlette classification (see Figure 89)	• Labs: no added value • Abdominal ultrasound: calcification, intraluminal lesions of the gallbladder, gallbladder polyps ≥10 mm, hepatic infiltration, thickened gallbladder wall • Abdominal contrast CT or MRCP in case of abnormal ultrasound findings • Histopathology of the surgically resected gallbladder: staging
Tx	• Curative: resection or liver transplantation, consider neo-adjuvant chemotherapy in borderline resectable tumour • Palliative: percutaneous or endoscopic bile duct stent for jaundice, coeliac plexus block for pain relief, chemotherapy	• Curative: cholecystectomy either with or without adjuvant chemotherapy, consider partial liver resection • Palliative: percutaneous or endoscopic bile duct stent for jaundice, coeliac plexus block for pain relief, chemotherapy
P	High mortality: approx. 70% of cholangiocarcinomas non-resectable at diagnosis	• It is often a chance histopathological finding after cholecystectomy • 5-year survival: 5-32%
!	Pathology specimens obtained from ERCP often produce false-negative results	Gallbladder carcinoma often goes unnoticed until it reaches an advanced stage

Table 62B // Bile duct and gallbladder carcinoma

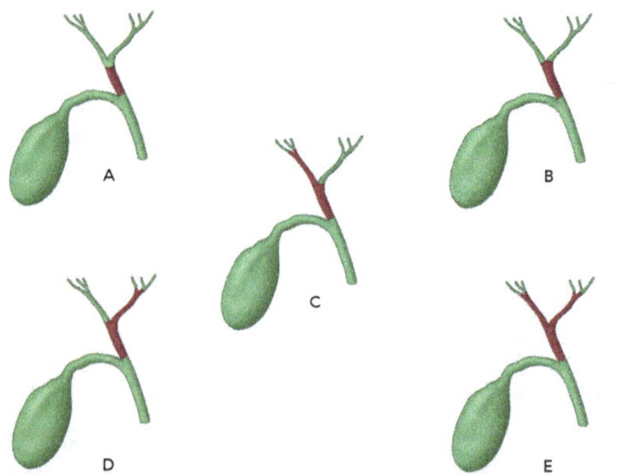

Figure 89 // Bismuth-Corlette classification for bile duct carcinoma
A: Type I **B:** Type II **C:** Type IIIa **D:** Type IIIb **E:** Type IV

Hepatocellular carcinoma (HCC)

D HCC is a primary liver tumour arising from hepatocytes in the liver parenchyma. The most commonly found hepatic malignancies in Western Europe are metastases from extrahepatic tumours.

E Incidence <2.7:100,000 per year, incidence rising, high incidence in Africa and East Asia, ♂:♀ 3:1, most common primary liver malignancy in adults

R Liver cirrhosis (++), advanced age (60-70), chronic HBV infection (+), HCV, alcohol, MASLD (+, also possible in absence of cirrhosis), haemochromatosis, East Asian or Sub-Saharan African descent

Hx
- Onset: asymptomatic (+)
- Advanced disease: fever, weight ↓, dyspnoea, epigastric pain, fullness, jaundice, increased abdominal girth (ascites)

PE T ↑, jaundice, stigmata of liver cirrhosis, RUQ tenderness, weight ↓, ascites

Dx
- Labs: alpha-foetoprotein (AFP) ↑
- Screening: abdominal ultrasound in patients at high risk of HCC (chronic liver disease) recommended every 6 mo
- Abdominal ultrasound (1st choice): intrahepatic mass
- Hepatic contrast MRI: ≥1 intrahepatic masses with macroscopic fat, mass effect, arterial enhancement, rapid wash-out, potential persisting ring enhancement
- Abdominal contrast CT: staging
- Biopsy when in doubt about diagnosis and treatment implications

Tx
- Curative:
  - Partial liver resection: only in early or very early HCC with max. 1 lesion and no portal hypertension
  - Local ablation, e.g. radiofrequency thermoablation (RFA), transcatheter arterial chemoembolisation (TACE), ultrasound-guided chemical ablation (ethanol injection), cryoablation, transarterial radioembolisation (TARE), or stereotactic radiotherapy (SRT)
  - Liver transplantation (Milan criteria)
- Palliative: systemic therapy with tyrosine kinase inhibitor (e.g. Sorafenib)

P
- Liver resection and transplantation have high morbidity and mortality
- 5-year survival: 20-30%

! Be aware of HCC in any patient with liver cirrhosis

The **Milan criteria** are used in considering patients with cirrhosis and HCC for liver transplantation. Scan the QR code for more information.

The **Barcelona Clinic Liver Cancer schedule (BCLC staging system)** is used to determine treatment options and prognosis. Scan the QR code for the latest update (2022).

Gastric carcinoma

D Over 90% of gastric carcinomas are adenocarcinomas (see Figure 90).

E
- Incidence 9:100,000 per year, ♂>♀
- Highest incidence in East Asia, South America, and Eastern Europe. The incidence of gastric carcinomas has been decreasing for several decades.

R Overweight, highly processed diet (high nitrates), smoking, hereditary factors (CDH1 mutation, Lynch syndrome), GORD, gastric polyps, chronic atrophic gastritis, *H. pylori* (+), alcohol use

Hx
- Onset: asymptomatic (+)
- Advanced disease: weight ↓ (++), appetite ↓, persistent epigastric symptoms (++), heartburn (+), oesophageal dysphagia, haematemesis, melaena, symptoms consistent with iron deficiency anaemia, horror carnis

PE Weight ↓, Virchow's lymph node (left supraclavicular)

Dx
- Upper endoscopy with biopsies (see Figure 90)
- Chest and abdominal contrast CT: staging, rule out peritoneal metastases prior to treatment
- Diagnostic laparoscopy in the absence of metastases: assess resectability

Tx
- Curative:
  - Tumour confined to the mucosa or submucosa: endomucosal resection. Invasive tumour: perioperative chemotherapy followed by total or subtotal gastric resection with lymph node dissection.
  - Perioperative chemotherapy, radiotherapy
- Palliative:
  - Oesophageal dysphagia: surgical or EUS-guided gastroenterostomy
  - Palliative systemic therapy (chemotherapy, targeted (e.g. hormonal)

therapy), future: immunotherapy. Haemorrhage or local pain: local radiotherapy.

P Prognosis is often poor because of late-stage detection: 40% have peritoneal metastases and 30% have liver metastases. 5-year survival: stage I 67%, stage II 46%, stage III 19%, stage IV 2%.

! Be aware that peritoneal carcinomatosis has a sensitivity of 100% but a specificity of 40% on abdominal contrast CT

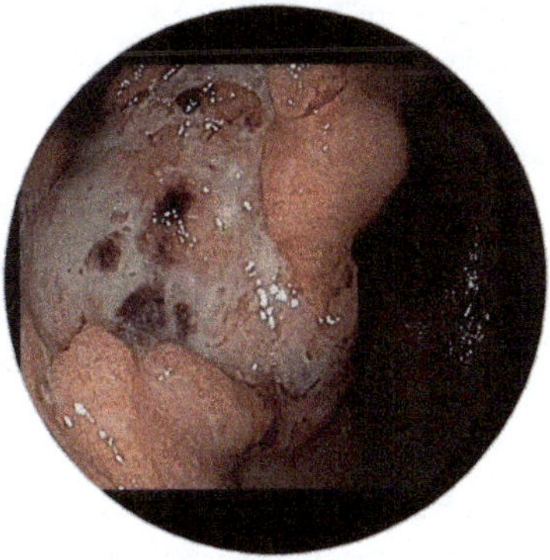

Figure 90 // Upper endoscopy: ulcerated tumour in gastric antrum

> The first descriptions of gastric cancer have been found in hieroglyphic inscriptions from ancient Egypt and date from 3000 BC.

Oesophageal carcinoma

D An oesophageal carcinoma is an adenocarcinoma or SCC arising from the oesophagus. Adenocarcinomas usually arise from glandular tissue in the mucosa of the lower $^{1}/_{3}$ of the oesophagus (see Figure 91).

E
- Incidence 10:100,000 per year, incidence rising, ♂>♀
- SCC is most common worldwide, in western and northern Europe, and in North America mainly adenocarcinomas

Ae Exposure to smoking and alcohol (SCC) or gastric acid (adenocarcinoma) → damaged oesophageal cells → continuous repair → DNA mutations in oncogenes/tumour suppressor genes → premalignancy/malignancy

R See Table 63

Hx
- Onset: asymptomatic ⊕
- Later stages are characterised by dysphagia (first solids, then also liquids, progressive) ⊕, often with weight ↓ ⊕, retrosternal pain (during eating) ⊕, hiccups, sometimes haematemesis, melaena, coughing, symptoms consistent with anaemia

PE Weight ↓, rectal exam: melaena

Dx
- Upper endoscopy with biopsies
- Chest and abdominal contrast CT: staging
- PET-CT in patients potentially eligible for curative treatment: more reliable assessment size of affected segment and distant metastases, not reliable in defining T-stage

Tx
- Curative:
  - Endomucosal resection, submucosal infiltration is an important prognostic factor. Submucosal infiltration is an indication for further resection or radiotherapy.
  - Endoscopic submucosal dissection (ESD) for tumours with submucosal infiltration
  - Neoadjuvant chemoradiotherapy followed by subtotal oesophageal resection and lymph node dissection
  - Incomplete pathological response after neo-adjuvant chemoradiotherapy and resection: adjuvant immunotherapy
- Palliative:
  - Systemic therapy depending on HER2 status and PDL-1 CPS score
  - Palliative radiotherapy for oesophageal dysphagia or haemorrhage

  Endoscopic stent placement for dysphagia (preferably not in conjunction with radiotherapy due to high risk of complications) if life expectancy <6 wk

P
- 5-year survival: stage I 66%, stage II 37%, stage III 28%, stage IV 3%
- After resection, 25% of patients have pulmonary complications

! Possible complications: tracheobronchial fistula or aortic involvement. Consider placing a feeding tube prior to the start of treatment.

RISK FACTOR	SQUAMOUS CELL CARCINOMA	ADENO-CARCINOMA
Smoking	++	+
Alcohol use	++	−
Barrett's oesophagus/reflux symptoms	−	++
Obesity	−	+
Corrosive oesophageal injury	++	−

Table 63A // Risk factors for oesophageal carcinoma

RISK FACTOR	SQUAMOUS CELL CARCINOMA	ADENO-CARCINOMA
Plummer-Vinson syndrome	++	−
Radiotherapy for mammary or lung carcinoma	++	++
Frequent, prolonged consumption of extremely hot beverages	+	−
♂	−	+
Familial	−	+
Descent	Asian	European and North American

Table 63B // Risk factors for oesophageal carcinoma

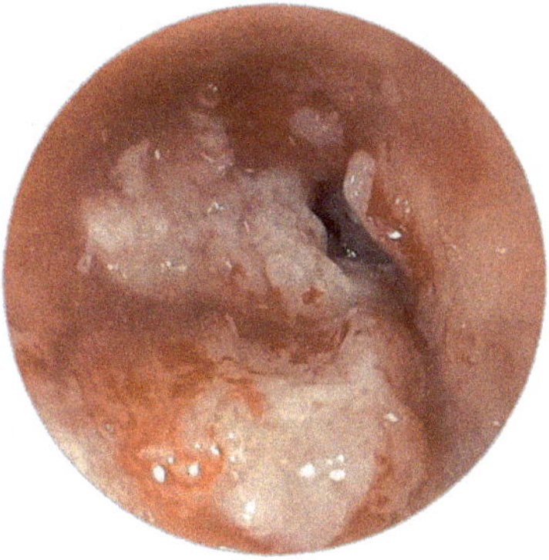

Figure 91 // Upper endoscopy: stenosing distal oesophageal carcinoma

> Barrett's oesophagus is a condition in which squamous epithelium transforms into columnar epithelium due to prolonged reflux and may be a preliminary stage of oesophageal carcinoma.

Pancreatic carcinoma

D A pancreatic carcinoma is a malignancy that originates from the pancreas (see Figure 92). Ductal adenocarcinomas are the most common; the majority of tumours are located in the pancreatic head, followed by the pancreatic tail and body.

E Highest incidence in Western countries, incidence has increased in recent years and will likely continue to rise

Ae Aetiology may be related to familial factors (e.g. Peutz-Jeghers syndrome, familial atypical multiple mole melanoma (FAMMM))

R Age >65, chronic pancreatitis, pancreatic cysts, smoking, alcohol, high caloric intake, high BMI

Hx Painless jaundice (++) (with itching, clay-coloured stools, dark urine), weight ↓ (++), general malaise (+), abdominal/epigastric pain (+), back pain (+), nausea, vomiting, diarrhoea (exocrine failure), increased abdominal girth (ascites) (−), fatigue

PE Jaundice, weight ↓, RUQ or epigastric pain, ascites in peritoneal carcinomatosis

Dx
- Labs: CA 19-9 ↑ (prognostic marker), in case of cholestasis: bilirubin ↑, ALP ↑, GGT ↑. Possibly glucose ↑ (endocrine pancreatic insufficiency).
- Faecal elastase ↓ (exocrine pancreatic insufficiency)
- EUS: to detect lesion, obtain pathology specimen
- ERCP: obtain pathology specimen, stent placement if needed
- Chest and abdominal contrast CT (pancreatic protocol): pancreatic mass, dilation of pancreatic duct, double-duct sign, atrophy of prestenotic pancreatic tissue, assess location and resectability based on local vascular and perivascular spread, and presence of metastases. Additional pancreatic MRI or PET-CT as needed.

Tx Consult dietitian: start pancreatic enzymes with meals
- Curative: surgical resection (pancreaticoduodenectomy, e.g. Whipple procedure), possibly in conjunction with neoadjuvant and/or adjuvant chemotherapy
- Palliative: endoscopic or percutaneous stent placement for bile duct obstruction, minimally invasive plexus coeliac block for pain relief, palliative chemotherapy

P
- 5-year survival: stage I 18%, stage II 11%, stage III 3%, stage IV 1%
- Median survival without therapy: 4-6 mo

! Consider IgG4-mediated disease in DDx, this may mimic pancreatic carcinoma (treat with prednisone)

> Pancreatic carcinomas are 'silent killers' because of their painless and insidious nature. Pancreatic tail carcinomas have the worst survival and the highest risk of metastases at diagnosis. This is partly because obstructive symptoms occur earlier in pancreatic head carcinoma, which is therefore discovered earlier. The 5-year recurrence rate is 95% even after curative surgery.

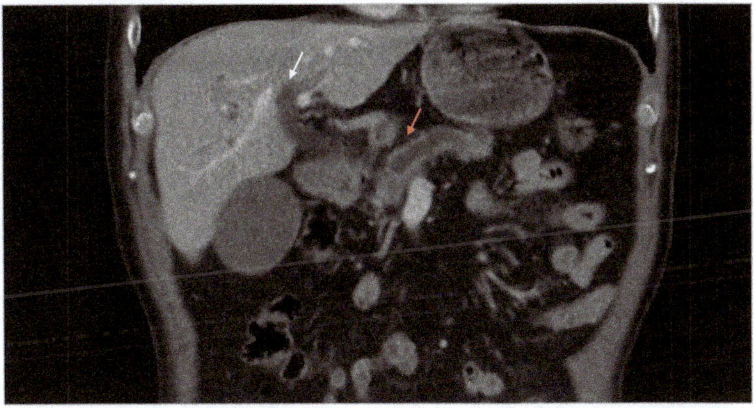

Figure 92 // Abdominal contrast CT: pancreatic carcinoma with dilated pancreatic duct (red arrow) and bile ducts (white arrow)

Vascular conditions

Angiodysplasia

D Angiodysplasias are acquired thin-walled vascular anomalies in the mucosal or submucosal layer of the GI tract and can bleed easily. Malformations may be present throughout the GI tract, particularly in the small intestine and caecum.

E Prevalence 8,000:100,000 after age 50. Most common cause of blood loss from the small intestine.

Ae Idiopathic, associated with obstructed submucosal veins and increased expression of angiogenetic factors

R Advanced age, end-stage kidney disease, von Willebrand disease, aortic stenosis (Heyde's syndrome), left ventricular assist devices (LVADs)

Hx Asymptomatic ⊕, haematemesis, melaena, or rectal blood loss after significant haemorrhage, symptoms consistent with anaemia. First clinical presentation often occurs after starting anticoagulants.

PE No added value, rectal exam may reveal blood loss/melaena

Dx
- Labs: Hb =/↓
- Endoscopy: small (2-10 mm), flat, cherry-red, fern-like lesions surrounded by pale mucosa with ectatic blood vessels radiating from a central vessel (see Figure 93). In patients with a negative endoscopy, capsule endoscopy can be performed to detect lesions in the small intestine.

Tx Isolated angiodysplasias (without evidence of GI haemorrhage or iron deficiency), usually found during screening colonoscopy: wait-and-see

- GI haemorrhage: endoscopic coagulation or clipping
- If endoscopic coagulation proves impossible or blood loss recurs despite successful coagulation: octreotide, thalidomide (note: prolonged thalidomide use is associated with frequent polyneuropathy)
- Chronic blood loss: iron supplementation, blood transfusion

P Most haemorrhages are self-limiting (90%), but 60% recurrence <2y

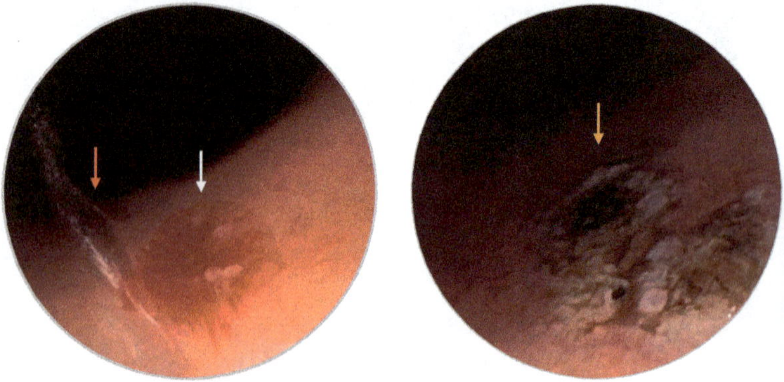

Figure 93 // Upper endoscopy: actively bleeding gastric angiodysplasia (white arrow) in the stomach being irrigated with water (red arrow). Right: haemostasis after coagulation (orange arrow).

Budd-Chiari syndrome

D Budd-Chiari syndrome is a condition characterised by hepatic venous outflow obstruction, regardless of the level or mechanism of obstruction. Obstruction due to cardiac disease, pericardial disease, or sinusoidal obstruction syndrome is ruled out.

E Prevalence 1-9:100,000

Ae
- Primary: primarily venous obstruction (thrombus or phlebitis)
- Secondary: compression/invasion of the hepatic veins and/or inferior vena cava (e.g. due to a malignancy)
- Hepatic vein obstruction (acute, chronic, or fulminant) → portal hypertension, if chronic: intrahepatic and extrahepatic venous collateral formation (see Figure 94)

R ♀, smoking, obesity, hypertension, acquired thrombophilia (e.g. myeloproliferative disease, polycythemia vera ⊕), inherited thrombophilia (e.g. factor V

Leiden), hormonal factors (e.g. pregnancy), medications (e.g. cytostatics, oral contraceptives)

Hx Asymptomatic (subacute or chronic), abdominal pain (RUQ), abdominal distension from ascites, GI haemorrhage due to varices or portal hypertensive gastropathy, fever ⊖, jaundice ⊖, hepatic encephalopathy ⊖, peripheral oedema ⊖

PE Ascites ⊕, hepatomegaly, splenomegaly, T↑ ⊖, jaundice ⊖, caput medusae ⊖, peripheral oedema ⊖

Dx
- Labs: diagnostics to reveal aetiology (complete blood count, coagulation tests)
- Abdominal ultrasound: absent, low, or reversed flow in hepatic veins ⊕, venous wall thickening, oedema/hyperechoic signal around the veins, hepatic venous collaterals, enlarged spleen, ascites
- Abdominal contrast CT/MRI according to liver protocol with inconclusive Doppler or high suspicion: delayed or absent filling of hepatic parenchyma, rapid clearance of contrast in the caudate lobe, changed liver segment ratio with hypertrophic caudate lobe, hepatic vein thrombus, collaterals, enlarged spleen, ascites
- Liver biopsy (not necessary for diagnosis): centrolobular congestion, necrosis, caudate lobe hypertrophy, fibrosis/cirrhosis

Tx Treat underlying cause (known in 80% of cases), treat complications of portal hypertension (if present), improve nutritional status, consider consulting Haematology

Start anticoagulant: LMWH or vitamin K antagonist (in the absence of CIs), consider thrombolysis or angiography with stenting (if thrombolysis is contraindicated)

If other strategies fail, consider surgical shunt, TIPS, liver transplantation

I Possible complications: portal hypertension (or associated complications), HCC (in liver cirrhosis). High mortality if untreated.

Patients developing acute, fulminant Budd-Chiari syndrome (5%) present with acute liver failure. When subacute, the syndrome (25%) does not present with acute liver failure, but can be accompanied by clinical manifestations such as ascites. Patients with the chronic form can present with complications of liver cirrhosis.

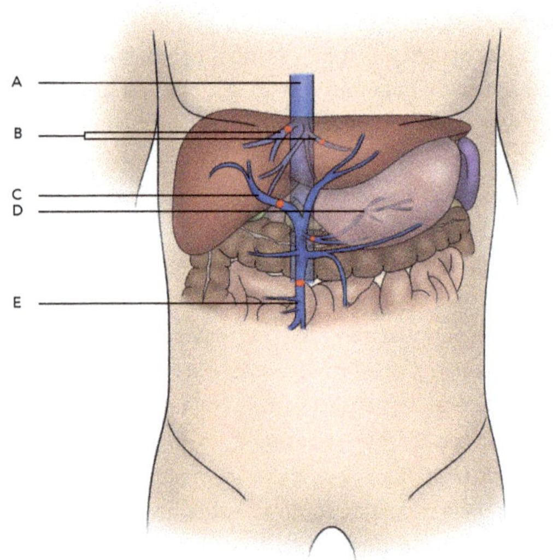

Figure 94 // Possible locations of thrombosis in Budd-Chiari syndrome
A: Inferior vena cava **B:** Hepatic veins **C:** Portal vein **D:** Splenic vein **E:** Mesenteric vein

Portal vein thrombosis (PVT)

D Portal vein thrombosis is characterised by the partial or complete occlusion of the portal vein by a blood clot (possibly affecting the mesenteric vessels or splenic vessels too, see Figure 95).

E Prevalence <1% in patients with compensated liver cirrhosis, prevalence 8-25% in patients on waiting list for liver transplantation

Ae Thrombus formation by different mechanisms (Virchow's triad: circulatory stasis, endothelial damage, hypercoagulation), esp. in the presence of multiple risk factors

R Idiopathic, liver cirrhosis (++), hepatobiliary or pancreatic malignancy (HCC (+)), acquired and hereditary coagulation conditions (+), intra-abdominal infection (e.g. acute pancreatitis or appendicitis), portal vein injury, hormonal factors (oral contraceptives, pregnancy)

Hx Asymptomatic, fever, abdominal pain (sudden onset or progressive over several days, often acute), nausea, abdominal distensions from ascites, splenic vessel occlusion: colicky abdominal pain

PE Not contributing ⊕, T ↑, signs of ascites, abdominal tenderness, if liver cirrhosis: stigmata of chronic liver disease

Dx
- Labs: acute phase reactants ↑, AST =/↑, ALT =/↑, if liver cirrhosis: bilirubin ↑, platelets ↑, INR ↑, if intestinal ischaemia: metabolic acidosis, D-dimer ↑, lactate ↑, WBC ↑
- Abdominal ultrasound: hepatomegaly, splenomegaly, hypertrophic caudate lobe, regeneration noduli in liver parenchyma, absent or reversed flow in hepatic veins, thrombus in inferior vena cava
- Abdominal contrast CT for high suspicion, inconclusive ultrasound, or thrombus using Doppler: diagnosis and extent of thrombus, presence of intra- and extrahepatic collateral vessels, caudate lobe enlargement, predisposing factors (e.g. intra-abdominal infection, malignancy)

Tx Treat triggering factor, repeat abdominal ultrasound/CT for follow-up

Anticoagulants for at least 3-6 mo (LMWH, followed by vit. K antagonist or DOAC), treat complications of portal hypertension, ABx in septic portal vein thrombosis

- Lower portal pressure: shunt, TIPS, thrombolysis
- Surgical exploration for acute portal vein thrombosis with infarction

P
- If treatment is started before intestinal infarction: good prognosis
- Untreated: risk of chronic portal vein thrombosis (with collateral formation) ↑, risk of intestinal infarction ↑ (risk of perforation, peritonitis, shock, organ failure, and mortality)

I
- Malignant portal vein thrombosis (malignant invasion or compression of the portal vein → thrombus formation) is a contraindication for liver transplantation
- Possible complications: related to portal hypertension (GI haemorrhage from oesophageal varices, ascites, hepatic encephalopathy), intestinal ischaemia, or acute pylephlebitis (fever, chills, painful liver)

The **portal vein** arises from the confluence of the superior mesenteric vein and the splenic vein, and supplies blood from the intestines and spleen to the liver. The vessel has an extrahepatic and an intrahepatic route.

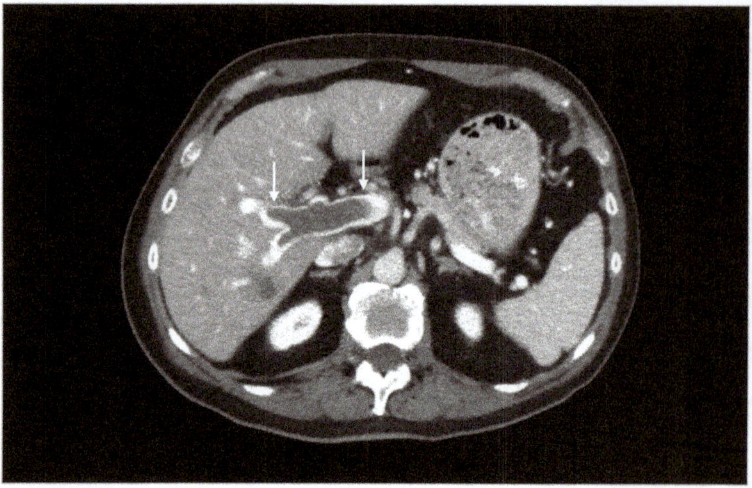

Figure 95 // Abdominal contrast CT: portal vein thrombosis extending into the left and right branches

Acute ischaemic colitis

D Acute ischaemic colitis is an inflammation of the large intestine resulting from reduced blood flow (see Figure 96).

E Incidence 16:100,000 per year

Ae
- Occlusive (e.g. thrombosis, embolism, aortic surgery, vasculitis)
- Nonocclusive/low blood flow ischaemia (e.g. heart failure, sepsis, vasoconstrictive medication, constipation, volvulus), leading cause of colonic ischemia (95%) and usually affecting areas of limited collateralisation (e.g. splenic flexure, rectosigmoid junction)

R Age >50, atherosclerosis, DM, vasculitis, systemic hypotension e.g. after myocardial infarction or resuscitation, dialysis, arrhythmias, digoxin, diuretics, vasopressin, shock/sepsis, iatrogenic (e.g. arterial reconstruction or cardiopulmonary bypass surgery)

Hx Non-specific, abdominal cramps (often left-sided) (++), urgent need to defecate (+), rectal bleeding/bloody diarrhoea (in right-sided ischaemia), nausea (−), vomiting (−)

PE
- T ↑, pulse ↑, BP ↓, left abdominal tenderness (++), abdominal guarding (−), rectal exam: blood on glove
- Severe cases may progress to intestinal necrosis and perforation with signs of septic shock

Dx
- Labs: no specific markers for ischaemia, D-dimer ↑, lactate ↑, LDH ↑, Hb ↓ (blood loss). WBC ↑ + albumin ↓ + metabolic acidosis + symptoms of ischaemia = suggestive of intestinal ischaemia with infarction.
- Colonoscopy: patchy, pale, oedematous, and fragile mucosa, in advanced stage: blue-purple translucent bulges in the intestinal mucosa, ulcers, haemorrhages
- Abdominal contrast CT (without contrast, CTA, and CTV): arterial occlusion, intestinal wall thickening, intestinal wall enhancement ↓ , air in the portal system and pneumobilia, thumb printing, intestinal pneumatosis, free fluid. Unlike colonoscopy, CT can identify transmural ischaemia.

Tx
Hospitalisation, NPO, NG tube if signs of ileus, IV fluid

Empiric broad-spectrum AB, stop blood pressure-lowering medication, consider anticoagulants for occlusive ischemia

In case of suspected necrosis, colon infarction, or persistent blood loss: consult surgeon for resection or interventional radiologist for endovascular revascularisation

P Usually reversible with improvement within 1-2d and complete resolution within 1-2 wk, but treatment can be challenging in older, debilitated patients with multimorbidity. Surgery is required in up to 20% of cases (resection of necrotic intestines).

! Beware of stricture formation or chronic colitis

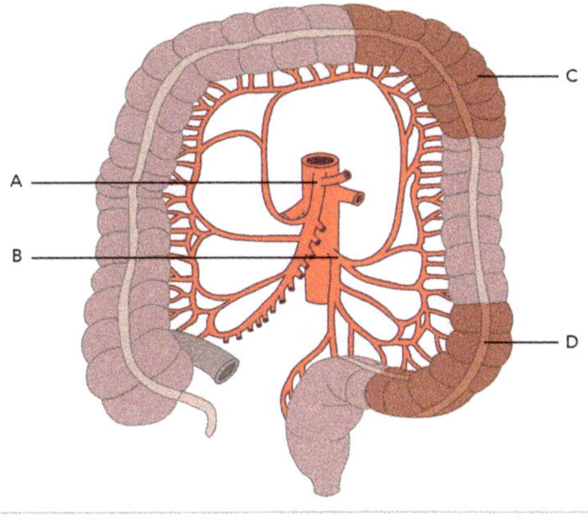

Figure 96 // Ischaemic colitis. The red areas highlight vulnerable parts of the colon as these are watershed regions of the blood supply.
A: Superior mesenteric artery **B:** Inferior mesenteric artery **C:** Splenic flexure **D:** Sigmoid colon

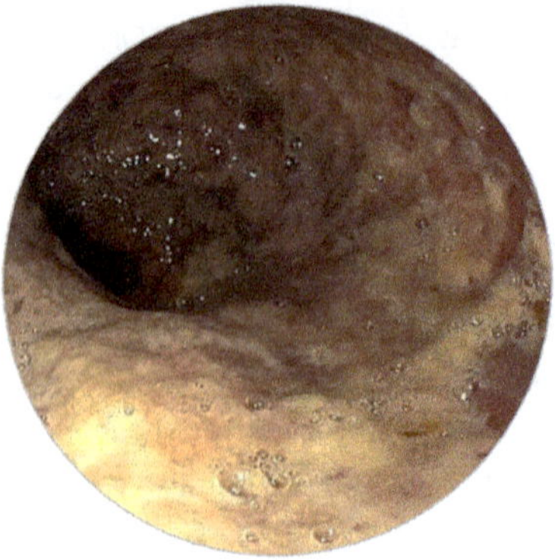

Figure 97 // Colonoscopy: ischaemic mucosa with necrosis of the colon

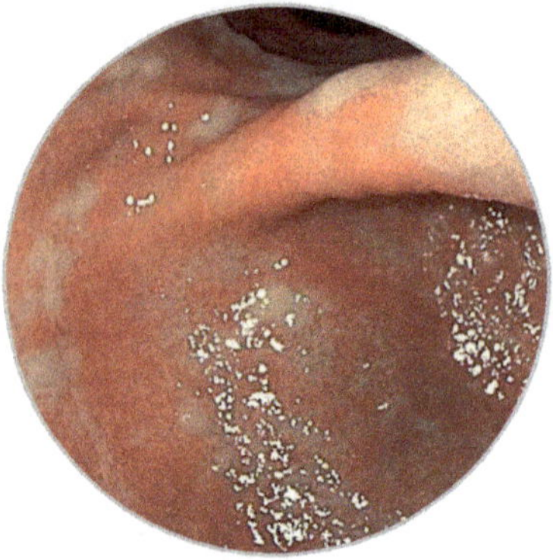

Figure 98 // Upper endoscopy: pale antral mucosa in chronic mesenteric ischaemia

Chronic mesenteric ischaemia (CMI) is chronic ischaemia of the stomach and intestines and often occurs secondary to atherosclerosis. There is always an indication for treatment in patients with two-vessel disease and a typical patient history.

- Typical history: unexplained postprandial abdominal pain, weight ↓ (>5% body weight), dietary changes (to avoid abdominal discomfort), or diarrhoea ⊖
- Risk factors: ♀, smoking, atherosclerosis, DM, hypercholesterolemia, peripheral vascular disease, age >60, positive FHx of CVD
- Additional diagnostics include abdominal ultrasound/contrast CT, upper endoscopy (see Figure 98) or colonoscopy (for diarrhoea in patients aged >50) to rule out alternative diagnoses. Abdominal contrast CT (without contrast, CTA and CTV) is used to detect stenosis/occlusion of the coeliac artery and superior mesenteric artery, subsequent intestinal ischaemia with intestinal pneumatosis, delayed/no enhancement of bowel wall and bowel wall thickening. In patients with single-vessel disease, perform visible light spectroscopy (VLS) or tonometry (functional tests) to detect mucosal ischaemia.

D-dimer is currently the most reliable biomarker for the diagnosis of ischaemic colitis with very high sensitivity. Low D-dimer thus virtually rules out ischaemic colitis, while normal **lactate** levels do not.

- **Thumbprinting** is a radiographic sign of ischaemic colitis. Ischaemia results in submucosal haemorrhages, causing localised swelling in the lumen and indentations on abdominal CT.
- **Intestinal pneumatosis** is characterised by the presence of gas in the walls of the GI tract, appearing on CT in patients with e.g. intestinal ischaemia.

See the Pocket *Cardiology and Vascular Medicine* for more information on vascular conditions.

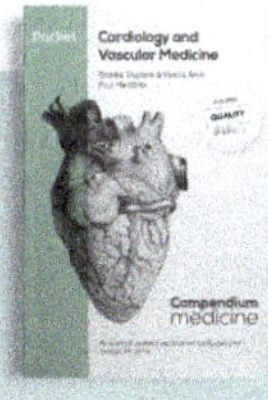

Alcohol-related conditions

See section *Management of alcohol-related conditions* for a systematic description of treatment recommendations.

Alcohol withdrawal syndrome (AWS)

D AWS is characterised by autonomic hyperactivity symptoms after quitting or reducing alcohol intake after a period of excessive use.

E Excessive alcohol consumption occurs in 10-20% of people at some point in their lives; the rate is double for hospitalised patients

Ae Alcohol is a CNS depressant (GABA-A ↑, NMDA receptor ↓), constant exposure results in a new equilibrium (downregulation of GABA-A, upregulation of NMDA). Abrupt cessation → autonomous hyperactivity. Reasons for varying severity of symptoms between individuals are unknown, genetic predisposition may be a factor.

R Excessive alcohol use, other alcohol-related conditions, history of complications from alcohol withdrawal syndrome (seizure, delirium, Wernicke), advanced age with severe somatic comorbidity, chronic use of GABAergic agents such as benzodiazepines, concomitant use of other drugs

Hx
- Symptoms consistent with autonomic hyperreactivity
- Last use, duration, quantity, frequency, previous episodes of withdrawal symptoms

- Rule out other illnesses that can present with similar symptoms, evaluate medications/drugs that can reduce alcohol withdrawal symptoms (e.g. benzodiazepines)

PE
- Pulse ↑, BP ↑, sweating
- Exploratory PE to detect possible complications of excessive alcohol consumption (e.g. arrhythmias, GI bleeding, ascites, infections, neurological damage)
- Neurological examination upon indication

Dx
- Labs: complete blood count, electrolytes, glucose, kidney function, liver panels. Typical findings include AST:ALT >2 in the absence of cirrhosis, Na ↓, macrocytosis.
- If indicated: check blood alcohol level (if alcohol use disorder is suspected: test carbohydrate-deficient transferrin (CDT)) ↑, ECG in patients with a history of cardiac conditions or bradycardia/tachycardia, consider brain CT for altered consciousness (e.g. rule out intracranial haemorrhage) or EEG: rule out neurological underlying cause

Tx See *Management of alcohol-related conditions* and Diagram 5

P 3-5% of patients hospitalised with AWS develop withdrawal delirium (consider adding antipsychotic if delirium is suspected)

> Early withdrawal symptoms (autonomic hyperreactivity) tend to occur 6-48h after cessation of alcohol intake. Typically, hallucinations or seizures occur after 48-72h, alcohol withdrawal, delirium after 72-96h. Patients who experience alcohol withdrawal-related seizures have an increased risk of developing alcohol withdrawal delirium.

> Definition of excessive alcohol consumption: ♀ >14 drinks/wk, ♂ >21 drinks/wk. Heavy drinkers: ♀ >7 drinks/wk, ♂ >14 drinks/wk or >3 drinks/d.

DSM-5 criteria for alcohol withdrawal:

A. Cessation/reduction of alcohol use that has been heavy and prolonged.

B. At least two of the following, developing within several hours to a few days after the cessation/reduction of alcohol use, listed under criterion A:

  1. Autonomic hyperactivity (e.g. sweating or pulse >100/min)
  2. Increased hand tremor
  3. Insomnia
  4. Nausea or vomiting
  5. Transient visual, tactile, or auditory hallucinations or illusions
  6. Psychomotor agitation
  7. Anxiety
  8. Generalised tonic-clonic seizures

C. The signs or symptoms in Criterion B cause clinically significant distress or impairment in social, occupational, or other important areas of functioning.

D. The signs or symptoms are not attributable to another medical condition and are not better explained by another mental disorder, not even intoxication or withdrawal from another substance.

Alcohol withdrawal delirium

D Alcohol withdrawal delirium, also known as delirium tremens, is an acute change in consciousness, attention, and cognition, with or without hallucinations, that occurs after cessation of excessive alcohol consumption.

E 5-10% of the patients with alcohol use disorder

Ae See *Alcohol withdrawal syndrome*

R CIWA-Ar score >15 (esp. with BP >150 mmHg or HR >100/min), previous withdrawal episode, advanced age, excessive substance abuse, comorbidities, underweight

Hx Symptoms consistent with autonomic hyperreactivity (psychomotor agitation, anxiety, restlessness, tremor, palpitations, headache), change in attention and consciousness (impaired memory, orientation, language, visual-spatial ability or perception), nausea, vomiting, appetite ↓. Symptoms of delirium often arise 3-4d after cessation and usually last 2-3d; may fluctuate throughout the day.

PE Pulse ↑, BP ↑, T ↑/↓, watch out for fluid underload due to sweating, fever, vomiting, and intake ↓

Dx
- Labs: electrolyte imbalances are common (Na ↓, K ↓, Mg ↓, P ↓), glucose ↓, also see Refeeding syndrome
- If indicated, diagnostics to rule out other underlying causes of delirium (e.g. urine sediment/culture for possible UTI, and chest X-ray for possible pneumonia)

Tx See *Management of alcohol-related conditions*

P Mortality 1-4%, mostly due to hyperthermia, cardiac arrhythmias, withdrawal seizures, or comorbidities

> The CIWA-Ar score assesses the risk in all patients suspected of being at risk for alcohol withdrawal. Any indication of daily alcohol use over several weeks or longer, irrespective of quantity, should prompt concern for potential alcohol withdrawal. Scan the QR code.

Wernicke encephalopathy

D Wernicke encephalopathy is a neurological syndrome caused by thiamine deficiency and usually accompanies excessive alcohol consumption.

E Western world: prevalence 1-3%, ♂>♀

Ae Thiamine plays a role in cerebral glucose metabolism, and a deficiency can cause neurological damage. Chronic: Korsakoff syndrome.

R Possible genetic predisposition, malnutrition/self-neglect, malabsorption, increased metabolism (e.g. disease), dialysis

Hx Non-specific symptoms, acute or subacute change in cognition/consciousness (++), eye movements (nystagmus, limited lateral eye movement, double vision (+)), and/or gait ataxia (+)

PE Neurological exam and exploratory PE to detect possible complications of excessive alcohol consumption (e.g. arrhythmias, GI bleeding, ascites, infections)

Dx
- Labs: electrolyte imbalances are common (Na ↓, K ↓, Mg ↓, P ↓), glucose ↓, also see Refeeding syndrome
- When in doubt: brain CT/MRI can rule out other neurological disorders, but must never delay the start of treatment with IV thiamine

Tx
- Consider NPO to prevent aspiration (impaired consciousness), consult dietician for dietary plan, preventive measures, consider consulting with Neurology when unsure about diagnosis, consider consulting

Psychiatry

- With increased risk or suspicion: start treatment, IV thiamine, correct electrolyte imbalances (if administering glucose: start patient on IV thiamine first to avoid Wernicke encephalopathy), see Management of alcohol-related conditions and Diagram 5

P Mortality 20%, surviving patients have 85% chance of developing Korsakoff syndrome, prognosis depends on time to IV thiamine administration

! Diagnostics should not delay treatment

The classic triad of Wernicke encephalopathy consists of: 1) acute changes in cognition; 2) abnormalities in eye movements; and 3) gait ataxia. However, this triad is rarely fully present, with most patients exhibiting only one or two of these symptoms.

Appendices

Appendix 1: Paracentesis

> This chapter only serves as an aid. How extensively and in what order issues are addressed varies per specialty (and hospital).

Ascites is the accumulation of fluid in the peritoneal cavity. It generally warrants a diagnostic paracentesis. This involves collecting a small amount of ascitic fluid and analysing e.g. the serum-to-ascites albumin gradient (SAAG) to distinguish between transudative or exudative ascites, and the presence of elevated WBC to rule out infections (e.g. SBP).

Large volumes of ascites may produce symptoms such as shortness of breath, abdominal pain, or difficulty bending over. A drain can be left temporarily or permanently in place to provide relief.

> Drains left in place during a diagnostic paracentesis must remain closed until SBP has been ruled out.

Procedure

Paracentesis should be performed in sterile surroundings. The classic site for paracentesis is the contralateral McBurney's point, located at two-thirds of the distance between the anterior superior iliac spine and the navel (see Figure 99). Paracentesis may also be performed at McBurney's point due to e.g. local tumour growth, an ostomy, or other obstructing factors. The chosen site is marked, and percussion is done to confirm the presence of ascitic fluid. Ultrasound can also be used to confirm the presence of ascitic fluid and rule out the presence of local tumours or other abnormalities. After the puncture site is disinfected, the ascitic fluid can be removed perpendicularly with a syringe, and a drain is left behind as needed (see Figure 100).

Complications

Possible complications of paracentesis include ascites leakage from the puncture site (very common), drain blockage (common), infection at the puncture site, bacterial peritonitis, bleeding, perforation of intestinal or bladder tissue (very rare, may result in bleeding or faecal peritonitis), and paracentesis-induced circulatory dysfunction (PICD). Administration of albumin is recommended for paracentesis volumes over five litres to prevent PICD.

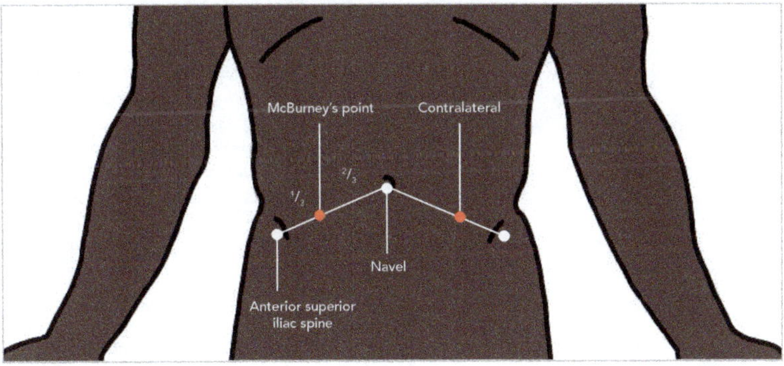

Figure 99 // Contralateral McBurney's point

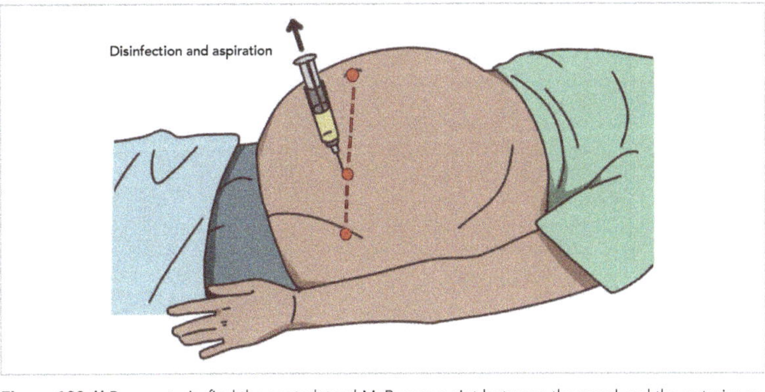

Figure 100 // Paracentesis: find the contralateral McBurney point between the navel and the anterior superior iliac spine for aspiration

Ascitic fluid analysis

> The SAAG can provide information on the origin of ascitic fluid. SAAG ≥11 g/L indicates transudative ascites (e.g. portal hypertension in cirrhosis). SAAG <11 g/L indicates exudative ascites (e.g. carcinomatous peritonitis). The serum-pleural effusion albumin gradient (SPAG) is the equivalent of SAAG for pleural effusion.

TEST	EXPLANATION	INTERPRETATION
Gross appearance	Visual features of ascitic fluid	• Clear: transudate (portal hypertension, heart failure) • Cloudy: exudate (infection, SBP, malignancy) • Pink/bloody: exudate (malignancy, infection, perforation, TB), perforated ulcer • Milky: triglyceride ↑ (chylous ascites), lymph obstruction (in malignancy/lymphoma), or after trauma • Brown: deeply jaundiced patients, biliary perforation, or perforated duodenal ulcer
Protein concentration	The total amount of protein in the ascitic fluid	↑ Indicates exudate ↓ Indicates transudate
Albumin	Protein produced by the liver that accounts for half of all serum proteins, important for osmotic pressure and transport	↑ SAAG ≥11 g/L (≥1.1 g/dL) indicates transudate/portal hypertensive ascites ↓ SAAG <11 g/L (<1.1 g/dL) indicates exudate/non-portal hypertensive ascites
Lactate dehydrogenase (LDH)	Important in cellular energy supply; also released following tissue damage	↑ Indicates exudate, >ULN for serum suggestive of bowel perforation instead of SBP ↓ Indicates transudate
Glucose	Carbohydrate that plays an important role in cellular energy supply	↓ Suggestive of presence of a bacterial cause or malignancy
Amylase	Enzyme produced by the pancreas and involved in carbohydrate digestion	↑ Suggestive of pancreatogenic cause (specifically pancreatitis, as well as pseudocyst leakage or pancreatic duct rupture)
Bilirubin	A breakdown product of haemoglobin that is conjugated in the liver and excreted with bile	↑ Suggestive of biliary or duodenal perforation
Carcinoembryonic antigen (CEA)	Protein produced by a fetus and found in very low concentrations in healthy adult blood	↑ • Suggestive of possibility of colorectal carcinoma • May also be elevated in patients with breast, lung, liver, pancreatic, gastric, and ovarian carcinomas
Triglycerides	Lipids that serve as sources and stores of energy in the body	↑ Suggestive of lymphatic anomalies, malignancy, cirrhosis, or infection

Table 64A // Ascitic fluid analysis

TEST	EXPLANATION	INTERPRETATION
Leukocytes	WBC, part of the immune system	↑ May indicate SBP, other bacterial peritonitis, or a malignancy (if there is a high percentage of foreign cells)
Neutrophil count	Specific type of white blood cell involved in fighting bacterial infections	>0.25 x 10^9/L/≥250/mm³: SBP in the context of cirrhosis or another form of peritonitis
Cytology and pathology	Microscopic examination of abnormal (malignant) cells, possibly with certain stains	• Malignant cells: consistent with carcinomatous peritonitis • Negative: does not rule out carcinomatous peritonitis • Positive Ziehl-Neelsen stain: consistent with peritoneal or non-peritoneal TB
Culture	Microbiological diagnostic method used to check for the presence of microorganisms	Results may prove the presence of a pathogen. Often negative in SBP.

Table 64B // Ascitic fluid analysis

In diagnostic paracentesis used to rule out SBP, the total leukocyte count is known before the differential blood count. At leukocyte counts >0.25 x 10^9/L, patients are often started on ABx before the differential blood count (the number of segmented neutrophils) is known, given that SBP has high mortality. If only a small proportion of leukocytes are found to be neutrophils (<0.25 x 10^9/L), an SBP has been ruled out.

ASCITIC FLUID	TRANSSUDATE (SAAG ≥11 G/L)	EXSUDATE (SAAG <11 G/L)
Causes	• Portal hypertension • Cirrhosis • Heart failure • Budd-Chiari syndrome • Myxoedema • Hepatic metastases • Alcoholic hepatitis	• Malignancy, e.g. peritoneal carcinomatosis • Infection, including peritoneal TB • Biliary ascites • Nephrotic syndrome • Pancreatitis • Serositis

Table 65 // Origin of ascitic fluid

Appendix 2: Commonly used calculators

Blatchford Bleeding Score

The Blatchford Bleeding Score identifies the risk of patients with an upper GI haemorrhage to determine whether intervention is indicated (endoscopy, transfusion, or admission). The chance that a patient will need an intervention (blood transfusion, endoscopy, or surgery) increases by 50% at scores ≥6. Patients with a score ≤1 are deemed low-risk and qualify for ambulatory monitoring. Scan the QR code for more information.

FACTOR	VALUE		SCORE
	♂	♀	
Urea (mmol/L)	<6.5		0
	6.5-7.9		+2
	8-9.9		+3
	10-24.9		+4
	≥25		+6
Hb (mmol/L)	>8	>7.5	0
	7.5-8.0	6.2-7.4	+1
	6.2-7.4	-	+3
	<6.2	<6.2	+6

Table 66A // Blatchford Bleeding Score

FACTOR	VALUE		SCORE
	♂	♀	
Systolic BP (mmHg)	≥110		0
	100-109		+1
	90-99		+2
	<90		+3
Other parameters	Heart rate >100/min		+1
	Melaena		+1
	Collapse		+2
	Liver disease		+2
	Heart failure		+2

Table 66B // Blatchford Bleeding Score

Child-Pugh Classification

The Child-Pugh Classification is used to estimate the 2-year survival of patients with chronic liver disease, particularly cirrhosis. A patient's Child-Pugh score can vary over time and should therefore be regularly recalculated. Scan the QR code for more information.

	VALUE	SCORE
Total bilirubin (μmol/L)	<35	+1
	35-51	+2
	>51	+3
Albumin (g/L)	>35	+1
	28-35	+2
	<28	+3
INR	<1.7	+1
	1.7-2.3	+2
	>2.3	+3

Table 67A // Child-Pugh Classification

	VALUE	SCORE
Ascites	Absent	+1
	Mild	+2
	Serious	+3
Encephalopathy	Absent	+1
	Mild (grade 1-2)	+2
	Severe/ comatose (grade 3-4)	+3

Table 67B // Child-Pugh Classification

SCORE	GRADE	INTERPRETATION	2-YEAR SURVIVAL
5-6	A	Mild cirrhosis	100-65%
7-9	B	Moderate cirrhosis	80-60%
≥10	C	Severe cirrhosis	45-35%

Table 68 // Interpretation Child-Pugh Classification

MELD score

The Model for End-Stage Liver Disease (MELD) score is used to estimate the prognosis of liver disease by predicting 3-month mortality. The score is based on serum creatinine, bilirubin, sodium, and INR, and is used as a scoring system for patients on the waiting list for liver transplantation. Scan the code for more information.

SCORE	3-MONTH MORTALITY
≥40	71-100%
30-39	52.6-74.5%
20-29	19.6-45.5%
10-19	6-20%
≤9	1.9-3.7%

Table 69 // Interpretation MELD score

Montreal Classification

The Montreal Classification is used to objectify and monitor the presentation and development of Crohn's disease and ulcerative colitis. For Crohn's disease: age at diagnosis, disease location, and disease behaviour are taken into account. 'L4' and 'p' are modifiers and can only be added to another score in the same factor category (see example). For ulcerative colitis, the classification system takes into account the extent and severity of the disease.

A patient diagnosed with Crohn's disease at age 22 with stricturing disease of the ileum and duodenum, as well as perianal disease, is classified as A2L1+4B2+p.

FACTOR	VALUE	SCORE
Age at diagnosis	≤16	A1
	17-40	A2
	≥40	A3
Disease location	Ileal	L1
	Colonic	L2
	Ileocolonic	L3
	Upper GI tract	L4
Disease behaviour	Non-stricturing and non-penetrating	B1
	Stricturing	B2
	Penetrating	B3
	Perianal disease	+p

Table 70 // Montreal Classification of Crohn's disease

FACTOR	VALUE	SCORE
Extent	Proctitis (limited to rectum)	E1
	Left-sided colitis (limited to area distal to splenic flexure)	E2
	Pancolitis (involvement extends proximal to splenic flexure)	E3
Severity	Remission (no symptoms)	S0
	Mild (≤4 bloody stools daily, no fever or tachycardia, Hb >6.5 mmol/L)	S1
	Moderate (>4-5 bloody stools daily, no systemic symptoms)	S2
	Severe (≥6 bloody stools daily, tachycardia, fever, Hb <6.5 mmol/L)	S3

Tabel 71 // Montreal Classification of ulcerative colitis

A patient diagnosed with ulcerative colitis at age 30, with the disease extending beyond the sigmoid but limited to the area distal to the splenic flexure, 5 bloody stools daily, an Hb of 6.9 mmol/L, and a temperature of 37.3 °C is classified as E2S2.

Travis Criteria

The Travis Criteria are used to predict the need for colectomy in patients with ulcerative colitis presenting with acute severe ulcerative colitis (ASUC). The score is usually calculated on day 3 of treatment for ASUC. Patients who meet both criteria have an 85% chance of undergoing a colectomy during the same admission.

CRITERION	THRESHOLD
Stool frequency	>8
CRP	>45 mg/L

Table 72 // Travis Criteria for acute severe ulcerative colitis

Truelove and Witts criteria

Truelove and Witts criteria are used to establish the severity of ulcerative colitis in adults. Scan the QR code for more information.

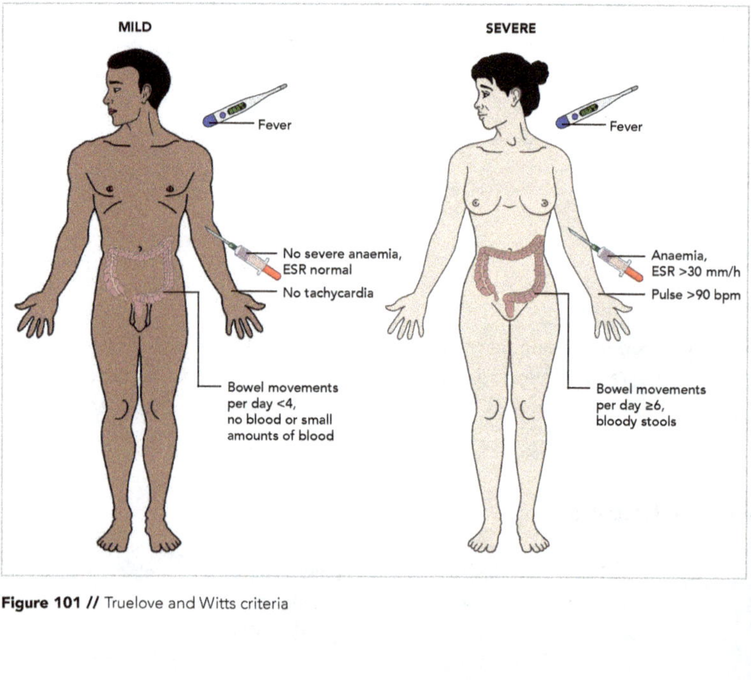

Figure 101 // Truelove and Witts criteria

Appendix 3: Hepatorenal syndrome (HRS): diagnostic and therapeutic algorithm

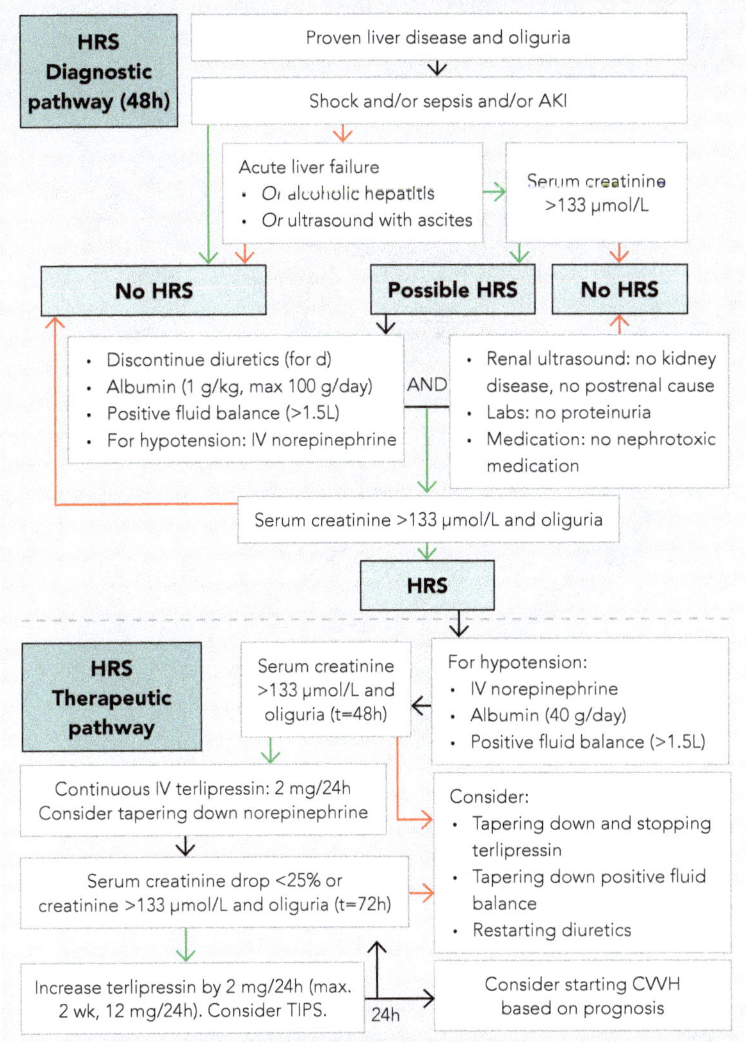

Diagram 13 // HRS: diagnostic and therapeutic algorithm
AKI: acute kidney insufficiency, CVVH: continuous veno-venous hemofiltration, HRS: hepatorenal syndrome, TIPS: transjugular intrahepatic portosystemic shunt

Appendix 4: Schematic overview entero-hepatic circulation

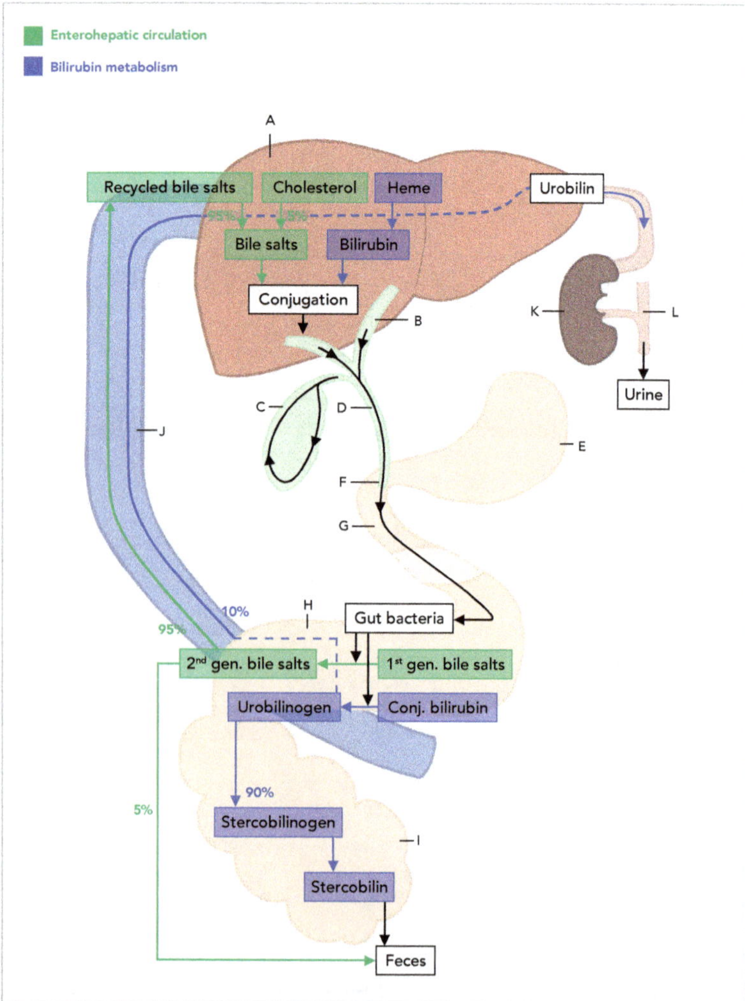

Diagram 14 // Enterohepatic circulation: bile salt and bile metabolism

A: Liver **B:** Intrahepatic bile duct **C:** Gallbladder **D:** Extrahepatic bile tract **E:** Stomach **F:** Major duodenal papilla **G:** Duodenum **H:** Small intestines **I:** Colon **J:** Portal vein **K:** Kidney **L:** Urinary tract

References

1. Åberg F, Byrne CD, Pirola CJ, Männistö V, Sookoian S. Alcohol consumption and metabolic syndrome: Clinical and epidemiological impact on liver disease. J Hepatol. 2023;78(1):191-206. doi:10.1016/j.jhep.2022.08.030. Available from: https://www.sciencedirect.com/science/article/pii/S0168827822030616.Basra S, Anand BS. Definition, epidemiology and magnitude of alcoholic hepatitis. World J Hepatol. 2011 May 27;3(5):108-13.
2. Afdhal NH. Acute cholangitis: clinical manifestations, diagnosis and management [Internet]. UpToDate. [2024]. Available from: https://www.uptodate.com/contents/acute-cholangitis-clinical-manifestations-diagnosis-and-management
3. Ahmed M. Acute cholangitis - an update. World J Gastrointest Pathophysiol. 2018;9(1):1-7. doi: 10.4291/wjgp.v9.i1.1.
4. Aithal GP, Palaniyappan N, China L, Härmälä S, Macken L, Ryan JM, et al. Guidelines on the management of ascites in cirrhosis. Gut. 2021 Jan;70(1):9-29. Available from: https://gut.bmj.com/content/70/1/9
5. Almadi MA, Lu Y, Alali AA, Barkun AN. Peptic ulcer disease. Lancet. 2024 Jul 6;404(10447):68-81. doi: 10.1016/S0140-6736(24)00155-7.
6. American College of Gastroenterology. ACG clinical guideline for the diagnosis and management of gastroparesis [Internet]. Am J Gastroenterol. 2022;117(1):14-31. Available from: https://journals.lww.com/ajg/fulltext/2022/01000/acg_clinical_guideline_for_the_diagnosis_and.14.aspx
7. American College of Gastroenterology. ACG clinical guideline: diagnosis and management of idiosyncratic drug-induced liver injury [Internet]. Am J Gastroenterol. 2021 May [cited 2025 Jan 27]. Available from: https://journals.lww.com/ajg/fulltext/2021/05000/acg_clinical_guideline__diagnosis_and_management.13.aspx
8. American College of Gastroenterology. ACG clinical guideline: gastroparesis [Internet]. Am J Gastroenterol. 2022;117(8):1233-45. Available from: https://journals.lww.com/ajg/Fulltext/2022/08000/ACG_Clinical_Guideline__Gastroparesis.15.aspx
9. American College of Gastroenterology. ACG clinical guideline: small intestinal bacterial overgrowth [Internet]. Am J Gastroenterol. 2020;115(2):165-78. Available from: https://journals.lww.com/ajg/Fulltext/2020/02000/ACG_Clinical_Guideline__Small_Intestinal_Bacterial.9.aspx
10. American College of Gastroenterology. ACG clinical guidelines: diagnosis and management of celiac disease [Internet]. Am J Gastroenterol. 2020;115(9):1420-35. Available from: https://journals.lww.com/ajg/Fulltext/2020/09000/ACG_Clinical_Guidelines__Diagnosis_and_Management.18.aspx
11. American College of Gastroenterology. ACG guidelines for gastroduodenal Crohn's disease [Internet]. Am J Gastroenterol. 2023;118(1):17-29. Available from: https://journals.lww.com/ajg/Fulltext/2023/01000/American_College_of_Gastroenterology_Guidelines.17.aspx
12. American College of Gastroenterology. Diagnosis and management of Barrett's esophagus [Internet]. Am J Gastroenterol. 2022;117(4):549-83. Available from: https://journals.lww.com/ajg/fulltext/2022/04000/diagnosis_and_management_of_barrett_s_esophagus_.17.aspx
13. American College of Radiology. ACR Appropriateness Criteria® Jaundice [Internet]. 2018 Jan 1. Available from: https://acsearch.acr.org/docs/69497/Narrative/
14. American Gastroenterological Association (AGA). Diagnosis and management of atrophic gastritis [Internet]. 2023. Available from: https://gastro.org/clinical-guidance/diagnosis-and-management-of-atrophic-gastritis/
15. American Gastroenterological Association (AGA). Management of eosinophilic esophagitis (EoE) [Internet]. 2023. Available from: https://gastro.org/clinical-guidance/management-of-eosinophilic-esophagitis-eoe/
16. American Gastroenterological Association (AGA). Management of refractory Helicobacter pylori infection [Internet]. 2023. Available from: https://gastro.org/clinical-guidance/management-of-refractory-helicobacter-pylori-infection/
17. American Gastroenterological Association (AGA). Medical management of colonic diverticulitis [Internet]. 2023. Available from: https://gastro.org/clinical-guidance/medical-management-of-colonic-diverticulitis/
18. American Gastroenterological Association (AGA). Pharmacological management of irritable bowel syndrome with diarrhea (IBS-D) [Internet]. 2023. Available from: https://gastro.org/clinical-guidance/pharmacological-management-of-irritable-bowel-syndrome-with-diarrhea-ibs-d/
19. American Gastroenterological Association (AGA). Update on gastric peroral endoscopic myotomy (G-POEM) for gastroparesis [Internet]. 2023. Available from: https://gastro.org/clinical-guidance/update-on-gastric-peroral-endoscopic-myotomy-g-poem-for-gastroparesis/
20. American Gastroenterological Association. AGA clinical practice update on the management of pancreatic necrosis [Internet]. Am J Gastroenterol. 2023;118(6):755-64. Available from: https://journals.lww.com/ajg/fulltext/2023/06000/american_gastroenterological_association_american.13.aspx
21. American Gastroenterological Association. Epidemiology, evaluation, and management of exocrine pan-

creatic insufficiency [Internet]. Available from: https://gastro.org/clinical-guidance/epidemiology-evaluation-management-exocrine-pancreatic-insufficiency/
22. American Gastroenterological Association. Initial management of acute pancreatitis (AP) [Internet]. Available from: https://gastro.org/clinical-guidance/initial-management-of-acute-pancreatitis-ap/
23. American Society of Addiction Medicine. The ASAM Clinical Practice Guideline on Alcohol Withdrawal Management. J Addict Med. 2020 May-Jun;14(3S Suppl 1):1-72. doi: 10.1097/ADM.0000000000000668.
24. American Society of Addiction Medicine. The ASAM Clinical Practice Guideline on alcohol withdrawal management. J Addict Med. 2020 May-Jun;14(3S Suppl 1):1-72. doi: 10.1097/ADM.0000000000000668.
25. Andrade RJ, Chalasani N, Björnsson ES, Suzuki A, Kullak-Ublick GA, Watkins PB, et al. Drug-induced liver injury. Nat Rev Dis Primers. 2019 Aug 22;5(1):58.
26. Antunes C, Tian C, Copelin EL II. Upper gastrointestinal bleeding. [Updated 2024 Aug 17]. In: StatPearls [Internet]. Treasure Island (FL): StatPearls Publishing; 2025 Jan–. Available from: https://www.ncbi.nlm.nih.gov/books/NBK470300/
27. Arizumi T, Tazuma S, Isayama H, Nakazawa T, Tsuyuguchi T, Takikawa H, Tanaka A; Japan PSC Study Group (JPSCSG). Ursodeoxycholic acid is associated with improved long-term outcome in patients with primary sclerosing cholangitis. J Gastroenterol. 2022;57:902–912. Available from: https://link.springer.com/article/10.1007/s00535-022-01914-3.
28. Arvanitakis, M., Dumonceau, J. M., Albert, J., Badaoui, A., Bali, M. A., Barthet, M., ... & van Hooft, J. E. (2018). Endoscopic management of acute necrotizing pancreatitis: European Society of Gastrointestinal Endoscopy (ESGE) evidence-based multidisciplinary guidelines. Endoscopy, 50(05), 524–546.
29. ASGE Standards of Practice Committee. ASGE guideline on the role of endoscopy in the evaluation and management of choledocholithiasis. Gastrointest Endosc. 2019;89:1075.
30. Azeem N. Choledocholithiasis: clinical manifestations, diagnosis and management [Internet]. UpToDate. [2023] Available from: https://www.uptodate.com/contents/choledocholithiasis-clinical-manifestations-diagnosis-and-management
31. Banks PA, Bollen TL, Dervenis C, Gooszen HG, Johnson CD, Sarr MG, et al.; Acute Pancreatitis Classification Working Group. Classification of acute pancreatitis—2012: revision of the Atlanta classification and definitions by international consensus. Gut. 2013 Jan;62(1):102-11.
32. Baronia AK, Ahmed A. Hypocalcemia in acute pancreatitis revisited. Indian J Crit Care Med. 2016 Mar;20(3):173-7. doi: 10.4103/0972-5229.178182.
33. Barton JC, Barton JC, Acton RT. Factors related to mean corpuscular volume in HFE p.C282Y homozygotes. eJHaem. 2024 Dec;6(1):e1063. doi: 10.1002/jha2.1063.
34. Bedene A, van Dorp ELA, Rosendaal FR, Dahan A, Lijfering WM. Risk of drug-related upper gastrointestinal bleeding in the total population of the Netherlands: a time-trend analysis. BMJ Open Gastroenterol. 2022;9(1):e000733. doi:10.1136/bmjgast-2021-000733. Available from: https://bmjopengastro.bmj.com/content/9/1/e000733.
35. Bhardwaj R, Vaziri H, Gautam A, Ballesteros E, Karimeddini D, Wu GY. Chylous ascites: a review of pathogenesis, diagnosis and treatment. J Clin Transl Hepatol. 2018;6(1):1-9. Available from: https://doi.org/10.14218/jcth.2017.00035
36. Bharucha AE, Parthasarathy G, Ditah I, et al. Temporal trends in the incidence and natural history of diverticulitis: A population-based study. Am J Gastroenterol. 2015;110(11):1589-1596. doi: 10.1038/ajg.2015.302.
37. Biggins SW, Angeli P, Garcia-Tsao G, Ginès P, Ling SC, Nadim MK, et al. Diagnosis, evaluation, and management of ascites, spontaneous bacterial peritonitis, and hepatorenal syndrome: 2021 practice guidance by the American Association for the Study of Liver Diseases. Hepatology. 2021 Aug;74(2):1014-48. Available from: https://aasldpubs.onlinelibrary.wiley.com/doi/10.1002/hep.31884
38. Bosma JW, van Meyel JJ, Siegert CEH. Het hepatorenaal syndroom. Ned Tijdschr Geneeskd. 2010;154:A1355.
39. Bots S, De Voogd F, De Jong M, Ligtvoet V, Löwenberg M, Duijvestein M, et al. Point-of-care intestinal ultrasound in IBD patients: disease management and diagnostic yield in a real-world cohort and proposal of a point-of-care algorithm. J Crohns Colitis. 2022;16(4):606-15.
40. Boxhoorn L, Timmerhuis HC, Besselink M, Bollen T, et al. Diagnosis and treatment of pancreatic duct disruption or disconnection: an international expert survey and case vignette study. Gastroenterology. 2020;158(6 Suppl):S-335.
41. Boxhoorn L, van Dijk SM, van Grinsven J, Verdonk RC, Boermeester MA, Bollen TL, et al.; Dutch Pancreatitis Study Group. Immediate versus postponed intervention for infected necrotizing pancreatitis. N Engl J Med. 2021 Oct 7;385(15):1372-81.
42. Brandt LJ. ACG clinical guideline: epidemiology, risk factors, patterns of presentation, diagnosis, and management of colon ischemia (CI). Am J Gastroenterol. 2015;110(1):18-44.
43. Bredenoord AJ, De Wit NJ. Wel of geen gastroscopie? Ned Tijdschr Geneeskd. 2021;165(48):D6179.
44. Brennan PN, Cartlidge P, Manship T, Dillon JF. Guideline review: EASL clinical practice guidelines: drug-induced liver injury (DILI). Frontline Gastroenterol. 2022;13(4):332-336. doi:10.1136/flgastro-2022-102112. Available from: https://fg.bmj.com/content/13/4/332.
45. British Society of Gastroenterology (BSG). NICE guidelines for pancreatitis [Internet]. 2023. Available from: https://www.bsg.org.uk/clinical-resource/nice-guidelines-pancreatitis/

46. Buxbaum JL, Abbas Fehmi SM, et al. ASGE guideline on the role of endoscopy in the evaluation and management of choledocholithiasis. Gastrointest Endosc. 2019;89:1075.
47. Capurso G, Traini M, Piciucchi M, Signoretti M, Arcidiacono PG. Exocrine pancreatic insufficiency: prevalence, diagnosis, and management. Clin Exp Gastroenterol. 2019;12:129-39.
48. Catharina Ziekenhuis. Referentiewaarden Algemeen Klinisch Laboratorium [Internet]. 2021 [cited 2022 Mar 7]. Available from: https://www.catharinaziekenhuis.nl/app/uploads/files/Verwijzer/Specialismen_en_afdelingen/Laboratorium_algemeen_klinisch/Referentiewaarden/20210708_appreferentiewaardenlijst_V39.pdf
49. Chaaban T, Kanj N, Bou Akl I. Hepatic hydrothorax: an updated review on a challenging disease. Lung. 2019;197:399-405.
50. Chalasani NP, Maddur H, Russo MW, Wong RJ, Reddy KR; Practice Parameters Committee of the American College of Gastroenterology. ACG Clinical Guideline: diagnosis and management of idiosyncratic drug-induced liver injury. Am J Gastroenterol. 2021 May 1;116(5):878-98. Available from: https://journals.lww.com/ajg/fulltext/2021/05000/acg_clinical_guideline__diagnosis_and_management.13.aspx
51. Chan AO, Wong BC. Epidemiology of gastric cancer [Internet]. UpToDate. 2024 Apr 10. Available from: https://www.uptodate.com/contents/epidemiology-of-gastric-cancer
52. Chang L, Chey WD, Imdad A, Almario CV, Bharucha AE, Diem S, Greer KB, Hanson B, Harris LA, Ko C, Murad MH, Patel A, Shah ED, Lembo AJ, Sultan S. American Gastroenterological Association–American College of Gastroenterology Clinical Practice Guideline: Pharmacological Management of Chronic Idiopathic Constipation. Am J Gastroenterol. 2023 Jun;118(6):936-954. doi: 10.14309/ajg.0000000000002227.
53. Chen Y-C, Malfertheiner P, Yu H-T, El-Omar EM, Wu M-S, Liou J-M, et al. Global prevalence of helicobacter pylori infection and Incidence of Gastric Cancer Between 1980 and 2022 [Internet]. Gastroenterology; 2024 [cited 2024]. Available from: https://www.gastrojournal.org/article/S0016-5085(23)05687-1/fulltext
54. Cleveland Clinic. Exocrine pancreatic insufficiency (EPI) [Internet]. 2021. Available from: https://my.clevelandclinic.org/health/diseases/21577-exocrine-pancreatic-insufficiency-epi
55. Crawford DHG, Ramm GA, Bridle KR, Nicoll AJ, Delatycki MB, Olynyk JK. Clinical practice guidelines on hemochromatosis: Asian Pacific Association for the Study of the Liver. Hepatol Int. 2023;17:522–541. Available from: https://doi.org/10.1007/s12072-023-10510-3.
56. Davis J, McDonald M. Pyogenic liver abscess [Internet]. UpToDate. 2020 [cited 2022 Mar 3]. Available from: https://www.uptodate.com/contents/pyogenic-liver-abscess
57. de Haan J. Leverfalen acuut op chronisch [Internet]. 2013 [cited 2022 Jan 31]. Available from: https://icv-erasmusmc.nl/protocol/leverfalen-acuut-op-chronisch/
58. De Jongh E, De Wit NJ, Numans ME, Smeink P, Van der Weele GM, Wesseler GH. Maagklachten [Internet]. Nederlands Huisartsen Genootschap; 2021. Available from: https://richtlijnen.nhg.org/standaarden/maagklachten
59. de-Madaria E, Buxbaum JL, Maisonneuve P, García García de Paredes A, Zapater P, Guilabert L, et al. Aggressive or moderate fluid resuscitation in acute pancreatitis. New England Journal of Medicine. 2022 Sept 14;387(11):989–1000. doi:10.1056/nejmoa2202884
60. den Hartog D. Compartimentsyndroom [Internet]. 2013. Available from: http://WES-rotterdam.nl/symposium_2013_files/compartimentsyndroom%2015-03-2013.pdf
61. Diabetes on the Net. At-a-glance factsheet: recognition and management of pancreatogenic type 3c diabetes [Internet]. Available from: https://diabetesonthenet.com/diabetes-primary-care/glance-factsheet-recognition-and-management-pancreatogenic-type-3c-diabetes/
62. Dietetics Department, UMC Utrecht. (2015). Richtlijn refeeding syndrome. Visited 15 March 2022, fromhttps://preview-assets-eu-01.kc-usercontent.com/546dd520-97db-01b7-154d-79bb6d950a2d/dadb2dd4-db12-4e58-81a9-17c07cabb2cf/Richtlijn-refeeding.pdf
63. Epstein J. Secretin stimulation test [Internet]. 2016. Available from: https://www.healthline.com/health/secretin-stimulation-test
64. European Association for the Study of the Liver (EASL); European Association for the Study of Diabetes (EASD); European Association for the Study of Obesity (EASO). EASL-EASD-EASO Clinical Practice Guidelines on the management of metabolic dysfunction-associated steatotic liver disease (MASLD). J Hepatol. 2024;81(3):492-542. Available from: https://www.journal-of-hepatology.eu/article/S0168-8278(24)00062-5/fulltext
65. European Association for the Study of the Liver (EASL). Diagnosis and management of gallstones: prevention, diagnosis, and treatment [Internet]. 2023. Available from: https://easl.eu/publication/prevention-diagnosis-and-treatment-of-gallstones/
66. European Association for the Study of the Liver (EASL). EASL Clinical Practice Guidelines on the prevention, diagnosis and treatment of gallstones. J Hepatol. 2016 Jul;65(1):146-181. doi: 10.1016/j.jhep.2016.03.005. PMID: 27085810.
67. European Association for the Study of the Liver. EASL Clinical Practice Guidelines: The diagnosis and management of patients with primary biliary cholangitis. J Hepatol. 2017 Jul;67(1):145-72. Available from: https://www.journal-of-hepatology.eu/article/S0168-8278(17)30186-1/fulltext
68. European Association for the Study of the Liver. EASL Clinical Practice Guidelines on haemochromatosis. J Hepatol. 2022 Aug;77(2):479-502. Available from: https://www.journal-of-hepatology.eu/article/S0168-

8278(22)00204-6/fulltext
69. European Association for the Study of the Liver. EASL Clinical Practice Guidelines for the management of patients with decompensated cirrhosis. J Hepatol. 2018 Aug;69(2):406-60.
70. European Association for the Study of the Liver. EASL Clinical Practice Guidelines: Management of alcohol-related liver disease. J Hepatol. 2018 Jul;69(1):154-81.
71. European Association for the Study of the Liver. EASL Clinical Practice Guidelines on the management of cystic liver diseases. J Hepatol. 2022 [cited 2025 Jan 27];S0168-8278(22)00347-6.
72. European Association for the Study of the Liver. EASL Clinical Practice Guidelines on sclerosing cholangitis. J Hepatol. 2022;77(2):507-26.
73. European Association for the Study of the Liver. EASL Clinical Practical Guidelines on the management of acute (fulminant) liver failure. J Hepatol. 2017 May;66(5):1047-81.
74. European Crohn's and Colitis Organisation. ECCO guidelines on therapeutics in Crohn's disease: medical treatment. J Crohns Colitis. 2020 Jan;14(1):4-22.
75. European Crohn's and Colitis Organisation. ECCO guidelines on therapeutics in Crohn's disease: surgical treatment. J Crohns Colitis. 2020 Feb;14(2):155-68.
76. European Crohn's and Colitis Organisation. European Crohn's and Colitis Organisation clinical guidelines: definition and management of Crohn's disease. J Crohns Colitis. 2019;13(2):144-59. Available from: https://academic.oup.com/ecco-jcc/article/13/2/144/5078195?login=true
77. European Crohn's and Colitis Organisation. European Crohn's and Colitis Organisation clinical guidelines: management of ulcerative colitis. J Crohns Colitis. 2019;13(3):273-96. Available from: https://academic.oup.com/ecco-jcc/article/13/3/273/5078200?login=true
78. European Crohn's and Colitis Organisation. European Crohn's and Colitis Organisation clinical guidelines: perianal fistulising Crohn's disease. J Crohns Colitis. 2022;16(2):179-200. Available from: https://academic.oup.com/ecco-jcc/article/16/2/179/6390023?login=true
79. European Society of Gastrointestinal Endoscopy (ESGE). Diagnosis and management of Barrett esophagus [Internet]. 2022. Available from: https://www.esge.com/diagnosis-and-management-of-barrett-esophagus
80. European Society of Gastrointestinal Endoscopy (ESGE). Endoscopic diagnosis and management of nonvariceal upper gastrointestinal hemorrhage: ESGE update 2021 [Internet]. 2021. Available from: https://www.esge.com/endoscopic-diagnosis-and-management-of-nonvariceal-upper-gastrointestinal-hemorrhage-esge-update-2021
81. European Society of Gastrointestinal Endoscopy (ESGE). Endoscopic management of Lynch syndrome and familial colorectal cancer risk: ESGE guideline [Internet]. 2023. Available from: https://www.esge.com/endoscopic-management-of-lynch-syndrome-and-of-familial-risk-of-colorectal-cancer-esge-guideline
82. European Society of Gastrointestinal Endoscopy (ESGE). Endoscopic management of polyposis syndromes [Internet]. 2023. Available from: https://www.esge.com/endoscopic-management-of-polyposis-syndromes
83. European Study Group on Cystic Tumours of the Pancreas. European evidence-based guidelines on pancreatic cystic neoplasms. Gut. 2018 May;67(5):789-804.
84. Evans KE, Leeds JS, Morley S, Sanders DS. Pancreatic insufficiency in adult celiac disease: do patients require long-term enzyme supplementation? Dig Dis Sci. 2010;55:2999-3004.
85. Federatie Medisch Specialisten. Coloscopie surveillance [Internet]. 2022. Available from: https://richtlijnendatabase.nl/richtlijn/coloscopie_surveillance/startpagina.html
86. Federatie Medisch Specialisten. Herkenning en diagnostiek bij acuut leverfalen [Internet]. 2020 [cited 2022 Aug 24]. Available from: https://richtlijnendatabase.nl/richtlijn/acuut_leverfalen/herkenning_en_diagnostiek_bij_acuut_leverfalen.html
87. Federatie Medisch Specialisten. Startpagina - Acuut leverfalen - Richtlijn - Richtlijnendatabase [Internet]. 2020 Dec 16. Available from: https://richtlijnendatabase.nl/richtlijn/acuut_leverfalen/startpagina_-_acuut_leverfalen.html
88. Fernandez-del Castillo C, Jimenez RE. Epidemiology and nonfamilial risk factors for exocrine pancreatic cancer [Internet]. UpToDate. 2024 Feb 8. Available from: https://www.uptodate.com/contents/epidemiology-and-nonfamilial-risk-factors-for-exocrine-pancreatic-cancer
89. Fontana RJ, Liou I, Reuben A, Suzuki A, Fiel MI, Lee W, Navarro V. AASLD practice guidance on drug, herbal, and dietary supplement-induced liver injury. Hepatology. 2023 Mar 1;77(3):1036-65. Available from: https://aasldpubs.onlinelibrary.wiley.com/doi/10.1002/hep.32728
90. Fowler K, Mucha J, Neumann M, Lewandowski W, Kaczanowska M, Grys M, et al. A systematic literature review of the global seroprevalence of cytomegalovirus: possible implications for treatment, screening, and vaccine development. BMC Public Health. 2022 Sep 1;22(1):1659.
91. Friedman SL. Alcoholic hepatitis: clinical manifestations and diagnosis [Internet]. UpToDate. 2021 [cited date unknown]. Available from: https://www.uptodate.com/contents/alcoholic-hepatitis-clinical-manifestations-and-diagnosis
92. Friedman SL. Management and prognosis of alcoholic hepatitis [Internet]. UpToDate. 2022 [cited 2022 Mar 7]. Available from: https://www.uptodate.com/contents/management-and-prognosis-of-alcoholic-hepatitis
93. Gallstone Disease: Diagnosis and Management of Cholelithiasis, Cholecystitis and Choledocholithiasis. London: National Institute for Health and Care Excellence (NICE); 2014 Oct. PMID: 25473723.

94. Garbuzenko DV, Arefyev NO. Hepatic hydrothorax: an update and review of the literature. World J Hepatol. 2017 Nov 18;9(31):1197-204.
95. Garcia-Pagán JC. Recent portal vein thrombosis in adults: clinical features, diagnosis, and management [Internet]. UpToDate. 2024 Sep 20. Available from: https://www.uptodate.com/contents/recent-portal-vein-thrombosis-in-adults-clinical-features-diagnosis-and-management
96. Gardner-Thorpe J, Love N, Wrightson J, Walsh S, Keeling N. The value of Modified Early Warning Score (MEWS) in surgical in-patients: a prospective observational study. Ann R Coll Surg Engl. 2006 Oct;88(6):571-5. doi: 10.1308/003588406X130615. PMID: 17059720; PMCID: PMC1963767.
97. Gardner, T. B., Adler, D. G., Forsmark, C. E., Sauer, B. G., & Taylor, J. R. (2020). ACG Clinical Guideline: Chronic Pancreatitis. The American Journal of Gastroenterology, 115(3), 322–339.
98. Geelkerken RH, Illuminati G, Jackson RW, Kärkkäinen JM, Kolkman JJ, Lönn L, et al. European guidelines on chronic mesenteric ischaemia. United European Gastroenterol J. 2020 May;8(4):371-95.
99. Gezondheidsenquête/Leefstijlmonitor, CBS with RIVM and Trimbos-instituut. 2020.
100. Gibson MK. Epidemiology and risk factors for esophageal cancer [Internet]. UpToDate. 2024 Dec 11. Available from: https://www.uptodate.com/contents/epidemiology-and-risk-factors-for-esophageal-cancer
101. Gjeorgjievski M, Cappell MS. Portal hypertensive gastropathy: a systematic review of the pathophysiology, clinical presentation, natural history, and therapy. World J Hepatol. 2016 Feb 28;8(4):231.
102. Goldberg E, Chopra S. Cirrhosis in adults: overview of complications, general management, and prognosis [Internet]. UpToDate. 2022 [cited 2022 Mar 3]. Available from: https://www.uptodate.com/contents/cirrhosis-in-adults-overview-of-complications-general-management-and-prognosis
103. Groome M, Robinson EM, Mowat C, Morieux AML, Allstaff S. Are patients in the IBD clinic at risk of proctitis secondary to sexually transmitted infections? Frontline Gastroenterol. 2017 Oct;8(4):267-71.
104. Grubel P. Colonic ischemia [Internet]. UpToDate. 2022 Aug. Available from: https://www.uptodate.com/contents/colonic-ischemia
105. Hennes EM, Zeniya M, Czaja AJ, Parés A, Dalekos GN, Krawitt EL, et al.; International Autoimmune Hepatitis Group. Simplified criteria for the diagnosis of autoimmune hepatitis. Hepatology. 2008 Jul;48(1):169-76.
106. Herkel J, Carambia A, Lohse AW. Autoimmune hepatitis: possible triggers, potential treatments. J Hepatol. 2020 Aug;73(2):446-8.
107. Hoffman RS, Weinhouse GL. Management of moderate and severe alcohol withdrawal syndromes [Internet]. UpToDate. 2021 Nov 4. Available from: https://www.uptodate.com/contents/management-of-moderate-and-severe-alcohol-withdrawal-syndromes
108. Hoffman RS, Weinhouse GL. Management of moderate and severe alcohol withdrawal syndromes [Internet]. UpToDate; 2021 Nov 4 [cited 2025 Feb 28]. Available from: https://www.uptodate.com/contents/management-of-moderate-and-severe-alcohol-withdrawal-syndromes?topicRef=1653&source=see_link.
109. Hollemans RA, Bakker OJ, Boermeester MA, Bollen TL, Bosscha K, Bruno MJ, et al.; Dutch Pancreatitis Study Group. Superiority of step-up approach vs open necrosectomy in long-term follow-up of patients with necrotizing pancreatitis. Gastroenterology. 2019 Mar;156(4):1016-26.
110. Holodinsky JK, Roberts DJ, Ball CG, Blaser A, Starkopf J, Zygun DA, et al. Risk factors for intra-abdominal hypertension and abdominal compartment syndrome among adult intensive care unit patients: a systematic review and meta-analysis. Crit Care. 2013;17:R249.
111. Holvoet T, Lobaton T, Hindryckx P. Optimal management of acute severe ulcerative colitis (ASUC): challenges and solutions. Clin Exp Gastroenterol. 2021 Mar 8;14:71-81. doi: 10.2147/CEG.S197719. Available from: https://www.ncbi.nlm.nih.gov/pmc/articles/PMC7955027/
112. Internisten Alrijne. Analyse en drainage van ascites bij patiënten met en zonder levercirrose [Internet]. 2018. Available from: https://www.internisten-alrijne.nl/ascites-analyse-en-drainage.html
113. Internisten Alrijne. Diagnostische ascitespunctie: uitvoering en bepalingen [Internet]. Available from: https://www.internisten-alrijne.nl/ascitespunctie-uitvoeren.html
114. Internisten Alrijne. Spontane bacteriële peritonitis, diagnose en behandeling [Internet]. Available from: https://www.internisten-alrijne.nl/spontane-bacteriele-peritonitis-sbp.html
115. Janczewski LM, Asare EA, Goodman KA. Updates on the Version 9 American Joint Committee on Cancer Staging System for Anal Cancer. Ann Surg Oncol. 2024 Jul;31(7):4155-4158. doi: 10.1245/s10434-024-15412-8. Epub 2024 May 12. PMID: 38735904.
116. Januszewicz W, Kaminski MF. Quality indicators in diagnostic upper gastrointestinal endoscopy. Ther Adv Gastroenterol. 2020;13:175628482091669.
117. Jensen PJ, Feldman M. Acute hemorrhagic erosive gastropathy and reactive gastropathy [Internet]. UpToDate. 2022 Mar 8 [cited 2022 Mar 11]. Available from: https://www.uptodate.com/contents/acute-hemorrhagic-erosive-gastropathy-and-reactive-gastropathy
118. Jurasz K, Podgórska D, Rzeska E, Sanecki M, Tomczyk K, Chojnacka N, Klarycki J, Cymer R. Gastric antral vascular ectasia, also known as watermelon stomach - diagnosis and treatment. J Educ Health Sport. 2024;52:012. doi:10.12775/JEHS.2024.52.012.
119. Kalayarasan R, Ananthakrishnan N, Kate V. Corrosive ingestion. Indian J Crit Care Med. 2019;23(Suppl 4):S282-6.
120. Kaplan DE, Bosch J, Ripoll C, et al. AASLD practice guidance on risk stratification and management of portal hypertension and varices in cirrhosis. Hepatology. 2023. doi: 10.1097/HEP.0000000000000647.

121. Katarey D, Verma S. Drug-induced liver injury. Clin Med (Lond). 2016 Dec;16(Suppl 6):s104-9.
122. Kindred Hospitals. Pathophysiology of diabetes mellitus [Internet]. 2013. Available from: https://www.kindredhealthcare.com/resources/blog-kindred-continuum/2013/11/07/pathophysiology-of-diabetes-mellitus
123. Kuiper JJ, de Man RA, van Buuren HR. Hepatische hydrothorax. Ned Tijdschr Geneeskd. 2006;150:1157-61.
124. Kwaliteitsinstituut voor de Gezondheidszorg CBO, Nederlands Huisartsen Genootschap (NHG). Multidisciplinaire richtlijn maagklachten [Internet]. 2004 [cited 2022 Mar 14]. Available from: https://www.mdl.nl/sites/www.mdl.nl/files/richlijnen/Multidiscplinaire_richtlijn_maagklachten_-_CBO_2004.pdf
125. Lai M. Budd-Chiari syndrome: epidemiology, clinical manifestations, and diagnosis [Internet]. UpToDate. 2024 Mar 1. Available from: https://www.uptodate.com/contents/budd-chiari-syndrome-epidemiology-clinical-manifestations-and-diagnosis
126. Lai M. Budd-Chiari syndrome: management [Internet]. UpToDate. 2024 May 22. Available from: https://www.uptodate.com/contents/budd-chiari-syndrome-management
127. Lambers WM, Kraaijenbrink B, Siegert CEH. Het 'refeeding'-syndroom. Ned Tijdschr Geneeskd. 2015;159:A8610.
128. Lankisch PG, Weber-Dany B, Maisonneuve P, Lowenfels AB. Pancreatic pseudocysts: prognostic factors for their development and their spontaneous resolution in the setting of acute pancreatitis. Pancreatology. 2012 Mar-Apr;12(2):85-90.
129. Larson AM. Drug-induced liver injury [Internet]. UpToDate. 2022 [cited 2022 Mar 7]. Available from: https://www.uptodate.com/contents/drug-induced-liver-injury
130. Larson AM. Drugs and the liver: metabolism and mechanisms of injury [Internet]. UpToDate. 2021 [cited date unknown]. Available from: https://www.uptodate.com/contents/drugs-and-the-liver-metabolism-and-mechanisms-of-injury
131. Laurent L, Vullierme M, Rebours V, Maire F, Hentic O, Francoz C, et al. Estimation of the prevalence of intraductal papillary mucinous neoplasm of the pancreas in the French population through patients waiting for liver transplantation. United European Gastroenterol J. 2017 Jun;5(4):499-503.
132. Leung KK, Hirschfield GM. Autoantibodies in primary biliary cholangitis. Clin Liver Dis. 2022 Nov;26(4):613-27. doi: 10.1016/j.cld.2022.06.004. PMID: 36270719.
133. Lindor KD, Bowlus CL, Boyer J, Levy C, Mayo M. Primary biliary cholangitis: 2021 practice guidance update from the American Association for the Study of Liver Diseases. Hepatology. 2022;75:1012-3.
134. Lindor KD, Bowlus CL, Boyer J, Levy C, Mayo M. Primary biliary cholangitis: 2018 practice guidance from the American Association for the Study of Liver Diseases. Hepatology. 2019 Jan;69(1):394-419.
135. Livzan MA, Mozgovoi SI, Gaus OV, Bordin DS, Kononov AV. Diagnostic principles for chronic gastritis associated with duodenogastric reflux. Diagnostics (Basel). 2023;13(2):186. doi:10.3390/diagnostics13020186.
136. Losie JA, Lam JC, Gregson CB, Parkins MD. Epidemiology and risk factors for pyogenic liver abscess in the Calgary Health Zone revisited: a population-based study. BMC Infect Dis. 2021 Sep 9;21(1):939.
137. Lowe RC, Anderson CD, Kowdley KV. Clinical manifestations and diagnosis of cholangiocarcinoma [Internet]. UpToDate. 2023 Jul 11. Available from: https://www.uptodate.com/contents/clinical-manifestations-and-diagnosis-of-cholangiocarcinoma
138. Lv Y, Han G, Fan D. Hepatic hydrothorax. Ann Hepatol. 2018;17:33-46.
139. Ma YB, Hu J, Duan YF. Acute pancreatitis connected with hypercalcemia crisis in hyperparathyroidism: a case report. World J Clin Cases. 2019 Aug 26;7(16):2367-73. doi: 10.12998/wjcc.v7.i16.2367.
140. Maag Darm Lever Stichting. Spijsverteringsziekten en -klachten [Internet]. 2022 [cited 2022 Mar 7]. Available from: https://www.mlds.nl/
141. Macias-Toro JD, Saurina-Sole A, Pou-Potau M, Esteve-Simo V, Duarte-Gallego V, Fulquet-Nicolas M, et al. Hydroelectrolytic disorders secondary to refeeding syndrome. Nefrologia. 2013;33(2):279-81.
142. Macrae FA. Epidemiology and risk factors for colorectal cancer [Internet]. UpToDate. 2025 Jan 7. Available from: https://www.uptodate.com/contents/epidemiology-and-risk-factors-for-colorectal-cancer
143. Manes G, Paspatis G, Aabakken L, Anderloni A, Arvanitakis M, Ah-Soune P, et al. Endoscopic management of common bile duct stones: ESGE guideline [Internet]. 2019. Available from: https://www.esge.com/endoscopic-management-of-common-bile-duct-stones-esge-guideline
144. Mansour D, McPherson S. Management of decompensated cirrhosis. Clin Med (Lond). 2018;18(Suppl 2):60-5.
145. Marciano S, Díaz JM, Dirchwolf M, Gadano A. Spontaneous bacterial peritonitis in patients with cirrhosis: incidence, outcomes, and treatment strategies. Hepat Med. 2019;11:13-22.
146. Mayo-Smith MF. Management of alcohol withdrawal delirium. An evidence-based practice guideline. Arch Intern Med. 2004;164(13):1405. doi: 10.1001/archinte.164.13.1405.
147. MDCalc. [Internet]. Available from: https://www.mdcalc.com/
148. MDCalc. Child-Pugh Score for Cirrhosis Mortality [Internet]. Available from: https://www.mdcalc.com/child-pugh-score-cirrhosis-mortality
149. MDCalc. Glasgow-Blatchford Bleeding Score (GBS) [Internet]. Available from: https://www.mdcalc.com/glasgow-blatchford-bleeding-score-gbs
150. MDCalc. MELD Score (Model For End-Stage Liver Disease) (12 and older) [Internet]. Available from: https://www.mdcalc.com/meld-score-model-end-stage-liver-disease-12-older
151. MDCalc. Montreal Classification for Inflammatory Bowel Disease (IBD) [Internet]. Available from: https://

www.mdcalc.com/montreal-classification-inflammatory-bowel-disease-ibd

152. MDCalc. Ranson's criteria for pancreatitis mortality [Internet]. [cited 2022 Feb 28]. Available from: https://www.mdcalc.com/ransons-criteria-pancreatitis-mortality#use-cases
153. Mehrotra B. Gallbladder cancer: epidemiology, risk factors, clinical features, and diagnosis [Internet]. UpToDate. 2025 Jan 7. Available from: https://www.uptodate.com/contents/epidemiology-risk-factors-clinical-features-and-diagnosis-of-gallbladder-cancer
154. Mellinger JL. Epidemiology of alcohol use and alcoholic liver disease. Clin Liver Dis (Hoboken). 2019 May 3;13(5):136-9.
155. Mohamed AA, Lu X, Mounmin FA. Diagnosis and treatment of esophageal candidiasis: current updates. Can J Gastroenterol Hepatol. 2019 Oct 20;2019:3585136.
156. National Institute on Alcohol Abuse and Alcoholism (NIAAA). Overview of alcohol consumption: moderate & binge drinking [Internet]. Available from: https://www.niaaa.nih.gov/alcohol-health/overview-alcohol-consumption/moderate-binge-drinking
157. Naveed M, Jamil LH, Fujii-Lau LL, Al-Haddad M, Buxbaum JL, Fishman DS, et al. American Society for Gastrointestinal Endoscopy guideline on the role of endoscopy in the management of acute colonic pseudo-obstruction and colonic volvulus. Gastrointest Endosc. 2020 Mar;91(3):721.
158. Nederlands Huisartsen Genootschap. Diabetes mellitus type 2 [Internet]. 2018. Available from: https://richtlijnen.nhg.org/standaarden/diabetes-mellitus-type-2#volledige-tekst
159. Nederlands Huisartsen Genootschap. Maagklachten [Internet]. 2021 Mar [cited 2025 Jan 27]. Available from: https://richtlijnen.nhg.org/standaarden/maagklachten
160. Nederlands Huisartsen Genootschap. NHG-Standaard Anemie [Internet]. 2014 [cited 2025 Jan 27]. Available from: https://richtlijnen.nhg.org/standaarden/anemie#volledige-tekst
161. Nederlandse Internistenvereniging. Child-Pugh Classificatie voor ernst leverziekte [Internet]. Available from: https://www.internisten.nl/jniv/calculator/child-pugh-classificatie-voor-ernst-leverziekte/
162. Nederlandse Internistenvereniging. Gastro-intestinale bloeding - Het Acute Boekje [Internet]. 2023. Available from: https://www.hetacuteboekje.nl/hoofdstuk/mdl/gastro-intestinale_bloeding.html
163. Nederlandse Vereniging van Maag-Darm-Leverartsen. Enterale toegang [Internet]. 2022 [cited 2025 Jan 27]. Available from: https://richtlijnendatabase.nl/richtlijn/enterale_toegang/startpagina_-_enterale_toegang.html
164. Nederlandse Vereniging van Maag-Darm-Leverartsen. Richtlijn Acuut Leverfalen [Internet]. 2020. p. 1–105. Available from: https://www.mdl.nl/sites/www.mdl.nl/files/richlijnen/Richtlijn%20acuut%20leverfalen_0.pdf
165. Nederlandse Vereniging van Maag-Darm-Leverartsen. Richtlijn Barrett-oesofagus [Internet]. Available from: https://www.mdl.nl/sites/www.mdl.nl/files/richlijnen/Richtlijnen%20Barrett%20oesofagus%20-%20jan%202018%20-%20tbv%20website.pdf
166. Nederlandse Vereniging van Maag-Darm-Leverartsen. Richtlijn bloedingen van de tractus digestivus [Internet]. 2017 [cited 2025 Jan 27]. Available from: https://www.mdl.nl/sites/www.mdl.nl/files/richlijnen/Richtlijn-bloedingen-definitief-mei2018.pdf
167. Nederlandse Vereniging van Maag-Darm-Leverartsen. Richtlijn bloedingen van de tractus digestivus [Internet]. 2017. Available from: https://www.mdl.nl/sites/www.mdl.nl/files/richlijnen/Richtlijnbloedingen-definitief-mei2018.pdf
168. Nederlandse Vereniging voor Klinische Chemie en Laboratoriumgeneeskunde. AFP [Internet]. 2010 [cited 2025 Jan 27]. Available from: https://www.nvkc.nl/zoek-een-test/?id=131
169. Nederlandse Vereniging voor Klinische Chemie en Laboratoriumgeneeskunde. CEA [Internet]. 2010 [cited 2025 Jan 27]. Available from: https://www.nvkc.nl/zoek-een-test/?id=176
170. Nederlandse Vereniging voor Klinische Chemie en Laboratoriumgeneeskunde. Chromogranine A [Internet]. 2010 [cited 2025 Jan 27]. Available from: https://www.nvkc.nl/zoek-een-test/?id=338
171. Newman RK, Stobart Gallagher MA, Gomez AE. Alcohol withdrawal. In: StatPearls [Internet]. Treasure Island (FL): StatPearls Publishing; 2022 Jan–. PMID: 28722912.
172. Newman RK, Stobart Gallagher MA, Gomez AE. Alcohol withdrawal. In: StatPearls [Internet]. Treasure Island (FL): StatPearls Publishing; 2022 Jan– [cited 2025 Feb 28]. Available from: https://www.ncbi.nlm.nih.gov/books/NBK28722912/.
173. Nguyen H, Le C, Nguyen H. Gastric antral vascular ectasia (watermelon stomach)—an enigmatic and often-overlooked cause of gastrointestinal bleeding in the elderly. Perm J. 2009;13(4):50-4.
174. NHG. Laboratoriumdiagnostiek Diarree (LESA) [Internet]. Nederlands Huisartsen Genootschap; 2020 [cited 2022 Mar 7]. Available from: https://www.nhg.org/themas/publicaties/laboratoriumdiagnostiek-diarree-volledige-tekst
175. Nishino K, Kawanaka M, Manabe N, Suehiro M, Kawamoto H, Haruma K. Portal hypertensive gastropathy in liver cirrhosis: prevalence, natural history, and risk factors. Intern Med. 2022;61(5):605-613. Available from: https://doi.org/10.2169/internalmedicine.7943-21.
176. Northup PG, Garcia-Pagan JC, Garcia-Tsao G, Intagliata NM, Superina RA, Roberts LN, et al. Vascular liver disorders, portal vein thrombosis, and procedural bleeding in patients with liver disease: 2020 practice guidance by the American Association for the Study of Liver Diseases. Hepatology. 2021 Jan;73(1):366-413. doi: 10.1002/hep.31646.
177. Oey RC, Buuren HR van, Man RA de. The diagnostic work-up in patients with ascites: current guidelines and

future prospects. Neth J Med. 2016;74(8):330-5.
178. Onnekink AM, Boxhoorn L, Timmerhuis HC, Bac ST, Dutch Pancreatitis Study Group. Endoscopic versus surgical step-up approach for infected necrotizing pancreatitis (extension): long-term follow-up of a randomized trial. Gastroenterology. 2022 Sep;163(3):712-22.e14.
179. Osna NA, Donohue TM Jr, Kharbanda KK. Alcoholic liver disease: pathogenesis and current management. Alcohol Res. 2017;38(2):147-61.
180. Othman MO, Harb D, Barkin JA. Introduction and practical approach to exocrine pancreatic insufficiency for the practicing clinician. Int J Clin Pract. 2018;72:e13066.
181. Oude Nijhuis RAB, Zaninotto G, Roman S, Boeckxstaens GE, Fockens P, Langendam MW, et al. European guideline on achalasia: UEG and ESNM recommendations. United European Gastroenterol J. 2020 Feb;8(1):13-33.
182. Pace C. Alcohol withdrawal: Epidemiology, clinical manifestations, course, assessment, and diagnosis [Internet]. UpToDate; 2022 Apr 5 [cited 2025 Feb 28]. Available from: https://www.uptodate.com/contents/alcohol-withdrawal-epidemiology-clinical-manifestations-course-assessment-and-diagnosis.
183. Pimentel M, Saad RJ, Long MD, Rao SSC. ACG Clinical Guideline: Small intestinal bacterial overgrowth. Am J Gastroenterol. 2020 Feb;115(2):165 78.
184. Reginelli A, Giacobbe G, Del Canto MT, Alessandrella M, Balestrucci G, Urraro F, Russo GM, Gallo L, Danti G, Frittoli B, Stoppino L, Schettini D, Iafrate F, Cappabianca S, Laghi A, Grassi R, Brunese L, Barile A, Miele V. Peritoneal carcinosis: What the radiologist needs to know. Diagnostics (Basel). 2023 Jun 5;13(11):1974. doi: 10.3390/diagnostics13111974.
185. Roche SP, Kobos R. Jaundice in the adult patient. Am Fam Physician. 2004 Jan 15;69(2):299–304. Available from: https://pubmed.ncbi.nlm.nih.gov/14765767/
186. Schuckit MA. Recognition and management of withdrawal delirium (delirium tremens). N Engl J Med. 2014;371(22):2109-2113. doi: 10.1056/nejmra1407298.
187. Sebghatollahi V, Parsa M, Minakari M, Azadbakht S. A clinician's guide to gallstones and common bile duct (CBD): A study protocol for a systematic review and evidence-based recommendations. Health Sci Rep. 2023 Sep 12. Available from: https://doi.org/10.1002/hsr2.1555.
188. Shaqran TM, Ismaeel MM, Alnuaman AA, Al Ahmad FA, Albalawi GA, Almubarak JN, AlHarbi RS, Alaqidi RS, AlAli YA, Alfawaz KS, Daghriri AA. Epidemiology, Causes, and Management of Gastro-esophageal Reflux Disease: A Systematic Review. Cureus. 2023 Oct 21;15(10):e47420. doi: 10.7759/cureus.47420. PMID: 38022211; PMCID: PMC10658748.
189. So YT. Wernicke encephalopathy [Internet]. UpToDate; 2020 Feb 11 [cited 2025 Feb 28]. Available from: https://www.uptodate.com/contents/wernicke-encephalopathy.
190. Stier EA, Clarke MA, Deshmukh AA, Wentzensen N, Liu Y, Poynten IM, Cavallari EN, Fink V, Barroso LF, Clifford GM, Cuming T, Goldstone SE, Hillman RJ, Rosa-Cunha I, La Rosa L, Palefsky JM, Plotzker R, Roberts JM, Jay N. International Anal Neoplasia Society's consensus guidelines for anal cancer screening. Int J Cancer. 2024 May 15;154(10):1694-1702. doi: 10.1002/ijc.34850. Epub 2024 Jan 31. PMID: 38297406.
191. TeachMeSurgery. Jaundice - Pre, intra, post-hepatic - management [Internet]. 2020 May 16. Available from: https://teachmesurgery.com/hpb/presentations/jaundice/
192. Wang Z, Shi Y, Xiong G, Han M, Chen X. The prognostic impact of preoperative CA19-9 on resectable cholangiocarcinoma: a comprehensive systematic review and meta-analysis. Discov Oncol. 2024;15:773. Available from: https://doi.org/10.1007/s12672-024-01683-w.
193. Wendon J, Cordoba J, Dhawan A, Larsen FS, Manns M, Nevens F, Samuel D, Simpson KJ, Yaron I, Bernardi M. EASL clinical practical guidelines on the management of acute (fulminant) liver failure. J Hepatol. 2017 May;66(5):1047–81. doi: 10.1016/j.jhep.2016.12.003
194. Wong GL. Updated Guidelines for the Prevention and Management of Chronic Hepatitis B-World Health Organization 2024 Compared With China 2022 HBV Guidelines. J Viral Hepat. 2024 Dec;31 Suppl 2:13-22. doi: 10.1111/jvh.14032. Epub 2024 Nov 6. PMID: 39503252.
195. World Health Organization. Global hepatitis report 2024: action for access in low- and middle-income countries. Geneva: World Health Organization; 2024. Available from: https://www.who.int/publications/i/item/9789240091672
196. Ye J, Cui L, Zhou Y, et al. "Gilbert's-like" syndrome as part of a spectrum of persistent unconjugated hyperbilirubinemia in post-chronic hepatitis patients. Sci Rep. 2018;8:2008. doi: 10.1038/s41598-018-19847-4

Are you missing a resource or topic? Or is there a new guideline that isn't yet listed here? Let us know! Together we can keep Compendium Medicine up to date.

Illustrations & figures

Illustrators

Yente S. Beentjes: *figure 45*
Hebe T.A. Boerhout: *figure 76*
Dagmar Bouwer: *figure 77*
Cas van Cruchten: *figure 89*
Susan Deelstra: *figure 43*
Maria van Doorn: *figures 2, 46, 59, and 68*
Lotte Dupuis: *figure 22*
Astrid A.H. Feikema: *figure 33*
Iza Hogenelst: *figures 29 and 37*
Jasmin Kaur: *figures 23, 24, and 25*
Koen L.C. Ketelaars: *figures 1, 67, 71, 72, 78, 81, 96, and right image of figure 101*
Rosalie C. Krijl: *figures 4, 5, 27, 28, 31, 32, 53, 54, 65, and 73*
Juliëtte M.E. Linskens: *figures 3, 39, and 94*
Kim A.M. van den Nobelen: *figures 51, 80, 82, and 83*
Laura Sanchez: *left image of figure 101*
Carlijn Sturm: *figures 79 and 99*
Isabel Versmissen: *figure 56*
Linda Xie: *figures 26, 55, 65, and 100*

Sources

01. Photos cover and About us: www.ivarpel.nl
02. Figures 6, 7, 8, 9, 10, 11, 12, 30, 50, 52, 66, 84, 92, and 95: Gwendolyn Vuurberg, MD, PhD
03. Figures 13, 36, 49, 60, 61, 86, and 90: Marcel Spanier, MD, PhD
04. Figures 14, 15, 16, 17, 18, 19, 20, 21, 24, 25, 34, 35, 38, 40, 41, 42, 44, 47, 48, 57, 58, 62, 63, 64, 69, 70, 74, 75, 85, 87, 88, 91, and 93: Suzanne Anije, MD, PhD Candidate
05. Figure 46, world map vector file: www.freepik.com
06. Figure 78 (Spider naevi): www.huidziekten.nl
07. Figure 78 (Palmar erythema): Erythema palmare - Journal of Online Hepatology
08. Figures 97 and 98: Duygu Harmankaya
09. Figure cover and beginning pages: Traité complet de l'anatomie de l'homme: comprenant la médicine opératoire 1831-1844 / Bourgery, Jean Baptiste Marc; Jacob, Nicolas Henri/ Public domain

Epilogue

Immersing ourselves in the content, connections, and practical applications has continually reminded us that Gastroenterology and Hepatology is a beautiful, multidisciplinary field. We have approached this work with an inclusive perspective, recognising that the field thrives through collaboration between diverse disciplines, specialties, and backgrounds – and that this diversity is precisely where its strength lies.

Through the collaborative effort of an incredible team consisting of students, illustrators, graphic designers, residents, and medical specialists, we have been able to turn our vision into reality with this pocket. Our goal was to ensure that you, as medical students and doctors, have access to essential information – literally at your fingertips, wherever in the world you may be.

To Niels and Jessica – what an incredible journey we have shared over the past years. Your dedication, ideas, and boundless, unwavering enthusiasm have shaped every step of this process. It has been intense, at times challenging, but above all deeply rewarding. We are especially grateful for your outstanding commitment and continued support. An earlier edition of this pocket formed the foundation for this work. We acknowledge Veronique and Linde, whose dedication and creativity laid the groundwork upon which we were able to build. This pocket would not have come together as it did without the outstanding support of Gwen. Your attentiveness, precision, and genuine motivation were invaluable – we truly could not have completed this project without you, and for that we are grateful.

We are enormously thankful to all the medical professionals who provided valuable feedback and content support, elevating the quality of this pocket. Your input was essential to achieving this result. This pocket would never have been as visually appealing without the work of all the illustrators – many of them also medical students – who collaborated on this pocket. We thank our team for their exceptional ability to clearly and creatively capture the essence of the specialty in their illustrations. We gratefully acknowledge our graphic hero, Maria, whose creative work has given this pocket guide its distinctive *Compendium Medicine* look. Special thanks also go to Laura, Pauline, Melanie, and Delano for ensuring the smooth functioning of the entire process.

Finally, a sincere thank you to all our colleagues who keep *Compendium Medicine* on their bookshelves. Your support has been indispensable in making our dreams a reality. We are incredibly proud of this team and hope to see you again soon, whether inside or outside the hospital!

Amsterdam, November 2025

Suzanne Anjie, MD & Romée Snijders, MD, PhD

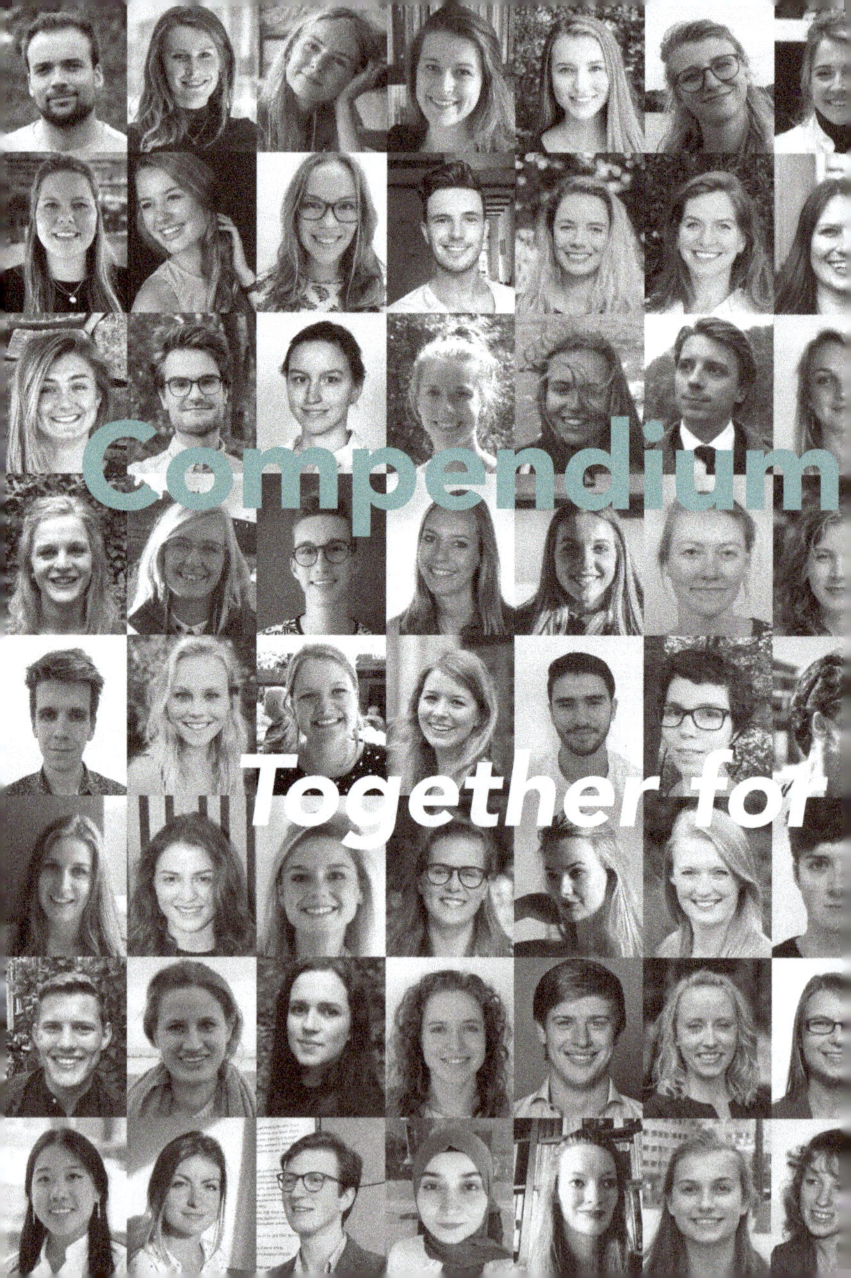
Compendium
Together for

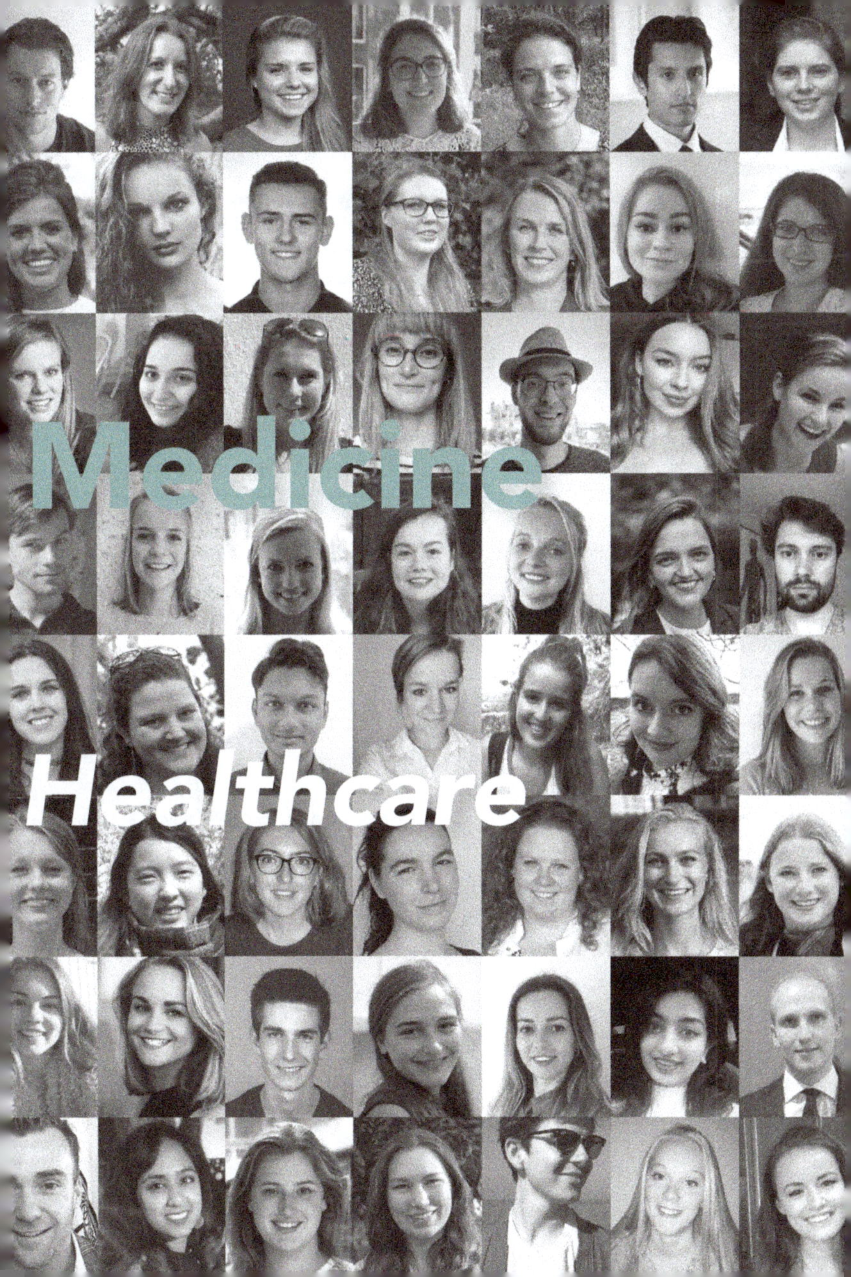
Medicine
Healthcare

About us

As medical students, we felt overwhelmed by the amount of medical knowledge available. An overview was lacking. Fueled by this need for change, we embarked on a journey that has now brought together over 500 students and doctors to create the entire *Compendium Medicine* book series. Our mission is to help and connect healthcare professionals globally by providing accessible knowledge.

The bigger picture

In 2015, at VU University in Amsterdam, the Netherlands, our paths crossed as we were both pursuing our medical educations. The vast sea of medical knowledge overwhelmed us, highlighting the need for a comprehensive overview. We were surprised by the isolated efforts of every hospital and university, each working on its own 'island', publishing individual books and reference works instead of fostering collaboration.

Motivated to make a difference, we envisioned a solution: a comprehensive guide encompassing all 36 subspecialties, enriched with figures, icons, charts, and mnemonics. Our vision was clear – our books had to be visual, concise, and to the point. With a dedicated team of students and doctors, we started writing an encyclopedia using our unique method. *Compendium Medicine* was born!

Book series

Following almost two years of dedicated effort, the first edition achieved sold-out status even before its official launch: a remarkable start to the ongoing rollercoaster journey. The most rewarding aspect of this experience has been – and still is – the overwhelmingly positive feedback from medical students and specialists. Our narrative caught the attention of prominent Dutch and Belgian newspapers and journals, leading to invitations to feature on popular talk shows on national television.

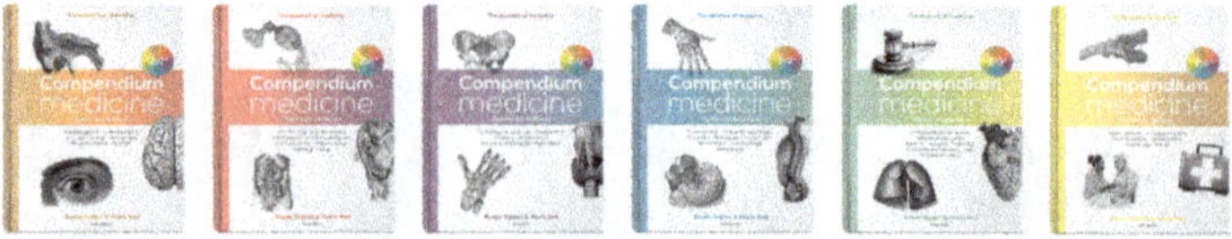

Compendium Medicine book series

Our white-coat pockets

One year later, both of us had started our clinical rotations. We recognized a common challenge faced by many peers: the need for quick and easy access to practical information. In response, we started creating our first series of pockets – concise yet comprehensive pocket-sized booklets designed to provide essential and practical information during a shift.

A period of many milestones followed. Our team expanded every month: from authors to medical specialists, from ambassadors to illustrators. With a growing number of followers on social media, a real community was born. With this team, we worked incredibly hard on new pockets as well as new additions like flashcards and pocket cards. As of now, we have launched a total of 20 different pockets!

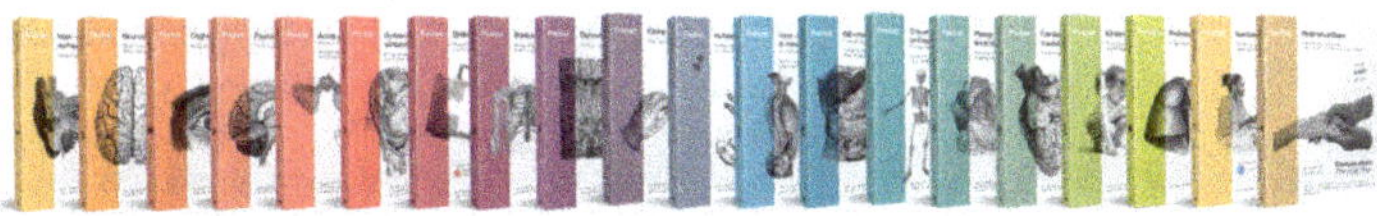

Compendium Medicine pockets

Expanding our mission globally

With the experience gained over the past years, we are committed to making a positive impact on medical students and healthcare professionals worldwide. This new phase kicked off with the distribution of our *Radiology* pocket to all continents. We were amazed to have reached readers from over 92 countries! Their positive feedback was instrumental in propelling us forward, and we are excited to present our eighth pocket in English: *Gastroenterology and Hepatology*. And this is just the beginning: we are actively working on bringing more pockets to you!

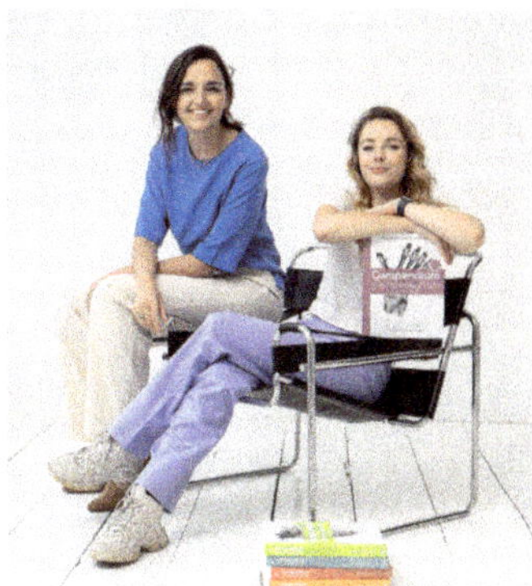

Romée Snijders & Veerle Smit

Doctors and founders of *Compendium Medicine*

Compendium Compass©

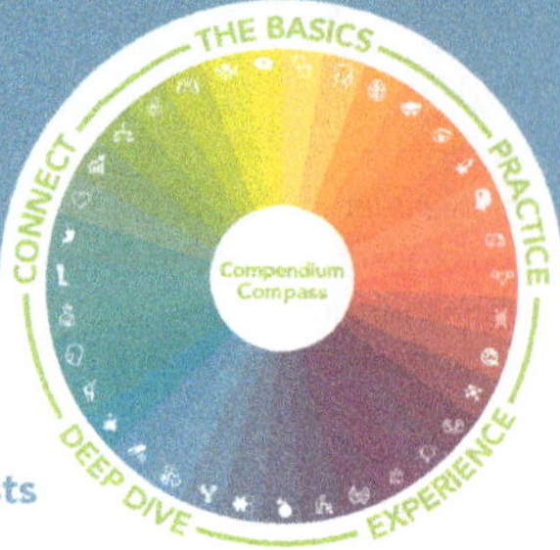

We believe that on your journey from medical student to retirement you continuously navigate these five steps. The Compendium Compass© assists you along the way.

1 THE BASICS

Start at the foundation. Explore all 44 medical specialisms through our comprehensive series, featuring clear diagrams, tables, and illustrations. Visit our website for additional details.

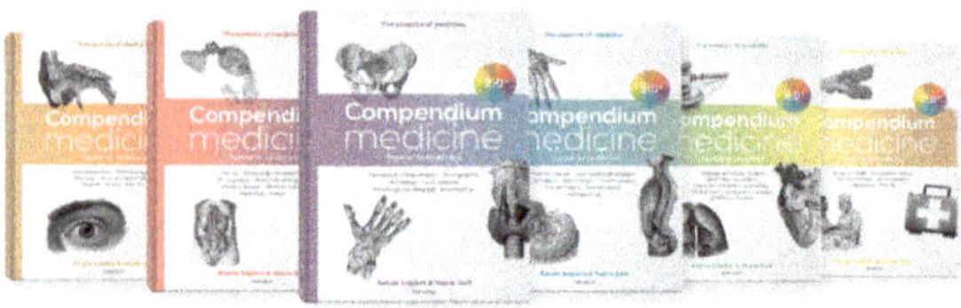

2 PRACTICE

Reinforce your foundational knowledge with our *Compendium Medicine* app and through our social media platforms! The app, which can be downloaded from the Apple and Android app stores, enables you to practice questions on a daily basis and participate in the monthly challenge.

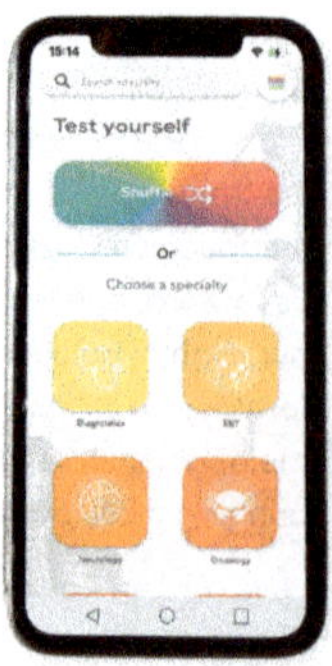

Scan this QR code for more information.

3 EXPERIENCE

Learn on-the-go by carrying our pockets and pocket cards with you on the ward, during your shifts and rounds, anytime. Our first pockets are already available worldwide, with many more to come. See below for details!

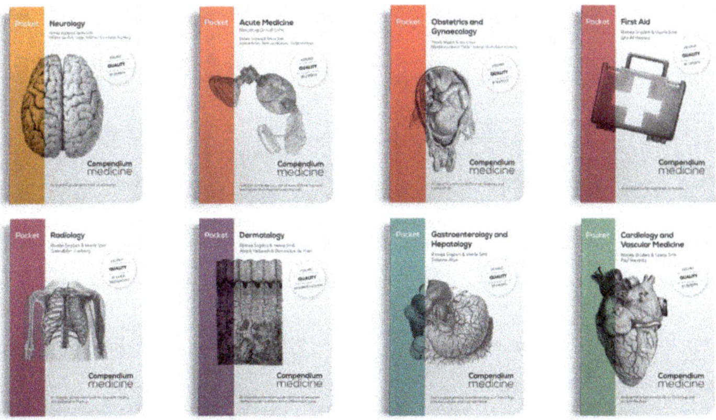

4 DEEP DIVE

Explore medical knowledge through extensive reading, immersing yourself in a variety of literature, guidelines, and the latest scientific articles.

5 CONNECT

Interested in connecting with individuals in your field? Become a member of our community through our social media platform – a network of students, physicians, specialists, and other healthcare professionals.

Abbreviations

AAA	abdominal aortic aneurysm
AB	antibiotics
ABG	arterial blood gas
ACE	angiotensin-converting enzyme
ACS	acute coronary syndrome
ADH	antidiuretic hormone
ADP	adenosine diphosphate
AF	atrial fibrillation
AFP	alpha-fetoprotein
AG	anion gap
AIH	autoimmune hepatitis
AIP	autoimmune pancreatitis
AKI	acute kidney injury
ALP	alkaline phosphatase
ALT	alanine transaminase
Ao-CLF	acute-on-chronic liver failure
AP	angina pectoris
APR	abdominoperineal resection
aPTT	activated partial thromboplastin test/time
ASA	acetylsalicylic acid
AST	aspartate aminotransferase
ASUC	acute severe ulcerative colitis
AVPU	Alert, Verbal, Pain, Unresponsive
AWS	alcohol withdrawal syndrome
BD-IPMN	branch-duct intraductal papillary mucinous neoplasm
BMI	body mass index
BP	blood pressure
CABG	coronary artery bypass graft
CAP	controlled attenuation parameter
CBD	common bile duct
CCA	cholangiocarcinoma
CEA	carcinoembryonic antigen
CHF	congestive heart failure
CI	contraindication
CIPO	chronic intestinal pseudo-obstruction
CKD	chronic kidney disease
CMV	cytomegalovirus
CNS	central nervous system
CO_2	carbondioxide
COPD	chronic obstructive pulmonary disease
COX	cyclooxygenase
CRP	C-reactive protein
CRT	capillary refill time

CSPH	clinically significant portal hypertension
CT	computed tomography
CVA	cerebrovascular accident
CVL	central venous line
CVP	central venous pressure
DAA	direct-acting antiviral
DDx	differential diagnosis
DEXA	dual-energy X-ray absorptiometry
DGBI	disorder of gut-brain interaction
DIC	disseminated intravascular coagulation
DILI	drug-induced liver injury
DM	diabetes mellitus
DNA	deoxyribonucleic acid
DOAC	direct oral anticoagulants
DOS	delirium observation screening
DPEJ	direct percutaneous endoscopic jejunostomy
DSM	diagnostic and statistical manual of mental disorders
DVT	deep vein thrombosis
EAEC	Enteroaggregative E. coli
EAUS	endoanal ultrasound
EBNA	Epstein-Barr nuclear antigen
EBV	Epstein-Barr virus
ECG	electrocardiogram
EDTA	ethylenediaminetetraacetic acid
EEG	electroencephalogram
EET	endoscopic eradication therapy
eFTR	endoscopic full thickness resection
EHEC	Enterohaemorrhagic E. coli
EIEC	Enteroinvasive E. coli
EMR	endoscopic mucosal resection
ENT	ear-, nose-, and throat
EPO	erythropoietin
ERCP	endoscopic retrograde cholangiopancreatography
ERT	emergency response team
ESBL	extended spectrum beta-lactamase
ESD	endoscopic submucosal dissection
ESR	erythrocyte sedimentation rate
ETEC	Enterotoxic E. coli
EUS	endoscopic ultrasound
FAMMM	familial atypical multiple mole melanoma
FAP	familial adenomatous polyposis

FDG	fluorodeoxyglucose
FHx	family history
FIT	faecal immunochemical test
FODMAP	fermentable oligosaccharides, disaccharides, monosaccharides, and polyols
GAVE	gastric antral vascular ectasia, gastrointestinal vascular ectasia
GCS	Glasgow coma scale
GFR	glomerular filtration rate
GGT	gamma-glutamyltransferase
GHB	gamma-hydroxybutyric acid
GI	gastro-intestinal
GIST	gastrointestinal stromal tumour
GORD	gastro-oesophageal reflux disease
GP	general practitioner
HAV	hepatitis A
Hb	haemoglobin
HBV	hepatitis B
HCC	hepatocellular carcinoma
HCV	hepatitis C
HDV	hepatitis D
HE	hepatic encephalopathy
HELLP	hemolysis, elevated liver enzyme levels, and low platelet levels
HEV	hepatitis E
HGD	high-grade dysplasia
HIT	heparin-induced thrombocytopaenia
HIV	human immunodeficiency virus
HNPCC	hereditairy nonpolyposis colorectal cancer
HR	heart rate
HRMO	highly resistant micro-organism
HRS	hepatorenal syndrome
Ht	Haematocrit
IBD	inflammatory bowel disease
IBS	irritable bowel syndrome
IBS-C	IBS with predominant constipation
IBS-D	IBS with predominant diarrhoea
IBS-M	IBS with mixed bowel habits
ICD	implantable cardioverter defibrillator
ICL	intercostal space left
ICR	intercostal space right
ICS	intercostal space
ICU	intensive care unit
IM	intramuscular
INR	international normalised ratio
IPMN	intraductal papillary mucinous neoplasm
IRC	infrared coagulation
ITP	immune thrombocytopaenia
IV	intravenous
LAR	low anterior resection
LDH	lactate dehydrogenase
LES	lower oesophageal sphincter
LGD	low-grade dysplasia
LIFT	ligation of intersphincteric fistula tract
LLQ	left lower quadrant
LMWH	low molecular weight heparin
LSD	lysergic acid diethylamide
LUQ	left upper quadrant
LVAD	left ventricular assist device
MALT	mucosa-associated lymphoid tissue
MAP	MUTYH-associated polyposis
MASH	metabolic dysfunction-associated steatohepatitis
MASLD	metabolic dysfunction-associated steatotic liver disease
MCH	mean corpuscular haemoglobin
MCHC	mean corpuscular haemoglobin concentration
MCU	medium care unit
MCV	mean corpuscular volume
MD-IPMN	main-duct intraductal papillary mucinous neoplasm
MetALD	metabolic dysfunction and alcohol-associated steatotic liver disease
MEWS	modified early warning score
MMA	methylmalonic acid
MRCP	MR cholangiopancreatography
MRE	magnetic resonance elastography
MRI	magnetic resonance imaging
MRSA	methicillin-resistant staphylococcus aureus
MT-IPMN	mixed-type intraductal papillary mucinous neoplasm
MTX	methotrexate
NBI	narrow band imaging
NEC	necrotising enterocolitis
NET	neuroendocrine tumour
NG	nasogastric
NPO	nil per os, nothing per mouth
NSAID	non-steroidal anti-inflammatory drug
NSBB	non-selective beta blocker
O_2	oxygen
OAC	oral anticoagulatioin
ORT	oral rehydration therapy

OTC	over-the-counter
PAD	peripheral arterial disease
PBC	primary biliary cholangitis
PCI	percutaneous coronary intervention
PDFF	proton density fat fractioni
PEG	percutaneous endoscopic gastrostomy
PERT	pancreatic enzyme replacement therapy
PET	positron emission tomography
Pgp	P-glycoprotein
PHG	portal hypertensive gastropathy
PICD	paracentesis-induced circulatory dysfunction
PID	pelvic inflammatory disease
PLT	platelet count
PMHx	previous medical history
PMI	point of maximum intensity
POCUS	point of care ultrasound
POEM	per oral endoscopic myotomy
PPE	personal protective equipment
PPI	proton pump inhibitor
PRG	percutaneous radiological gastrostomy
PSC	primary sclerosing cholangitis
PT	prothrombin time
PTC	percutaneous bile duct drainage
PTH	parathyroid hormone
PVT	portal vein thrombosis
RAAS	renin-angiotensin-aldosterone system
RBC	red blood cell
RBL	rubber band ligation
RDW	red blood cell distribution width
RFA	radiofrequency ablation
RLQ	right lower quadrant
RNA	ribonucleir acid
RR	respiratory rate
RTIC	reticulocyte count
RUQ	right upper quadrant
SAAG	serum-to-ascites albumin gradient
SBP	spontaneous bacterial peritonitis
SCAD	segmental colitis associated with diverticulosis
SCC	squamous cell carcinoma
SIADH	syndrome of inappropriate antidiuretic hormone secretion
SIBO	small intestinal bacterial overgrowth
SIRS	systemic inflammatory response syndrome
SOL	space-occupying lesion
SpO_2	oxygen saturation
SPS	serrated polyposis syndrome
SRT	stereotactic radiotherapy
SSRI	selective serotonin reuptake inhibitor
STEC	Shiga-toxic-producing E. coli
STI	sexually transmitted infection
SWE	shear wave elastography
T	temperature
TACE	transcatheter arterial chemoembolisation
TARE	transarterial radioembolisation
TB	tuberculosis
TCA	tricyclic antidepressants
TEM	transanal endoscopic microsurgery
TIA	transient ischaemic attack
TIBC	total iron-binding capacity
TIPS	transjugular intrahepatic portosystemic shunt
TME	total mesorectal excision
TPMT	thiopurine methyltransferase
TPN	total parenteral nutrition
TSH	thyroid stimulating hormone
UDCA	ursodeoxycholic acid
US	ultrasound
UTI	urinary tract infection
VARD	video-assisted retroperitoneal debridement
VAS	visual analogue scale
VCA	viral capsid antigen
VCTE	vibration-controlled transient elastography
VKA	vitamin K antagonist
VLS	visible light spectroscopy
VTE	venous thromboembolism
WBC	white blood cell
WON	walled-off necrosis

Index

www.ingramcontent.com/pod-product-compliance
Lightning Source LLC
Chambersburg PA
CBHW050522240926
51846CB00003B/662
* 9 7 8 9 0 8 3 3 7 4 0 8 6 *